Nutrition Policy
Implementation
Issues and Experience

Nutrition Policy Implementation
Issues and Experience

Edited by

NEVIN S. SCRIMSHAW

Institute Professor, Massachusetts Institute of Technology
Director, MIT/Harvard International Food and Nutrition Program
Senior Adviser, World Hunger Program, United Nations University

and

MITCHEL B. WALLERSTEIN

Associate Director, MIT/Harvard International Food and Nutrition Program
Lecturer, Departments of Political Science and Nutrition
Massachusetts Institute of Technology

Sponsored by the United Nations University, Tokyo, Japan

PLENUM PRESS • NEW YORK AND LONDON

Library of Congress Cataloging in Publication Data

Main entry under title:

Nutrition policy implementation.

Includes bibliographical references and index.
1. Nutrition policy. I. Scrimshaw, Nevin S. II. Wallerstein, Mitchel B.
TX359.N886 1982   363.8'56   82-9137
ISBN-13: 978-1-4684-4093-5   e-ISBN-13: 978-1-4684-4091-1
DOI: 10.1007/978-1-4684-4091-1

© 1982 Plenum Press, New York
Softcover reprint of the hardcover 1st edition 1982

A Division of Plenum Publishing Corporation
233 Spring Street, New York, N.Y. 10013

Preface

The MIT International Nutrition Planning Program (INP) was initiated in the fall of 1972 with a grant from the Rockefeller Foundation, later supplemented by funds from USAID under the 211D Program. Conceived as a multidisciplinary undertaking, the INP was a joint effort of the Department of Nutrition and Food Science and the Center for International Studies at MIT that also included representatives of the Departments of Economics, Political Science, Urban Studies, Humanities (Anthropology), and Civil Engineering. It has been successful in attracting graduate students and conducting research on various international food and nutrition problems, including the design of intervention programs.

A condition of the original grant from the Rockefeller Foundation was the organization of a meeting to summarize and evaluate the progress of the program. It was ultimately decided that the best approach would be a workshop that would attempt to assess what had been learned about the implementation of food and nutrition policies since the start of the INP. Out of concern for food and nutrition policy issues, the World Hunger Programme of The United Nations University (UNU) and the Ford Foundation also agreed to cosponsor the workshop.

The interest of the UNU stemmed from an expert group meeting in 1975 that identified research and training in food and nutrition policy and planning as a major subprogram priority. In 1977 the UNU signed an agreement of association with a consortium consisting of the MIT-INP and the Center for International Health of the Harvard School of Public Health, with the resulting program to be known as the International Food and Nutrition Program (IFNP). At the time of the workshop, a total of 20 UNU Fellows, drawn from all parts of the world, had participated in the IFNP advanced study program, taking advantage of the resources of both institutions. The workshop itself drew upon faculty and staff members at MIT and Harvard, as well as individuals from instituions both within and outside the United States to discuss, in various categories, the implementation of nutrition policies.

Because the conference marked the end of the first phase of the program at MIT, the moment was considered particularly auspicious for merging the UNU-sponsored IFNP and the MIT-sponsored programs, both to avoid confusion and duplication of effort and to indicate that concern with planning activities and field studies necessarily involves policy analysis across a broad range of disciplines. From the beginning, the INP approach has been multidisciplinary, and the involvement of the Harvard School of Public Health brought into the program yet another group of disciplines. Students entering the program through either Harvard or MIT may take part in courses in both institutions through cross-registration and participate in a weekly Food Policy Seminar. It is intended that the present volume will be a reference source on the kinds of food and nutrition issues that occupy IFNP students and staff.

The IFNP has benefited greatly from the participation in this workshop of individuals from other institutions in the United States and abroad. This has been possible through the support of the Rockefeller and Ford Foundations and The United Nations University World Hunger Programme. Thanks are extended to these institutions for making this volume possible.

NEVIN S. SCRIMSHAW
MITCHEL B. WALLERSTEIN

Contents

Introduction

Selection of the most effective and appropriate format for this conference presented a number of organizational dilemmas. First, unlike the October 1971 MIT Conference on "Nutrition, National Development, and Planning," which first served to focus international attention on the need for explicit attention to nutrition policy and planning activities, the present meeting was intended to identify and evaluate the progress achieved in specific programmatic areas during the ensuing 8-year period. For this reason, six substantive topics were selected as the basis for workshop discussions after an initial session on the latest scientific evidence on the synergistic relationship between nutrition and infection, and the impacts of nutrition on learning and behavior and on work performance, providing a "rationale" for investment in nutrition programs. Subsequent workshops then assessed the status of programming in the areas of: (1) food fortification; (2) supplementary feeding and formulated foods; (3) integrated, multisectoral, village-level interventions; (4) small-farm agricultural systems; (5) food conservation and post-harvest food loss, and (6) food price controls and consumer subsidies.

A second major concern was how to organize the flow of the discussion so that it would focus effectively on the most critical problem (or problems) now facing the international nutrition community. Interestingly, there was near-unanimous agreement among the conference organizers that the problem of implementation—and, more specifically, the "interface" between the rhetorical statement of policy and the actual operation of programs—was the most serious obstacle impeding progress on the reduction of hunger and malnutrition.

In order to facilitate further the flow of discussion within a 4½-day meeting, the conference theme was approached from two different directions: one highlighting the most salient issues and problems within each of the six topical areas cited above and the other providing specific, in-depth country case experience with specific programs. Accordingly, in addition to "issue papers" prepared for each of the workshops, 16 "country case study" papers were contributed, illustrating experience in different national settings.

For the purposes of this volume, the material has been organized into eight sections, beginning with the current "rationale" for investment by national governments in nutrition programming. This is followed by presentation of the six topical areas, each including an issue paper, two or more country case studies, and a summary of relevant workshop discussion. A substantial effort has been made in all cases to present only the most salient and insightful workshop discussions that supplemented the material contained in the papers.

The final section of the book records the efforts of the final plenary session to deal in an explicit fashion with the conference theme. It includes a summary of general plenary discussions, a rapporteur's summary of the conference, and five concluding afterthoughts contributed by certain participants in the period immediately following the meeting.

The editors wish to express sincere appreciation and thanks to Mr. David Sahn and Miss Jane Dittrich for their invaluable assistance in the editorial development of these proceedings.

N.S.S.
M.B.W.

The Rationale for Investment in Nutrition

Policies and plans to improve human nutrition must have strong justification before resources allocated in competition with other development needs can be solicited and obtained. The strongest rationale is that adverse functional consequences ensue when people are not able to obtain enough of the right kinds of food. The three main consequences are decreased cognitive and physical performance, increased frequency and severity of infections, and increased mortality. The papers in this first section, each presented by a world authority, provide strong evidence that susceptibility to, and death from, infectious disease are increased by even mild degrees of deficiency of specific nutrients, that physical and mental growth and development are impaired, and that physical activity in children and work performance in adults are decreased by caloric inadequacy and iron deficiency. Each of the three papers in this section represents an authoritative state-of-the-art summary of current knowledge, and each includes some new data.

Brozek's presentation is based on the extensive published review of field studies of malnutrition, learning, and behavior. Viteri, who has done outstanding original work on the effects of nutrition on behavior, provides convincing evidence that nutrition interventions can increase work production. The third paper, by Chandra, is an authoritative state-of-the-art review of the present information on the relationship between malnutrition and resistance to infection. The comments on these papers also present additional valuable information and insight.

The editors wish to acknowledge the contribution of Daniel Bankson and Judith McGuire, who served as rapporteurs for this workshop.

Nutrition and Work Performance

FERNANDO E. VITERI

INTRODUCTION

Intuitively, one accepts the hypothesis that optimal work performance and socioeconomic function require adequate nutrition and that, consequently, an altered nutritional status should result in some impairment of those complex human endeavors. Data and many observations are available that demonstrate clearly that *severe* nutritional deficiencies and excesses can seriously hamper work performance and social function. However, these extremes, which are actually disease states, must be treated as such, and, if they are abundant within a social group, emergency actions must be established to prevent death (i.e., interventions in famine situations). Work performance under these circumstances becomes a secondary matter. The questions that I believe need answers from the nutrition policy planner's point of view, and that are directed toward facilitating the elaboration and implementation of policies, concern population groups defined as mild to moderately undernourished. I will address the subject from the standpoint of undernutrition, recognizing that the consquences of overnutrition (such as early establishment of obesity, diabetes, and cardiovascular disease) may be as serious in terms of work performance and productivity as those afflicting undernourished populations.

FERNANDO E. VITERI • Division of Human Nutrition and Biology, Institute of Nutrition of Central America and Panama (INCAP), Guatemala City, Guatemala.

QUESTIONS

The *first* question to be asked is: What is meant by mild to moderately undernourished populations?

Generally, a population has been identified as suffering from undernutrition on the basis of infant and preschool child mortality statistics, growth retardation in the paediatric population, clinical evidence of severe malnutrition in a certain number of children, prevalence of diarrheal diseases, poverty, and, last but not least, estimates of dietary intake. Only recently have indicators of functional performance been looked at as sensitive indicators of inadequate nutrition, particularly in the adult population. Among these indicators reproductive and lactative performance in the female population, physical work performance in the male population, and possibly social behavioral patterns of population groups should be mentioned. Still, dietary surveys and estimates at the population level are often utilized to define whether populations are undernourished, referring adequacy of intakes to requirement figures in the case of energy, and to recommended allowances for protein and other nutrients (1). There is no doubt that populations who, for multiple reasons, chronically consume limited amounts of food, primarily based on roots, tubers, and cereals, are more at risk of being undernourished than others who consume a more abundant and varied diet. However, within limits still not well established, the human "adapts" to a range of food intakes, thus making a diagnosis of mild to moderate undernutrition (especially of energy and protein) on the basis of only mild to moderate inadequacy of food intake essentially impossible.

In the case of physical work and activity that demand energy expenditure, the question of adequacy of energy intake becomes particularly important. We have shown that adult male populations engaged in agricultural energy-demanding activities "adapt" their energy expenditure to their intake and maintain stable body weights at mean intakes that range between 2700 kcal/day and 3550 kcal/day (2–4). If we compare these mean intakes with the calculated "adequate" intakes computed from energy requirement estimates, some populations would be deficient and others would exceed their energy requirements. Consequently, if this were the case, the deficient populations should be losing weight and would eventually die in an emaciated state, while the others would be gaining weight and would become obese. The fact that all populations maintained their weight throughout several years and that body composition studies did not disclose obesity in the high-intake groups clearly demonstrates a remarkable adaptation to chronic energy intakes by these population groups. These facts, however, need further in-depth analyses in terms of the characteristics of the populations, their similarities and differences, and the "adaptation" mechanisms set in motion.

The pertinent characteristics of the populations were that they were composed of healthy males 16 years of age and older engaged in agricultural activities that demanded physical effort and endurance, who were paid or benefitted according to the product or amount of work performed, and who lived at sea level or in the highlands (up to 1800 m above sea level) in Guatemala (Table 1). No migratory workers were studied; the ethnic groups were Caucasian, Mayan, and mixed. Their cultural patterns were predominantly occidental (vs. Mayan). Agricultural labors included sugar cane care and cutting (5); coffee plantation work and harvesting of coffee (6); corn, rice, bean, and forage cultivation; and care of animals (mostly cows) (4). I would like to stress the fact that their earnings depended on their work output, executing energy-demanding tasks requiring endurance.

Two of the five populations studied received supplements: one a food supplement (SI), and the other an energy-rich drink (HES). One other population, matched to the one receiving the energy-rich drink, received an identical drink except that it did not contain any calories (LES). The other two populations did not receive any nutritional benefit (SAP and C). All of the populations received medical care.

The main anthropometrical and work performance data are presented in Table 2. It is evident that the lightest group was SAP. The SI group was the heavier of these two groups. In terms of adiposity, the SAP was leaner than the SI. Accurate determinations of lean body mass

TABLE 1. Summary Information of the Core Studies Performed at INCAP in the Area of Nutrition and Work Performance

Population	No.	Age (years)	Location	Occupation	Intervention	Energy intake (kcal/day)
SAP	20	18.6[a] (2.6)	Highlands	Agriculture (varied)	None	2693 (592)
SI	19	25.8 (9.0)	Highlands	Agriculture (varied)	Food supplement (3 years)	3550 (423)
HES	92	35.5 (11.5)	Lowlands	Sugar cane	Energy-rich drink (14 months)	3023 (579)
LES	59	34.4 (10.2)	Lowlands	Sugar cane	Energy-poor drink (14 months)	2891 (524)
C	20	31.6 (6.6)	Lowlands	Coffee, agriculture (varied)	None	2466 (760)

[a] Mean (S.D.).

TABLE 2. Pertinent Anthropometric and Functional Characteristics of the
Subjects in the Studies Shown in Table 1

Population	Height (cm)	Weight (kg)	Weight/height (kg/cm)	Adiposity (% body weight)	Skinfold (triceps) (mm)	$\dot{V}_{02}$ max (liters/min)
SAP	158.5[a]	50.8	0.32	8.1	3.8	2065
	(5.1)	(4.1)	(0.02)	(3.8)	(1.2)	(234)
SI	161.2	57.8	0.36	12.6	7.4	2480
	(4.1)	(4.5)	(0.02)	(3.2)	(2.2)	(216)
HES	159.0	53.5	0.34	—	4.8	2570
	(6.4)	(6.0)	(0.03)	—	(1.6)	(473)
LES	160.4	52.6	0.33	—	4.6	2581
	(5.8)	(5.4)	(0.03)	—	(1.6)	(628)
C	166.6	57.3	0.34	—	5.4	2674
	(6.8)	(6.0)	(0.03)	—	(1.6)	(412)

[a] Mean (S.D.).

and muscle mass were done only in the SI and SAP (2) groups, the former showing greater muscle mass. All groups can be considered physically fit according to population standards; their maximal physical working capacity (maximal aerobic power or $\dot{V}_{02}$ max.) was also excellent and identical in the two extreme groups (SI and SAP) when expressed per unit of body protein or "cell residue." Maximal aerobic power ($\dot{V}_{02}$ max.), however, was proportional—in absolute terms—to the total lean body mass. That is, heavier, nonobese individuals will have larger maximal aerobic power. This measurement is important because populations engaged in energy-demanding activities usually work at about 50% of their $\dot{V}_{02}$ max.; therefore, it conditions, to an extent, the work output and performance of individuals. Attention must be paid to the variability within population groups of all the above measurements, indicative of different levels of adaptation, and energy equilibrium at which individuals function.

The main mechanisms by which these populations manage to maintain long-term energy equilibrium appears to be by changing their activity patterns at work, when this is possible, and out of work. Indeed, we have been able to show that the members of the SAP group worked at lesser intensity and for shorter periods of time than did members of the SI group while performing the same chores. The net result was that members of the SI group accomplished more work per unit of time and earned more. Moreover, these subjects remained active after work, while those in the SAP group essentially collapsed at home after work, taking long naps and barely moving until bedtime. They also slept slightly longer at night than did those in the SI group. In terms of relative effort in the performance of similar chores, the men in the SAP group worked at 87% mean intensity of the SI workers. In terms of work efficiency, it took the SAP workers 389 min to do what SI men did in 202 min, that is, 1.9 times as long. These figures may explain some of the employment patterns in developing countries, where people are preferentially hired to do a specific job or task rather than by day or week.

Other possible adaptive mechanisms include a change in the efficiency of coupling, in the magnitude of wasteful metabolic pathways, in the conversion of energy to physical work, and in dexterity in the performance of specified tasks (7,8). The data regarding these mechanisms are still very scanty, and it is difficult to attribute a magnitude or an efficiency ratio, although there are suggestions that the relative efficiency of work output may have a coefficient of variation as high as 30% (9).

The original question of what is meant by mildly to moderately undernourished populations, when applied to energy intake and its evaluation, therefore requires careful consideration of two different situations that I will describe as physiological energy needs (PEN) and recommended energy allowances (REA).

PEN would be the energy intake that is considered adequate to meet the minimum energy needs compatible with health for a person in a specified age/sex category allowing him/her to maintain sedentary activity. These needs depend on three variables that are interrelated in a complex way: (1) age, (2) body size and composition, and (3) climate and other microecological factors. PEN should allow for an adequate rate of growth (based on currently accepted standards) and satisfactory mental and biological functions, such as immune mechanisms, pregnancy, and lactation. Levels of intake below PEN mean that weight cannot be maintained and inadequate functioning will become apparent. There is an intraindividual variability that probably amounts to a coefficient of variation of 15–20% (10,11). These figures should apply in a universal fashion to "healthy reference populations." Those segments of a population whose intakes fall below PEN should be considered undernourished even if they are able to maintain body weight, because this will most probably occur at the expense of lean body mass, and they will have functional defects.

REA, on the other hand, is the sum of PEN and the extra energy considered necessary for the following: (1) facilitating activity beyond sedentary living, (2) insuring the available energy to meet the demands expected from his/her way of life as may be perceived by his/her society, and (3), replenishing an individual's or a population's energy deficit, should the occasion arise. REA should aim at allowing population groups to reach a desirable quality of life and social function within a cultural setting. REA is the goal that the socially aware nutrition planner should aim for, and it should not be used in defining "undernourished" populations. When an REA is not met, the result should be lower productivity than desirable for the sociocultural setting where energy-demanding activities are indispensable for survival and development.

The *second* question to be asked is: What can be accomplished, in terms of physical work performance, by improving the nutrition of population groups?

This question requires the analysis of two situations: (1) the effects of past, and (2) the effects of present nutritional conditions. Improving the nutritional condition of populations will result in greater physical work capacity, at least by improving the chances of children to achieve greater height and, with it, greater lean body mass and absolute aerobic power ($\dot{V}_{0_2}$ max.) when they reach adulthood. This potential benefit is translated into two actual conditions:

1. An agricultural worker's $\dot{V}_{0_2}$ max. correlates significantly ($r = 0.57$) with height, and stepwise regression analysis, which also includes weight-for-height, age, dietary intake, and hematocrit as predictors of $\dot{V}_{0_2}$ max., consistently points to height as the most significant predictor (12).
2. Work performance, measured as cane cut per unit of time and total daily productivity, has been shown to be significantly correlated with the height of the worker (5,13). In both communities engaged in sugar cane cutting, the taller workers (163–174 cm) cut a mean of 6% more cane than the shorter ones (144–156 cm) throughout adulthood (17–60 years of age), independent of energy intake (5).

Past nutrition appears to have a negative effect on adult productivity if it diminishes adult height. The mental development and intellectual consequences of early malnutrition on work performance in adulthood can only be speculated upon (14).

Improving present nutritional conditions has been shown to benefit work performance and productivity by several mechanisms under different circumstances, all of which must be analyzed. Three are discussed in the following paragraphs.

The first mechanism is an increase in energy intake for three years by means of food supplementation that supplied 250 kcal/day and 5.5 g of protein/day. This resulted in a clear superiority in body composition of the workers in the SI group in relation to unsupplemented workers of similar backgrounds (2). SI men had significantly more muscle mass per unit height (7–18%), while adiposity remained on the low side (mean 12.6% of body weight). SAP workers had only 8.1% mean adiposity, which was lower than that of other "normal" peasants or that of cadets (a reference population). These last two groups had 12.9 and 12.4% adiposity, respectively.

The SI workers had a mean daily intake of 3550 kcal/day, which allowed a mean of 1956 kcal to be spent in activity daily, in comparison to the SAP men who could only spend an average of 1167 kcal/day in physical activity and still maintain energy equilibrium, with a mean intake of 2690 kcal/day. This indicates that SAP men had only 60% of the food energy available for work that the SI workers had. This assumes no differences in efficiency of energy conversion to work between the two groups. Detailed energy balance studies suggest that this is a sound assumption (4).

Under the conditions of life and work of these two groups of agricultural laborers, present improvement of energy intake allows greater energy expenditure and physical activity, not only during work but also after work, as indicated previously. Protein intake by the SI and SAP groups was ample even before supplementation of the former group, so that the 5.5 g/day increase in protein intake is considered inconsequential.

The second circumstance arises in the analysis of the sequence of events during energy supplementation of agricultural workers; a study involving two groups of cane cutters (HES and LES groups) was carried out. After a period of basal evaluation, the HES group received a high-energy supplement (sucrose-containing drink) under direct supervision in the field, while the LES group received, under identical conditions, a drink that supplied only 24 kcal/day. The high-energy drink provided 560 kcal/day. The supplementation period lasted over two years, but at present only data on the first 13 months of supplementation are available (5).

The effects of supplementation can be summarized as follows:

1. Body weight remained stable.
2. Total energy intake in the HES group was, on the average, 281 kcal/day higher than in the LES group (S.D. ± 621 kcal/day), because of a lower home energy intake in the HES group during supplementation. Daily energy intake in this group was 3023 ± 579 kcal (mean ± S.D.).
3. Workers' productivity, maximal aerobic capacity, and home

energy intake progressively decline after age 35, so that by age 62 productivity has dropped to approximately 83% of that at the peak age (20–27 years). This effect appears to be offset by increasing the energy intake to at least 2600 kcal/day. The decline in maximal aerobic power with age also appears to be annulled when the worker's intake allows for continued physical activity up to the fifth decade of life (12).

4. There appears to be a different pattern of energy expenditure related to age in the HES group. The younger workers did not significantly increase their productivity with increasing energy intakes; after-work activities (leisure activities) apparently account for most of the necessary increase in energy expenditure to maintain energy balance. In older workers, energy supplementation resulted in increased work performance and output, as indicated in point 3.

5. The supplemented workers as a group did increase daily output in a proportionate fashion to daily increments in intake. Younger workers appeared more efficient in that, as a mean, older workers spent more energy cutting the same amount of cane. For example, at age 55, the efficiency had dropped 12% compared to that at age 18.

These results show a marginal effect of energy supplementation on productivity, which, however, is significant primarily in its positive effect among workers whose intake is lower (older workers in this population). Among younger workers, increased energy intake was primarily utilized in leisure activity.

Parallel studies have demonstrated that correction of anemia results in greater capacity to perform tasks that demand near maximal aerobic power (15,16). Even mild anemia reduces physical fitness. Moreover, correction of anemia, and possibly of iron deficiency *per se*, appears to be able to increase the productivity of workers engaged in energy-demanding tasks (17). Our interpretation of the combined results regarding chronic, inadequate energy intake and anemia as they relate to work performance and productivity is expressed as follows: Limitations in energy intake, below REAs, lead to an energy equilibrium at activity levels that can limit work performance and productivity. The presence of anemia further hampers these functions, at least by blunting the peak activities required in most agricultural occupations. It may be that anemia also reduces the activity level, which is usually set at near 50% of aerobic power. This may occur as a consequence of generalized dysfunction caused by severe iron deficiency (18,19).

The *third* question to be asked is: What nutritional aspects and other behavioral and social conditions influence work performance, energy balance, and productivity?

The data to answer this question in a quantitative manner are very scarce, except for the interesting work done by Kraut and co-workers with regard to industrial production and calorie intake in Germany during World War II and immediately thereafter (20,21).

In our explorations of the complex area of nutrition and productivity, we have found some interesting interrelations that partially answer this third question.

First, from the work already referred to, it would appear that population groups maintain energy equilibrium primarily by modulating energy expenditure and physical activity. However, the fact that the HES group of cane cutters reduced their energy intake at home when they were receiving an energy supplement in the field, and achieved energy equilibrium with a mean intake of 3023 kcal/day and a standard deviation that amounted to a coefficient of variation of 19% suggests the following: among populations who depend on physical fitness to be able to work, the development of obesity is as undesirable as is the loss of lean body mass (muscle) for energy purposes, since both result in poor work performance. Therefore, a careful system of feedback is constantly in operation, regulating activity levels and energy expenditure on the one hand, and energy intake on the other, when extraneous conditions set a limit to energy expenditure in the face of abundant energy availability. These conditions may be sociocultural work patterns, agroindustrial administration subtleties, or motivational aspects.

Second, studies we have conducted with recruits who came from agricultural environments (2) demonstrate that energy balance can be easily disrupted when enforced limitations in energy expenditure occur in the face of abundant food. Indeed, after 16 months in the army, a group of recruits who entered the army with 8% adiposity had doubled this percentage, while muscle mass had fallen by 5%. Mean energy intake in the army had increased by about 300 kcal/day in relation to previous intake, while expenditure was reduced. The change in intake was detrimental under that special setting, while it had proven beneficial to the SI workers.

Many other questions come to mind in the area of nutrition, work performance, and productivity that are only beginning to be answered. Unfortunately, it is too early to provide further answers to the questions that plague the nutrition planner, and that could be of help in implementing food and nutrition policies. Whole areas of agronomic practices, employment theory, community development, and policy integration (to name but a few) that influence decisions at governmental levels have not even been considered in this paper, but are addressed by others in this volume.

ACKNOWLEDGMENTS. Close collaborators in much of the work discussed here are Drs. B. Torún and M. D. C. Immink, and Lic. R. Flores. Their contributions to these studies are hereby acknowledged with sincere appreciation. This work has been partially supported by grants from the W. K. Kellogg Foundation, the U.S. Army Research and Development Command, and the Government of Guatemala.

REFERENCES

1. World Health Organization Tech. Rep. Ser. No. 522, *Energy and Protein Requirements.* Report of a joint FAO/WHO ad hoc expert committee, WHO, Geneva, 1973.
2. Viteri, F. E. Considerations on the effect of nutrition on the body composition and physical working capacity of young Guatemalan adults. In: *Amino Acid Fortification of Protein Foods*, N. S. Scrimshaw and A. M. Altschul (Eds.), MIT Press, Cambridge, Massachusetts, and London, England, 1971.
3. Viteri, F. E., B. Torún, J. C. Galicia, and E. Herrera. Determining energy cost of work of agricultural activities by respirometer and energy balance techniques. *Am. J. Clin. Nutr.* 24:1418, 1971.
4. Viteri, F. E., and B. Torún. Ingestión calórica de trabajo físico de obreros agrícolas en Guatemala: Efecto de la suplementación alimentaria y su lugar en los programas de salud. *Bol. Of. Sanit. Panam.* 78:58, 1975.
5. Immink, M. D. C. Human energy supplementation and worker productivity: A case study of sugarcane cutters in Guatemala. Ph.D. Dissertation, University of Hawaii, 1978.
6. Viteri, F. E., R. Flores, F. Hernandez, and B. Torún. Food intake and energy expenditure in an agricultural cooperative in the Guatemalan lowlands. In preparation (INCAP), 1982.
7. Hegsted, D. M. Energy needs and energy utilization. *Nutr. Rev.* 32:33, 1974.
8. Miller, D. S., P. Mumford, and M. J. Stock. Gluttony 2: Thermogenesis in overeating man. *Am J. Clin. Nutr.* 20:1223, 1967.
9. Edmunson, W. Individual variations in work output per unit energy intake in East Java. *Ecol. Food Nutr.* 6:147, 1977.
10. Robertson, J. M., and D. D. Reid. Standards for the basal metabolism of normal people in Britain. *Lancet* i:940, 1952.
11. Wedgewood, R. J., D. E. Bass, J. A. Klimas, C. R. Kleeman, and M. Quinn. Relationship of body composition to basal metabolic rate in normal man. *J. Appl. Physiol.* 6:317, 1953.
12. Flores, R., B. Torún, and F. E. Viteri. Ciclo Agrícola, Estado nutricional y capacidad de trabajo físico de trabajadores de una cooperativa agrícola en la Costa de Guatemala. *Arch. Latinoam. Nutr.* in preparation, 1982.
13. Spurr, G. B., M. Barac-Nieto, and M. G. Maksud. Productivity and maximal oxygen consumption in sugar cane cutters. *Am. J. Clin. Nutr.* 30:316, 1977.

14. Selowsky, M., and L. Taylor. The economics of malnourished children: An example of disinvestment in human capital. *Econ. Develop. Cult. Change* **22:**17, 1973.
15. Viteri, F. E. Physical fitness and anemia. *Proceedings of the International Symposium on Malnutrition and Function of Blood Cells,* Kyoto, Japan, 1972, pp. 559–583, National Institute of Nutrition, Tokyo, 1973.
16. Viteri, F. E., and B. Torún. Anaemia and physical work capacity. *Clin. Haematol.* **3:**609, 1974.
17. Basta, S. S., Soekirman, D. Karyadi, and N. S. Scrimshaw. Iron deficiency anemia and the productivity of adult males in Indonesia. *Am. J. Clin. Nutr.* **32:**916, 1979.
18. Finch, C. A., L. R. Miller, A. R. Inamdar, R. Person, K. Seiler, and B. Mackler. Iron deficiency in the rat: Physiological and biochemical studies of muscle dysfunction. *J. Clin. Invest.* **58:**447, 1976.
19. Dallman, P. R., E. Beutler, and C. A. Finch. Annotation: Effects of iron deficiency exclusive of anaemia. *Br. J. Haematol.* **40:**179, 1978.
20. Kraut, H. A., and E. A. Muller. Calorie intake and industrial output. *Science* **104:**495, 1946.
21. Keller, W. D., and J. A. Kraut. Work and nutrition. *World Rev. Nutr. Diet.* **3:**65, 1962.

Comment

HARRY L. JACOBS

The data Viteri summarizes are an excellent example of the usefulness of combining techniques of work physiology, metabolic physiology, and clinical nutrition with some aspects of psychology and sociology. The questions of energy balance, adaptation, performance, and productivity in mild to moderate malnutrition, raised by Viteri, are part of a general recognition of the need for a broader approach in nutrition, one in which the biological and social sciences are blended to form a *functional approach* in which food supply is a major variable and nutritional limits are set within the boundaries to which man can adapt (1). The work of Viteri's group over the last decade is an outstanding example of that trend.

Although I have not labeled my own work "functional nutrition" as such, my interests in sensory and metabolic responses to energy deficits in animal models (2–6) and in food preferences and feeding systems as they influence fitness and performance in the military (7,8) do fit into the same trend. I have begun to consider questions of energy deficits and excesses of over- and undernutrition and of developing and developed societies as two sides of the same coin.

Problems of undernutrition occur when food supply lags behind physical work requirements. Thus, an economy of scarcity produces a limited food choice for the individual. When this is combined with a labor-intensive work force in the economy, producing a heavy work load for the individual, it leads to problems of health, performance, and behavioral effectiveness. In extreme cases of under- or overnutrition, we can easily evaluate health and fitness effects in terms of longevity, morbidity, and the kinds of measures of physiological status referred to by

HARRY L. JACOBS • Behavioral Sciences Division, Department of the Army, U.S. Army Natick Research and Development Command, Natick, Massachusetts.

Viteri. As we shift from the extremes to mild malnutrition, the problem of measuring productivity effects becomes more difficult; there has been progress, however, in measuring the quantity and efficiency of work patterns, as Viteri illustrates.

Transition to an economy of plenty increases food supply and provides *ad libitum* food choice within the framework of the society's food distribution system. When this is combined with a shift from a heavy workload to a sedentary workload, a new set of health and performance problems must be faced. The factors relevant to the transition from undernutrition to overnutrition are also critical in the shift from a developing to a developed society.

Until recently, I have looked at the development of problems of overnutrition in the U.S. Armed Forces as an example indigenous to highly developed Western society, where the military are subject to the same sociocultural forces experienced by their civilian counterparts. Viteri's observations on the military in Guatemala suggest that the military in developing countries could provide a useful tool to study the transition from problems of undernutrition to problems of overnutrition.

First, Viteri studied soldier recruits from peasant stock, who left their agricultural work setting where they were all energy-deficient but quite fit. On entering the army they were given an "energy supplement" of about 300 cal/day for 16 months, with a sedentary workload. Over the 16-month period they gained weight, mostly fat, and became *less* fit. On the other hand, another group of cadets coming into the army from elite families *increased* their fitness without a supplement, because rigorous exercise was a part of their officer's training program.

These studies show that energy deficit, body weight, and fitness depended upon the initial ratios of energy input to output. In agricultural workers with a high workload, extra calories are a nutrition supplement; in agricultural workers with a low workload (the soldier recruits), extra calories may simply be excess calories. Recent studies by Spurr and his co-workers in Colombian agricultural workers demonstrate the same points (9). They compared Colombian agricultural workers with migrant workers in Florida and with U.S. Civil Service workers. Both of the latter two were much less fit in terms of work capacity and efficiency; in addition, the Civil Service personnel had much more adipose tissue.

It would be most instructive to compare Viteri's studies with data on groups of peasant laborers, soldiers, and elite groups in countries like India, Brazil, and Argentina that are more industrialized than Guatemala. Studies of the military in these countries could provide an excellent model of the transition between undernutrition and overnutrition in developing countries, as well as help us understand the phenomenon within Western society.

References

1. Calloway, D. H., C. Wood, R. Beall, and D. J. Cattle. Collaborative research program on intake and function. Final report, AID Contract No. AID/DSAN-C-002, 1980.
2. Jacobs, H. L. Sensory and metabolic regulation of food intake: Thoughts on a dual system regulated by energy balance. In: *Proceedings of the VII International Congress of Nutrition*, Vol. II. *Regulation of Hunger and Satiety*, pp. 17–29, F. Vieweg, Braunschweig, 1966.
3. Jacobs, H. L. Taste and the role of experience in the regulation of food intake. In: *Chemical Senses and Nutrition*, M. R. Kare and O. Maller (Eds.), p. 187, Johns Hopkins, Baltimore, Maryland, 1967.
4. Shetty, P. S., and S. Dua-Sharma. Clinical-metabolic profiles and taste preferences in undernourished subjects. In: *Symposium on Food Habits and Energy Balance in Man*, H. L. Jacobs (Ed.), Proceedings of the XXVI Congress of Physiological Sciences, Delhi, India, 1974.
5. Sharma, K. N., H. L. Jacobs, V. Gopal, and S. Dua-Sharma. Nutritional state/taste interactions in food intake: Behavioral and physiological evidence for gastric/taste modulation. In: *Chemical Senses and Nutrition*, M. Kare and O. Maller (Eds.), p. 169, Academic Press, New York, 1977.
6. Morgane, P. J. and H. L. Jacobs. Hunger and satiety. In: *World Rev. Nutr. Diet.* **10**:100, 1969.
7. Jacobs, H. L. National ferment in dietary goals: Challenge and opportunity for the defense department's food program. *Act. Rep. Res. Dev. Assoc. Mil. Food Packag. Syst.* **30**:69, 1978. (From Fall Meeting, 1977, held at U.S. Army Natick Laboratories, Natick, Massachusetts).
8. Jacobs, H. L. Behavioral sciences, consumer decisions, and food system evaluation: The Natick Labs food program and military feeding as prototypes. In: *New England Conference on Food, Nutrition, and Health*, Vol. II, Federal Regional Council of New England, Final Report, p. 150, 1980.
9. Spurr, G. B., M. Barac, and M. G. Maksud. Clinical and subclinical malnutrition: Their influence on the capacity to do work. Final report, US Agency for International Development, Project No. AID/CSD, 2943, 1975.

Discussion

Among the major issues addressed in the general discussion was the need to pay greater attention to research on the energy needs and expenditures of women. Beyond the fact that women have special energy needs associated with pregnancy and lactation, their active involvement in agricultural and domestic work also markedly increases their energy expenditure. The problem is that planners and economists alike have traditionally disregarded the role of women in the food-production sector, and hence, overlooked their increased dietary-energy requirements.

The discussion attempted to clarify whether energy intakes below recommended allowances initiate biological adaptative mechanisms, and/or behavioral changes that enable the individual to adapt to chronically low intakes of energy. Some argued that there is a linear relationship between energy intake and physical output; the more one works, the more calories one needs. However, others pointed to the accumulating evidence that, besides adaptations in work practices that decrease energy expenditure, metabolic adaptations do take place.

The Impact of Malnutrition on Behavior

Josef Brožek

Introduction

The central concerns in the area of malnutrition and behavior can be grouped under three categories: facts, theories, and modes of intervention.

In an effort to obtain comparative, factual information regarding the major recent longitudinal studies on malnutrition and development carried out in the Western Hemisphere, predominantly in Latin America (Colombia, Mexico, and Guatemala), a working conference was held in Cali, Colombia, in 1975. The following features of each study were considered: the starting and completion dates, the scheduled periods of observation, the populations under study, their home diets, nutritional supplements (if any), behavioral stimulation (if any), and the procedures and measurements used (1). Partial aspects of these studies have been described in journal articles, contributions to conference proceedings, and book chapters. There is an urgent need for comprehensive, systematic, monographic presentations of each of these studies. Some general conclusions will be noted in the next section of this paper. Theoretical considerations will be limited primarily to the problem of modeling.

"Intervention," in a broad sense, refers to the way in which the phenomena under consideration can be altered. Here we are concerned with

Josef Brožek • University of Würzburg, Würzburg, Federal Republic of Germany. *Present address:* Department of Psychology, Lehigh University, Bethlehem, Pennsylvania.

medical, nutritional, and behavioral modes of intervention. These, in turn, must be considered in a wider socioeconomic context.

It is useful to differentiate between interventions applied in the context of clinical and subclinical malnutrition. Children with clinical malnutrition receive medical and nutritional (and, at times, special behavioral) treatment in the hospital. Behavioral intervention may be continued through home visits after discharge, although this is done very rarely (2).

In the case of subclinical malnutrition, the forms and conditions of both nutritional and behavioral intervention are more diversified. In communities in which the risk of malnutrition is high, we may start with food supplementation during pregnancy, continue to supplement the mother's food intake for a period of time, begin to supplement the child when called for, and continue to do so for varying lengths of time, in accordance with the design of the study. The supplementation may be initiated in preschool children or provided in the form of school breakfast, or, more typically, school lunch.

DOES NUTRITION (AND MALNUTRITION) MAKE A DIFFERENCE?

It is difficult and, in fact, impossible to provide categorical answers to this question. We begin by separating the issues into two broad categories:

- Does nutrition affect behavior?
- Does improved feeding, including various forms of supplementary feeding, improve mental function and performance?

Unfortunately, performance (P) is a function of capacity (C) and motivation (M), $P = f(C \times M)$. Thus, that which might appear to be a very simple question at the onset quickly becomes a series of complex questions.

The fundamental issue is not whether malnutrition makes a difference, but rather what *kind* of "malnutrition" we have in mind, i.e., a deficit in calories, or a surplus of calories leading to obesity; or a deficit of energy, or of protein, or a combined energy–protein deficiency leading to generalized malnutrition. Or are we concerned with one of the particularized forms of malnutrition resulting from deficits of, for example, iron or iodine? Even in areas of severe, clinical energy–protein malnutrition we must state whether we are referring to nutritional marasmus, kwashiorkor, or marasmic kwashiorkor. Of course, in the area of subclinical, chronic deficiency we must specify the *magnitude* of the deviation of the criterion variable from the reference standard, whether we study the effects of depressed linear growth (stunting) or of underdevelopment (or actual loss) of soft tissues (wasting). In other words, we must specify not only the qualitative aspects of the nutrient deficit, but also the number of quantitative features (including the severity and duration of the deficit) and of qualitative indicators, such as the subject's sex. To generalize is difficult.

While a "cumulative record" of research on malnutrition and behavior can be provided fairly readily (3), endeavors aimed at a synthesis of information have been few. This review notes three such efforts, referring to (1) selected longitudinal studies, dealing primarily with chronic, subclinical malnutrition; (2) sequelae of clinical malnutrition; and (3) effects of both clinical and subclinical malnutrition.

LONGITUDINAL STUDIES

The general conclusions, based on a review of the major (primarily Latin American) studies on the effects of malnutrition, nutritional stimulation, and behavioral stimulation (1, pp. 246–247), are not very definitive. This is due, in part, to high diversity among research designs and in part to the fact that only partial, and in some cases preliminary, results from these projects were available. The conclusions bear on three sets of outcomes: birth weight, child growth, and behavior.

The available data indicate that birth weight can be increased by nutritional supplements provided to the pregnant mother, although this finding is not universal. The nutrients that are critically involved appear to depend upon the specific situation, with energy supply being dominant in some areas, whereas in other regions the protein content of the supplement seems to be the important factor. Finally, birth weight correlates with a number of environmental and socioeconomic factors. Their effects must be controlled before the etiology of low birth weight can be fully understood.

Nutritional supplementation of young, malnourished children increases their rates of growth. While gain in height may parallel that of more favored populations, the question remains open as to whether (and under what conditions) a true catch-up growth is possible that would bring previously malnourished children to the level considered "normal" for their age group.

The studies under consideration have indicated that child behavior is affected positively by nutritional supplementation of the undernourished mother during pregnancy and following delivery, as well as by supplementation of undernourished children or children "at risk" of malnutrition. More definite conclusions must await completion of several of these studies, or analysis of the data already at hand. At the time of the Cali conference (1975), it appeared that the earlier supplementation begins, the greater the likelihood of a positive outcome (1). The positive effects reported tended to be more definitive for motor than for cognitive functions. However, this was a tendency, not a consistent finding. It was stressed that the behavioral outcomes interact, in complex ways, with the characteristics of the child's macroenvironment (including socioeconomic conditions) and its microenvironment (such as the amount of behavioral stimulation available to the child).

SEQUELAE OF CLINICAL ENERGY–PROTEIN MALNUTRITION

Lloyd-Still (4) summarized, in tabular form, 13 studies on the sequelae of infant malnutrition. In children who varied in age at follow-up from 1 to 5 years, the performance of the index children was poorer than that of the controls. The acquisition of language skill seems to have been affected most, although this was not observed in all studies. In one study the fine motor functions appeared to be particularly sensitive to the stress of malnutrition in infancy.

In results obtained from 10 groups of children who were older (over 5 years) at follow-up, the findings concerning sequelae of infant malnutrition were not consistent. In five studies the intelligence of the index children was significantly lower. In two studies the difference was in the expected direction but was marginal, and in three other studies it was not statistically significant.

MALNUTRITION—SUBCLINICAL AND CLINICAL

An extensive, though not exhaustive, analysis and tabular presentation of the results reported in the literature was undertaken by Pollitt and Thomson (5), which summarizes three retrospective, observational (noninterventional) studies on mild to moderate malnutrition (5, Table 7). This leaves out a number of other studies reported in the literature (3, pp. 163–164). Furthermore, the use of varying criteria of nutritional status makes comparative analysis of the results difficult, if not impossible. Several prospective Latin American studies are discussed in the text, but not summarized in tabular form. Two general conclusions are offered: (1) Among populations where malnutrition is endemic, both indicators of human growth (stunting) and socioeconomic variables (such as income or maternal education) correlate with measurements of mental development; assessment of their independent contribution to the variance of the test scores calls for further research. (2) Upgrading the quality of life through infancy and the preschool years enhances mental development.

Briefly noted are five studies, summarized in the authors' Table 6, on severe undernutrition secondary to neonatal disorders. These conditions provide a welcome opportunity to study the effects of malnutrition uncomplicated by poverty, infection, and parasitism. However, the results are not uniform. The body of this review deals with primary clinical malnutrition. Pollitt and Thomson's Table 3 summarizes six behavioral studies of children who recovered from nutritional marasmus, Table 4 refers to six studies of children who had kwashiorkor, and Table 5 covers nine studies on the behavioral effects of mixed or undifferentiated clinical energy–protein malnutrition.

Typically, in nutritional marasmus, the process of wasting is initiated very early, during the first year of life—a period of peak velocity in brain growth. The weight deficit is both severe and chronic, producing a lengthy impairment of the child's interaction with the environment. The condition results in a deficit of intellectual function that tends to persist. By contrast, infants who eventually develop kwashiorkor tend to grow satisfactorily during the first year. This severe but acute malnutrition occurs during the second year of life—a period of lessened brain vulnerability. The impairment of a child's interaction with the environment is shorter in duration and the chances for psychological rehabilitation are better.

Pollitt and Thomson summarize the results of the studies they reviewed as follows (5, p. 283): (1) Nutritional marasmus, characterized by a protracted, severe deficit of expected weight-for-age during the first year of life, results in severe impairment of intellectual function. (2) Kwashiorkor may, but generally does not, leave measurable retardation in intellectual function.

Malnutrition, Socioeconomic Status, and Mental Function

In the laboratory, where environmental conditions can be rigorously controlled, we can operate with a simple model according to which nutrition (N) has a direct impact on the organism, including the organism's behavior (B):

$$N \rightarrow B$$

This is a simple and, one can argue, an overly simple model. It does not imply that the environmental factors (E) do not play a role, but that they are controlled. Thus, we might write more properly:

$$N[E] \rightarrow B$$

"Control" refers to the uniformity of conditions maintained in experiments performed in a given laboratory with given personnel. With E constant, we can study the effect of variations in N on B.

A more generally applicable model:

$$N \searrow \atop E \nearrow \quad B$$

indicates that both nutritional and socioenvironmental variables can affect behavior.

One may build into the first model the concept that the interaction between nutrition and behavior is a two-way process:

$$N \rightleftarrows B$$

This would account for the fact that food habits (a behavioral variable) importantly affect food intake.

A more complex model (6, p. 16) takes into account the interactions between diet, environment, and the organism (with its metabolic, structural, physiological, and behavioral aspects):

$$\text{Diet} \leftarrow \text{Environment}$$
$$\searrow \qquad \swarrow$$
$$\text{Organism}$$

The crucial point is that socioeconomic factors interact with nutritional factors when affecting behavior. This fact is of theoretical importance in that it is relevant to our understanding of behavioral deficits in malnourished children. It is also of practical significance for increasing the effectiveness of medical and nutritional treatment of children suffering from clinical malnutrition, and for the rehabilitation of chronically malnourished children.

Our principal concern is with the human condition. Nevertheless, it may be useful to recall that, in their review of the literature on the effects of perinatal malnutrition on later behavior of the rat, Levine and

Wiener (7) pointed out that the results of animal studies are not free from contaminating environmental (psychosocial) variables. These variables interact with early malnutrition and may contribute to, or even account for, the behavioral changes observed in nutritionally rehabilitated animals.

Levitsky (8) stresses the need for strict environmental controls in animal studies because variation in environmental conditions can have significant effects, negative (stressful) as well as positive (ameliorative). Levitsky believes that a failure to control for such factors as housing conditions of the animals may account (at least in part, we would add) for the inability of investigators to replicate one another's findings. Levitsky specifically mentions that, in most of the studies in which long-term effects of early malnutrition were demonstrated, the animals were housed individually with a minimum of experimenter interaction with the animals, while in studies in which such an effect could not be demonstrated, the animals were reared in group cages. He refers to earlier studies from Cornell in which it was shown that " . . . raising malnourished animals in a 'stimulating' environment greatly ameliorates the behavioral effects of malnutrion," and reports that " . . . raising animals in an environment consisting of only two animals to a cage is sufficient to over-ride most of the effects of early malnutrition" (8, p. 271).

In Cynomolgus monkeys reared under conditions of severe protein depletion, Hiroshi Wako (personal communication, 1977) observed such patterns of disturbed behavior as excessive fear and aggression, self-clasping, huddling, stereotyped rocking, head-knocking, and autoeroticism. He noted that monkeys fed by a caretaker tended to develop these symptoms in a less severe form than did animals who nursed from bottles attached to the sides of the cages. These observations provide additional evidence that environmental deprivation (isolation) and malnutrition tend to act synergistically in producing disturbances in behavior.

SUBCLINICAL MALNUTRITION

NUTRITIONAL AND SOCIOECONOMIC FACTORS

The fact that both the socioeconomic level of the family and the severity of chronic undernutrition influence children's measured intelligence was documented in Delhi, India by Gupta et al. (9). When the degree of underweight was moderate and was held constant (at 70–90% of the reference weight), the children's mean IQ decreased with the level of socioeconomic status of the family (based on income, education, and occupation): from 105.3 for social class II, to 95.3 for social class III, and 85.1 for social class IV. At the same time within a given social class (specifically, class IV), the mean IQ decreased with the severity of chronic, subclinical malnutrition. The mean IQs were 88.1 for subjects in the range of weight between 71 and 90% of the norm, 76.6 for the weight class between 60 and 70%, and 66.0 for severe undernutrition (relative weight between 51 and 60% of the reference weight).

Using correlational analysis, Klein *et al.* (10) examined the relationship between selected indicators of nutritional status (stature and head circumference) and scores on seven psychological tests in a group of 311 boys and 321 girls measured at 5 and 7 years of age. The median value of statistically significant coefficients of correlation for height was 0.23, and for head circumference it was 0.21. The significant *r*s between an index of the families' socioeconomic status were in the same range, with a median *r* of 0.21.

NUTRITIONAL SUPPLEMENTATION AND PSYCHOEDUCATIONAL STIMULATION

McKay *et al.* (11,12) carried out a study in Cali, Colombia that was aimed at assessing the effectiveness of health care, nutritional supplementation, and psychoeducational stimulation in improving cognitive ability of chronically malnourished preschool children. The study children, drawn from poor urban families, had both low weight values (below the 25th percentile of North American norms) and low height values (below the 50th percentile). Two hundred and forty of the children were assigned at random to treatments differing in nature (i.e., nutritional supplementation with or without psychoeducational stimulation) and in duration (i.e., 1, 2, and 3 years). A control group of 60 children, drawn from the same socioeconomic stratum, received health care only. The food supplement, prepared and served at the center at which the psychoeducational stimulation was provided, was designed to meet 100% of the children's protein needs and 80% of their calorie needs. The children not receiving psychoeducational stimulation consumed the supplementary food at home.

When tested in verbal reasoning, the group receiving the comprehensive treatment (i.e., health care, nutritional supplementation, and psychoeducational stimulation) showed significant improvement between scores earned at ages 3.5 and 5 years, while the group receiving health care and nutritional supplement maintained its low level of performance, and the group receiving health care alone showed a decrement. The improvement seen in verbal reasoning in the group receiving the comprehensive treatment was not present in all psychological functions measured. Specifically, the treatment failed to produce significant improvement in performance on a test of short-term memory.

At 5 years of age, the performance on the Wechsler test of intelligence and on a test involving recognition of colors and objects was highest in the supplemented and stimulated group, lower in the group receiving food supplements, and lowest in the group that received health care only.

CLINICAL MALNUTRITION

REHABILITATION: EFFECTS OF PSYCHOSOCIAL STIMULATION

When infants of Lebanese Arab families of low socioeconomic status, hospitalized for energy–protein malnutrition of the marasmic type, were divided into two matched groups, the subjects who received psychosocial stimulation in addition to standard nutritional and medical care showed a greater improvement in terms of scores on the Griffiths Mental Development Scale (13) than found in the control group. However, the effects of extra psychosocial stimulation received during rehabilitation in the hospital did not persist when the children returned home (14).

Mönckeberg (15) reported positive results in a study similar to that carried out in Lebanon, in that it included the addition of psychosensory stimulation and affective support to medical–nutritional treatment of infants with nutritional marasmus. The children were housed and treated in a special, small treatment center equipped with 30 beds. In addition to adequate diet, each child was given one-half hour of psychosensory stimulation twice a day and an additional one-half hour of physical exercise, also twice a day. Affective stimulation was provided by volunteers throughout the day.

Mönckeberg reported data on 80 infants receiving the "integral treatment," compared with 80 infants receiving standard medical–nutritional treatment in a pediatric hospital in Santiago, Chile. The two groups were matched in age and weight at admission and in marked retardation in psychomotor development. After about four months, the "special treatment" children gained significantly more in height and weight than was achieved by the "standard treatment" group. Over a period of five months, the average quotient of psychomotor development rose from 55 to 85, versus a change from 56 to 65 in the "standard treatment" group.

TABLE 1. Effects of Clinical Malnutrition (CM) in Infancy, Height at Follow-up as Indicator of Nutritional Status (Stunting), and Background History on the Mean IQ of Jamaican Boys

	Mean IQ			
	Tall		Short	
Social background	CM absent	CM present	CM absent	CM present
Favorable	71	69	65	62
Unfavorable	62	55	58	49

FOLLOW-UP STUDIES: EFFECTS OF FAMILY SOCIAL ENVIRONMENT

Follow-up studies of Jamaican boys hospitalized in infancy (age range 6–24 months) indicated that at school age the index children, as a group, were significantly smaller in height and head circumference than their unrelated classmates and neighbors, matched for age and sex, had a lower level of intelligence, did significantly less well in school, and tended to be rated more often by their parents as backward and unsociable (16,17).

Two facts are of particular relevance in the present context: (1) The caretakers' level of capacity, the quality of home furnishings, and the intellectual stimulation received by the index cases indicate that the infants who developed clinical malnutrition came from more disadvantaged families than did their peer controls. (2) The data obtained at follow-up, at ages from 6 to 10 years, suggest that episodes of clinical malnutrition in infancy have had different consequences for intellectual development, depending on social background and on nutrition (and health) during the years preceding the follow-up examinations. The data are summarized in Table 1. The mean IQs of comparison children (free of clinical malnutrition in infancy) and index children with favorable social background and who are tall, are almost identical. The difference is largest for children whose social background is unfavorable and who are short.

FERREIRA'S MODEL

Unaware of Richardson's data (16,17), Maria Ferreira (18,19) developed a semiquantitative model relating nutrition, socioeconomic status of the family, and mental development. Its basic assumption is that biological stress factors, such as malnutrition, interacting with unfavorable socioeconomic conditions, hinder mental development.

The model (Table 2) considers the joint effects at three age levels: 1 year, 3 years, and school age. At the youngest age, the effect of malnutrition is independent of the socioeconomic level of the family. The differential effect of the social background increases with age: at the higher economic level the measured psychological impact of malnutrition (Δ) decreases; at the lower economic level the impact increases.

It may be of interest to test the model using Richardsons' data (16,17) and Table 1, even though figures for only one age group—school age (6–10 years)—are available. As indicated in Table 3, and in agreement with Ferreira's model, the effect of early clinical malnutrition is larger in children with a poorer socioeconomic background than in children of better-situated families. Richardson's data indicate, furthermore, that chronically poor nutritional status, judged by the amount of stunting (reflecting nutrition and health in the preceding years), has a small additional effect.

Ferreira offers an auxiliary hypothesis that specifies the underlying mechanism to be interference with the establishment of "syntonic," "synchronic," and "reciprocal" relationships between the child and the mother (19). Born into an impoverished social environment, the child is less likely to find in its family a person ready to "syntonize," to "tune in," to be stimulating and responsive to the child's behavior. In turn, because of malnutrition and frequent ill health, the child is likely to be less able to be stimulating and responsive to the care-giver. The typical

TABLE 2. Effects of Biological (e.g., Nutritional) and Social Factors on Mental Development[a]

Approximate age	Socioeconomic level	
	Higher	Lower
1 year	Δ[b]	Δ
3 years	Δ	Δ
School age	~	Δ

[a] From Reference 18, p. 39.
[b] The size of the delta symbol (Δ) indicates the magnitude of the mean differences in scores on developmental scales and tests of intelligence between better-nourished and poorly nourished children at a given socioeconomic level.

TABLE 3. Mean Difference between
Intelligence Scores of the Comparison
Group and of School-Age Children Who
Experienced Clinical Malnutrition in
Infancy, Taking into Account Nutritional
Status at Follow-up and Social Background[a]

	Socioeconomic level	
Chronic nutritional status	Higher	Lower
Higher	2[b]	7
Lower	3	9

[a] See Table 1 for original data.
[b] IQ difference.

malnourished child is apathetic, has little or no interest in his/her social
environment, and is irritable. The combination of these factors creates,
in Ferreira's terminology, an "interactional deprivation" that, when present throughout the child's early years, inhibits intellectual development.

The concept of "interactional deprivation" is similar to the concept
of "functional isolation" of malnourished animals, formulated by Barnes
with Levitsky (8), as the mechanism involved in malnutrition's long-
term effects on behavior. According to the isolation hypothesis, malnutrition does not affect the "hardware" of the learning mechanism, but
alters the "program," i.e., "The well nourished, healthy, growing animal
is . . . programmed with a hunger to learn all about its environment, not
just the essential features. This is dramatically inhibited by malnutrition.
The malnourished animal, apparently, responds only to those features of
the environment that are of immediate biological significance." (8, p.
176). We welcome the interactionally oriented concepts (interactional
deprivation, isolation hypothesis) as important components of a comprehensive model of the mechanisms through which deficits of nutrients
yield alterations in behavior. A polarization between morphological–
physiological changes in the organism (including the central nervous,
hormonal, and muscular systems) and sociopsychological mechanisms is,
we believe, counterproductive.

Ferreira's model may be tested (and made more quantitative and
more specific) independently of the author's auxiliary hypotheses, one
of which postulates that a socioeconomically deprived environment
affects the child's experience of the "locus of control," making the child
feel externally controlled and unable to develop a sense of its own power
for making effective decisions.

In Ferreira's view, the implementation of effective intervention programs must incorporate " . . . an improvement of the social and economic conditions of the poor through a more just remuneration for their work, which will allow them to have decent nutrition and will make it possible for them to gain a sense of their own power over the future" (18, pp. 37–48). We agree, but see the problem of the eradication of malnutrition as much more complex. Complexity does not justify—and we wish to make this clear—governmental passivity and inactivity.

CLOSING COMMENT

The etiology of endemic energy–protein malnutrition is complex, with poverty as a subsoil, the deficiency of specific nutrients as a frequent complicating factor, and infection and parasitism as added stresses. Endemic poverty, in turn, has its own complex set of socioeconomic, political, and behavioral determinants. Inadequate food intake—the primary factor in malnutrition—is the last link in a long chain of factors. Furthermore, "chain" is an inappropriate metaphor because it suggests a linear model, whereas we deal with an interactive system. The "war on hunger" is such a difficult task because it is inseparable from the "war on poverty."

The biological and psychological effects of severe malnutrition are also complex, even when we restrict our attention to deficits of energy (calories) and protein. The effects include retardation of the growth of the body and of the central nervous system, disordered metabolism and organ function, and changes in the various facets of behavior—motor functions, intelligence, and personality. The presence of specific effects and their magnitude depend on a variety of conditions: nutritional (nature, duration, and severity of nutritional deficits), organismic (age, sex, state of health), and environmental.

One of the pressing needs in research on malnutrition and behavior is to develop a comprehensive, yet workable, mathematical model, or, more likely, a set of models of various forms of malnutrition, their etiology, and their impact. Whereas in the past the emphasis has been placed on clinical energy–protein malnutrition, i.e., the forms of malnutrition calling for hospitalization of the malnourished child, in recent years the emphasis has shifted to the study of chronic, subclinical malnutrition. This is justified because the number of children suffering from less severe, chronic forms of malnutrition greatly exceeds the number of children exhibiting symptoms of severe, clinical, acute energy–protein malnutrition. Yet, for how many behavioral functions can we draw a "dose-response" curve that would indicate the presence and magnitude of the

effects of different degrees of malnutrition throughout the whole range
of severity of chronic malnutrition?

REFERENCES

1. Brožek, J., D. B. Coursin, and M. S. Read. Longitudinal studies on the effects of malnutrition, nutritional supplementation, and behavioral stimulation. *Bull. Panam.
   Health Org.* **11**:237–249, 1977.
2. Grantham-McGregor, S. M., M. E. Stewart, and P. Desai. A new look at the assessment
   of mental development in young children recovering from severe malnutrition. *Dev.
   Med. Child Neurol.* **20**:773–778, 1978.
3. Brožek, J. Nutrition, malnutrition, and behavior. *Ann. Rev. Psychol.* **29**:157–177, 1978.
   (In Spanish: *Bol. Oficin. Panam.* **85**:506–529, 1978; in Portuguese: *Cadernos de Pesquisa*
   29:11–30, 1979.)
4. Lloyd-Still, J. D. Clinical studies on the effects of malnutrition during infancy on subsequent physical and intellectual development. In: *Malnutrition and Intellectual Development*, J. D. Lloyd-Still (Ed.), pp. 103–159, Publishing Sciences Group, Littleton, Massachusetts, 1976.
5. Pollitt, E., and C. Thomson. Protein-calorie malnutrition and behavior: A view from
   psychology. In: *Nutrition and the Brain*, R. J. Wurtman and J. J. Wurtman (Eds.), pp.
   261–306, Raven Press, New York, 1977.
6. Subcommittee on nutrition, brain development, and behavior. The Relation of Nutrition to Brain Development and Behavior: A Position Paper, National Academy of Sci-
   ences/National Research Council, Washington, D.C., 1973.
7. Levine S., and S. Weiner. A critical analysis of data on malnutrition and behavioral
   deficits. *Adv. Pediatr.* **22**:113–136, 1976.
8. Levitsky, D. Comment. In: *Malnutrition, Environment, and Behavior*, D. A. Levitsky (Ed.),
   p. 271, Cornell University Press, Ithaca, New York, 1979.
9. Gupta, S., D. C. Dhingra, M. V. Singh, and K. Anand. Impact of nutrition on intelligence. *Indian Pediatr.* **12**:1079–1082, 1975.
10. Klein, R. E., C. Yarbrough, R. E. Lasky, and J.-P. Habicht. Correlations of mild to mod-
    erate protein-calorie malnutrition among rural Guatemalan infants and preschool
    children. In: *Early Malnutrition and Mental Development*. J. Cravioto, L. Hambraeus, and
    B. Vahlquist (Eds.), pp. 168–181, Almqvist & Wiksell, Uppsala, 1974.
11. McKay, H. E., A. McKay, and L. Sinisterra. Intellectual development of malnourished
    preschool children in programs of stimulation and nutritional supplementation. In:
    Early Malnutrition and Mental Development. J. Cravioto, L. Hambraeus, and B. Vahlquist
    (Eds.), pp. 226–232, Almqvist & Wiksell, Uppsala, 1974.
12. McKay, H., L. Sinisterra, A. McKay, H. Gómez, and P. Lloreda. Improving cognitive
    ability in chronically deprived children. *Science* **200**:270–278, 1978.
13. Yatkin, U. S., and D. S. McLaren. The behavioural development of infants recovering
    from severe malnutrition. *J. Ment. Defic. Res.* **14**(1):25–31, 1970.
14. McLaren, D. S., U. S. Yatkin, A. A. Kanawati, S. Sabbagh, and Z. Kadi. The relationship
    of severe marasmic protein-energy malnutrition and rehabilitation in infancy to sub-
    sequent mental development. In: *Protein-Calorie Malnutrition*, R. E. Olson (Ed.), pp.
    107–112, Academic Press, New York, 1975.
15. Mönckeberg, F. Recovery of severely malnourished infants: Effects of early sensory-
    affective stimulation. In: *Behavioral Effects of Energy and Protein Deficits*, J. Brožek (Ed.),
    pp. 121–130, DHEW Publication No. (NIH) 79-106, Washington, D.C., 1979.

16. Richardson, S. A. The influence of severe malnutrition in infancy on the intelligence of children at school age: An ecological perspective. In: *Environment as a Therapy for Brain Dysfunction*, R. N. Walsh, and W. T. Greenough (Eds.), pp. 256–275, Plenum Press, New York, 1976.
17. Richardson, S. A. The relation of severe malnutrition in infancy to the intelligence of school children with differing life histories. *Pediatr. Res.* **10:**57–61, 1976.
18. Ferreira, M. C. R. (Ed.), *Desnutrição, Pobreza e Desenvolvimiento Mental*. A special issue of *Cadernos de Pesquisa* (Fundação Carlos Chagas, São Paulo, Brazil) No. 29, 1979.
19. Ferreira, M. C. R. Malnutrition and mother-infant asynchrony: Slow mental development. *Int. J. Behav. Dev.* **1:**207–219, 1978.

Comment

Ernesto Pollitt

In considering Brožek's paper, it is quite clear that the data generated from studies conducted on malnutrition and mental development have reached the ears of policy makers. As a consequence, there is now great interest in looking at the significance of these data in terms of policy. Two important events are taking place. One is that a number of governments are already implementing programs on behalf of children, especially preschool children. Many of these programs are based on data that emerged from studies on malnutrition and mental development. Similarly, other governments are interested in becoming involved in these kinds of programs and are currently exploring such possibilities and their implications for national development. Therefore, it is essential to provide conclusions from existing data that are relevant to policy makers.

We now know that malnutrition is a significant cause of cognitive deficiency. For example, as Brožek pointed out, the malnourished child who lives in poverty has a much higher probability of suffering from cognitive deficits than the nonmalnourished child who also lives in poverty. Second, it is also clear that protein–calorie malnutrition is not the only type of nutritional deficiency that affects behavior or cognition. Data exist that show iron deficiency to have a very specific impact on selective cognitive processes. Even in its milder forms, iron deficiency affects attention span and concentration.

The third conclusion I would stress is that cognitive function is extremely plastic in the young child, who is affected by the adverse as well as the beneficial effects of the environmental conditions in which he lives. This fact has two important implications. The first is that interventions can have significant beneficial impact on the child. However,

Ernesto Pollitt • University of Texas Health Science Center at Houston, School of Public Health, Houston, Texas.

due to the plasticity of the central nervous system and behavior, if the child is involved in the intervention for only a short period, the benefits that were accrued from treatment will be lost.

The fourth conclusion is that these interventions can be implemented even as late as 36 months after birth. The earlier hypothesis was that if an intervention was begun after the first 12 or 24 months in a child's life, damage to cognitive development would be irreversible. This does not seem to be true, although the optimal time for intervention is between 18 and 36 months. Important beneficial effects are seen even if the intervention begins at as late as 36 or 48 months, and such a strategy can bring a child to an almost normal level of development.

The next point to stress is that the cognitive benefits accrued to the child will be greater if nutrition supplementation is provided in the context of a multifactorial intervention, including such components as medical care. In other words, if the intervention is restricted to nutrition supplementation, it is not going to bring the kinds of results that come from a multifaceted intervention.

My final comment is that the socioeconomic factors that interact with malnutrition are probably more potent threats to cognition than nutritional deficiency itself. The conclusions outlined above can be used in formulating policy. A government can act upon these findings, and it is time to utilize all the information that has accumulated to date in the context of policy-making.

Discussion

Following the comment by Pollitt, attention focused on the optimal age at which to intervene in order to reduce the deleterious effects of malnutrition on behavior and mental development. A question was raised as to whether intervention during prenatal and early postnatal periods was not more valuable than during the 18- to 36-month period. Pollitt responded that the types of behaviors developed before 18 months of age are not necessarily important precursors or antecedents of those kinds of behaviors essential to problem-solving, although it is recognized that the kinds of psychomotor or sensory motor behavior that enhance the child's adaptation to his environment are developing in the first 12 months of life. What is important, however, is that, according to the data, even under conditions of prenatal undernutrition followed by postnatal undernutrition, the child will develop normally, given the right kinds of stimulation.

A final question addressed to Pollitt concerned how planners can deal with the problems of the behavioral consequences of malnutrition. Are the only viable answers either to change the fundamental socioeconomic structure of the family and society, or to remove the child from a low-class environment to an atmosphere more conducive for learning and development?

Pollitt pointed out that there is a lack of research and experience about potential administrative infrastructures to affect low-income families and raise the quality of their environment. However, the use of well-operated institutionalized child-care facilities represents a viable strategy for affecting the child's environment without disrupting family structures. The problem with the child-care strategy is that obviously it is not applicable to isolated populations.

It was suggested, in summary, that relevant interventions are as varied as the countries, cultures, and communities experiencing malnutrition. They range from economic reinforcement for the family to specific programs to benefit the individuals who are at greatest risk. It is neither desirable nor possible, however, to attempt to put these in a priority order for implementation, nor to suggest that any have higher or lower potential for success; the ultimate choice will depend on the circumstances and politics found in specific situations.

Some participants felt that Pollitt had been too conservative in his interpretation of the available data. Specifically, it was argued that prolonged, severe protein–energy malnutrition in early life leads to irreversible alterations in behavioral and psychological development; the consequences are greater if the mother is undernourished during pregnancy. Similarly, most of the data from studies of chronic undernutrition in childhood leading to marked growth retardation also indicate subsequent impaired behavioral development, depending on the nature of the social environment in which the child lives. Studies of educational rehabilitation following malnutrition do not support the blanket contention that the deficits can be overcome or reversed by providing mental stimulation. Whether or not there is long-term impairment in the learning ability of the child was therefore viewed as an issue demanding further attention and clarification.

In response to the expression of concern about the strength of previous statements about the relationship between prenatal and early postnatal malnutrition and behavioral impairment, Pollitt clarified his position by stating that he was referring only to moderate malnutrition as opposed to the case of the marasmic child who suffers prolonged, severe deprivation. Another participant also suggested that even in "normal" populations there is very poor correlation between scores on early childhood behavior scales and later behavioral development. It was noted, for example, that the relationship between walking at 19 versus 27 months of age (i.e., late maturation of simple behaviors) and intellectual function later in life is tenuous at best.

The assertion that the socioeconomic factors that interact with nutritional factors are a more significant determinant of behavior and development was also raised in terms of its policy implications. Specifically, it was asked whether it is sufficient to concentrate solely on socioeconomic variables. In response, a study was cited from Cali, Colombia, that tested the differential impacts of health care and/or nutrition with or without psychoeducational stimulation. With the three treatments combined, the child's cognitive function improved; with only nutritional and health intervention, the same level of impairment was maintained; with only medical assistance, the problem worsened. Unfortunately, there was no group receiving only stimulation, so the results of such an approach cannot be compared to nutritional intervention alone.

Malnutrition and Infection

R. K. CHANDRA

INTRODUCTION

The ability of individuals to achieve their full potential depends upon an optimal interaction of genes and environment. Adverse factors that can retard such an achievement in underprivileged populations are legion. These are interlinked (Fig. 1). The prominent factors include poverty, malnutrition, infection, illiteracy, poor sanitation, sociocultural handicaps, and large sibships competing for limited resources. Malnutrition itself has a complex etiology. Food availability and nutrient intake are important determinants. However, many other factors play a significant role, including environmental contamination, absorption, and infectious disease. Changes in nutritional status can alter susceptibility to disease, manifestations of pathological states, and final outcome in terms of work capacity, morbidity, and survival.

Malnutrition and infection rank among the most pervasive and serious of health problems in the world today. The relationship of nutrition and infection at first blush seems straightforward and easily testable. Clinicians believe that the frequency and severity of infectious illness in malnourished individuals are increased, and that infection can precipitate or worsen nutritional deficiency. Even though the general thrust of this interaction is established (1), the precise quantitative and qualitative relationships remain to be defined. The underlying mechanisms of pathogenesis and interplay defy easy analysis. Recent studies have revealed impaired function of a variety of host-protective factors in malnourished individuals (2,3). It is possible that the clinical problem of repeated and severe infections in undernourished persons is the result, to a major

R. K. CHANDRA • Clinical Research Center, Massachusetts Institute of Technology, Cambridge, Massachusetts.

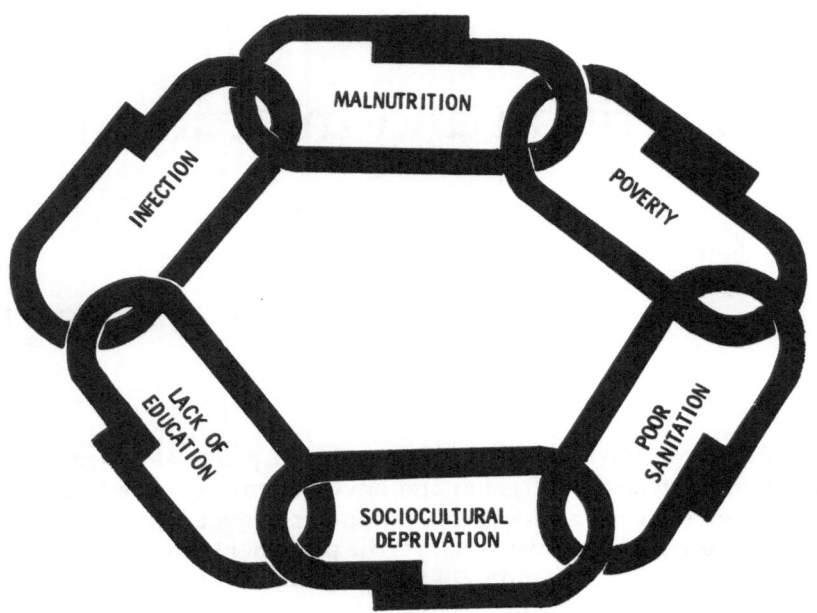

FIGURE 1. Important interlinked factors that can strangle the growth, development, and survival of underprivileged individuals. Reprinted with permission from Reference 3.

extent, of a summation of variable individual abnormalities in several critical cellular and humoral immunological functions. Infection itself can result in significant deficits in immunity function and in nutrition (4).

Clinical and epidemiological observations of the common association of malnutrition and infection have led to investigations employing sophisticated techniques of molecular and cellular biology. These studies have yielded interesting data of fundamental importance. Animal models of nutritional deficiency syndromes have been used to study interactions in strictly controlled—quantitatively and qualitatively— conditions. However, the extrapolation from the relationships examined at microlevel research to the expanded horizon of the individual and the population is complicated by a sharp diminution in scientific purity. This is because a multitude of ecologic and social factors impinge on the diet–health nexus.

As in other areas of clinical research, scientific inquiry into malnutrition–infection relationships must not remain centripetally confined. It is imperative that we look for relevance and application of knowledge to policy with the ultimate objective of alleviation of human suffering caused by the malnutrition–infection complex. Based on existing knowledge, we should plan strategies for successful interventions. The task is formidable, but that is no reason for not trying.

INFECTIONS IN UNDERNOURISHED INDIVIDUALS

The common association of malnutrition and infection does not necessarily imply a causal relationship. It must be recognized that the same economic, sociocultural, and ecological factors that contribute to the genesis of undernutrition may well maintain a high frequency of infectious diseases. Evidence to support the hypothesis that nutritional deficiency increases susceptibility to infection has been acquired in three main ways (1): clinical studies in out-patient and in-patient settings, the epidemiological approach through observation of disease as it occurs in the population, and controlled experiments in laboratory animals subjected to nutritional deprivation and challenged with pathogens. Results of field surveys in several regions of the world have confirmed the intimate association of malnutrition, growth failure, infection, and diarrheal disease.

Many diseases run a more severe course in malnourished individuals (5). Measles and herpes simplex produce life-threatening illness in children with kwashiorkor; undernourished infants without gross protein deficiency do not fare so badly. Gram-negative septicemia and *Pneumocystis carinii* are seen more frequently in malnourished individuals (6). There is a heavier load of parasites and a higher prevalence of tuberculosis. However, these may be the cause and/or the consequence of undernutrition. Chronic mucocutaneous candidiasis is often complicated by iron deficiency, and the correction of the latter is associated with clinical and immunologic improvement. The frequency of respiratory infection in iron-deficient groups appears to be higher than in iron-replete groups (7). Animals deprived of iron generally succumb more easily to infectious challenge (8). Similar information is available for a variety of other nutrients (3). Occasionally, selected nutrient deficits may increase resistance to challenge with a microorganism or a transplantable tumor.

IMMUNOCOMPETENCE IN UNDERNUTRITION

The body of core knowledge of the effects of protein–malnutrition on immunity has grown phenomenally in the past ten or so years (2,3,9). Even though various studies employed different methods and the extent of nutritional deficiency varied, a thread of fairly consistent observations runs through many of the reports. There is a reduction in the proportion and absolute number of circulating T lymphocytes, as detected by rosette formation with sheep red cells (10). This change in T-cell number is promptly reversed within a few weeks of nutritional supplementation and it may serve as an early sign of nutritional recovery. The proportion of T cells with a receptor for IgM-Fc (the "helper" cells) is reduced, whereas T cells with a receptor for IgG-Fc (the "suppressor" cells) is increased (Fig. 2). B lymphocytes are largely unchanged in number. The number of "null" cells mediating spontaneous cytotoxicity is increased; many of these null cells may be undifferentiated T-cell precursors. In protein – energy malnutrition, serum thymic hormone activity is reduced, and the levels of terminal deoxynucleotidyl transferase enzyme found in large amounts in the early stages of T-cell differentiation are increased and correlate with the proportion of null cells (11). Skin tests for delayed hypersensitivity response are impaired in malnourished individuals (12). The release of soluble mediators of the inflammatory response may be reduced.

Antibody response to an adequate antigenic challenge is generally normal in distribution. Antigens requiring the help of T cells fare less well. Secretory IgA antibody responses are decreased (13,14); this may be the consequence of the reduced number of IgA-producing plasma cells

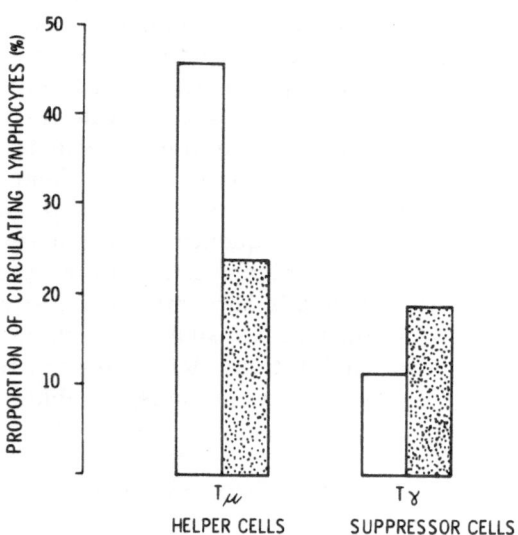

FIGURE 2. T-lymphocyte subsets. Data of Chandra (11).

in the submucosa, decreased synthesis of secretory component by flattened villi, and few intraepithelial lymphocytes. Impaired mucosal immunity may facilitate the occurrence of Gram-negative septicemia and the production of antibodies to luminal protein antigens. Data on antibody affinity are conspicuously lacking. In animal models of protein deficiency, there is a marked reduction in affinity of antibody, poorer and slower clearance of administered antigens, and increased incidence of immune complexes.

Ingestion of particles by polymorphonuclear leukocytes is normal, but intracellular killing of bacteria and fungi is reduced in protein–energy malnutrition (15,16). Chemotaxis is generally normal. Opsonic activity of the plasma depends upon complement components and antibody and other ill-defined factors; it is reduced in malnourished children when tests are conducted using serum at lower than 10% concentration. Both the classical and the alternate pathway of complement are less competent. The serum levels of C3, factor B, and other components are reduced; this may be the combined result of reduced synthesis and increased consumption. Experimental protein–calorie malnutrition in rats was associated with depression of phagocytosis-induced oxygen consumption and hexose monophosphate shunt activity, as well as marked impairment of humoral chemotactic factors.

Many other nonspecific protective factors are influenced by nutritional deficiency, including lysozyme and interferon (2,3). Furthermore, tissue changes may promote colonization and reduce local resistance. The main effects of malnutrition on immunity are summarized in Fig. 3.

Nutritional and Immunologic Effects of Infection

Infection itself can produce significant changes in nutritional status and in immune function (Table 1). The extent of such alterations is determined by the severity and duration of illness, by the nature of the microbe, and by the health status of the individual prior to infection. Febrile illnesses increase tissue catabolism and nutrient loss in the urine, reduce appetite, decrease absorption, or cause protein loss in the gastrointestinal tract. In addition, the rapid sequestration of nutrients and their utilization in the production of acute-phase reactant proteins, antibodies, complement, and other host-protective factors result in further deficits (4). Infection also suppresses many aspects of immunity, possibly by alterations in hormonal balance, by invasion of lymphoid tissues, by endotoxemia, by altered ratios of lymphocyte subsets, or by increased levels of C-reactive protein. Measles is associated with a prolonged

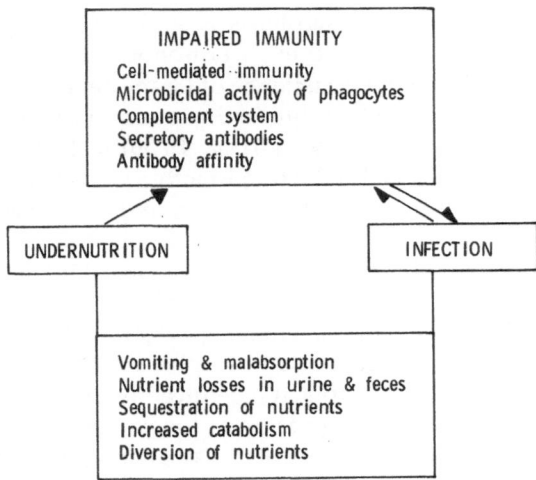

FIGURE 3. Main immunologic deficits in protein–energy malnutrition and mechanisms of infection-induced nutritional deficiency. Reprinted with permission from Reference 3.

TABLE 1. Nutrient Consequences of Infection[a]

I. Absolute losses
   Increased urinary nitrogen
   Loss of electrolytes, minerals, and proteins in vomiting and diarrhea
   Proteinuria
   Negative balance of cations, minerals, and trace elements
II. Functional wastage
   A. Overutilization
      Increased usage of metabolic substrates
      Depletion of glycogen stores
      Diversion of amino acids for gluconeogenesis
      Mobilization of fat from depots
      Increased synthesis of cholesterol and triglycerides
   B. Diversion
      Hepatic uptake of plasma nutrients, e.g., amino acids
      Synthesis of acute phase reactants
      Increased hepatocytic synthesis of enzymes
   C. Sequestration
      Uptake of minerals (Fe, Zn) into hepatocytes and phagocytes
      Uptake of trace elements by liver and other organs

---

[a] Reprinted from Reference 2.

period of negative nitrogen balance and impaired cell-mediated immunity (2); in these circumstances, kwashiorkor may be precipitated, and secondary infections such as tuberculosis may supervene. In addition, infection-induced granulocyte dysfunction may adversely influence the outcome of infectious illness.

The effects of recurrent, chronic infections and inadequate dietary intake are negatively additive or even perhaps synergistic. This concept of synergism of malnutrition and infection derived considerable support from field studies in Guatemala (1). Manifest nutritional disease is often preceded by an episode of infectious disease, especially acute gastroenteritis, diarrhea, measles, or whooping cough. On the other hand, the majority of deaths due to diarrhea and respiratory infection were seen in malnourished children. Poor nutrition is a major determinant of diarrhea and it is strongly associated with poor weaning practices.

INTERVENTIONS

The correction of the high morbidity associated with the twin problems of malnutrition and infection requires a multifaceted approach. A single-factor approach is not satisfactory. The main pillars of interventions include promotion of breast-feeding, effective immunization, selected short-term nutritional supplementation, prevention of low birth weight, family planning, increased agricultural production, and improved sanitation (Fig. 4).

The rapid decline in breast-feeding has taken the heaviest toll in developing countries where it is almost impossible to ensure that the infant will receive adequate amounts of hygienically prepared formula. Artificial feeding is associated with a higher risk of diarrhea, respiratory disease, and ear infection, and there is a higher rate of occurrence of life-threatening complications, such as dehydration and septicemia. The beneficial effects of breast-feeding are also seen in industrialized countries (Table 2).

Immunization schedules should be made more effective by modifying the dose of antigen, the number of doses, the timing in relation to nutritional status, and the type of adjuvant used. In addition, short-term nutritional supplements given before immunization may enhance effectiveness. Such supplements are justified before and during impending stress, such as infection and surgery. Specific nutrients may be required for individual subjects.

Immunodeficiency secondary to low birth weight may be severe and prolonged (17). Appropriate prepregnancy, antenatal, and perinatal mea-

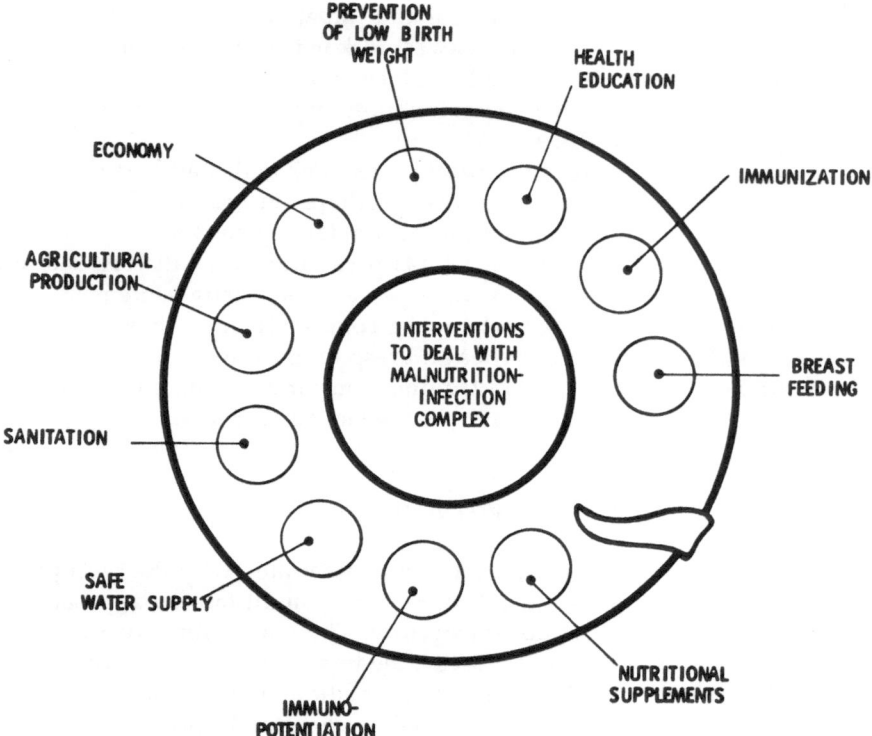

FIGURE 4. Interventions to deal with malnutrition and infection. Reprinted with permission from Reference 3.

TABLE 2. Effect of Type of Feeding on Growth and Incidence of Infection[a]

	India		Canada	
	Breast milk	Milk formula	Breast milk	Milk formula
Number	50	50	30	30
Growth failure[b]	11	34	0	0
Obesity[b]	1	1	2	9
Respiratory infection[c]	87	156	31	77
Otitis[c]	37	79	5	41
Diarrhea[c]	108	326	3	9

[a] Reprinted from References 5 and 20.
[b] Number of children affected.
[c] Number of episodes of illness for the group over 12 months.

sures will reduce the incidence of small-for-gestation births. The strategies dealing with this problem must necessarily take into account the prevalence of various risk factors causing low birth weight (preterm, small-for-gestation, or both) and the magnitude of risk associated with each of these factors.

Immunopotentiation using transfer factor and levimasole can improve immune function for a short period (5). The value of immunopotentiation may lie in providing short-term benefit before imminent stress, such as infection or surgery.

The past record of intervention programs is less than satisfactory. John Field has observed that " . . . the documentary evidence concerning nutrition programs and specific interventions is long on descriptions . . . adequate—if unsophisticated—on costs, weak on impact, and limited on process."* These intervention programs should be interlinked with health services. It is recognized that curative and preventive services also have an impact on nutritional status, largely through their bearing on the incidence and severity of disease.

OBESITY AND IMMUNITY

The positive linear relationship between nutrient intake and disease may be understood to imply the less the worse, the more the better. However, nothing could be farther from the truth. There are critical thresholds and levels of optimal interactions. If we widen the scope of malnutrition to include the state of excess intake and obesity, then immune responses are again observed to be impaired. Obese adolescents and adults show an increased incidence of infections, including postoperative sepsis; infection-associated mortality is increased. A proportion of obese individuals show a variable decrease in cell-mediated immunity and intracellular killing of bacteria (18). In an analogous situation, genetically obese mice demonstrate reduced numbers of antibody-forming cells in the spleen and show alterations in natural-killer-cell activity and antibody-dependent, cell-mediated cytotoxicity (19). The generation of cytotoxicity following *in vivo* immunization is decreased, whereas it is unaltered after *in vitro* immunization, suggesting a deleterious microenvironment that may include hormonal changes and metabolic factors, among others.

*Background paper: Workshop on Nutrient Intake and Disease Response, Hyannis, Massachusetts, September 1978.

IMPLICATIONS

The wide-ranging effects of malnutrition on immunity may have several clinical implications. Defense against many microorganisms is decreased, promoting serious complications and prolonged illness. Impaired mucosal immunity can result in septicemia. The efficacy of prophylactic immunization has to be carefully assessed in malnourished populations. There is a need to recognize the frequent occurrence of secondary malnutrition in hospitalized patients and in those with chronic disease, including cancer. Individuals receiving total parenteral nutrition may develop deficits of specific nutrients with consequences on immunity and susceptibility to infection. Increased awareness of the problem, critical analysis of existing information, and planned studies will lead to the development of cost-effective intervention programs with the ultimate objective of eradicating malnutrition and infection.

REFERENCES

1. Scrimshaw, N. S., C. E. Taylor, and J. E. Gordon. *Interactions of Nutrition and Infection.* WHO Monograph No. 57, WHO, Geneva, 1968.
2. Chandra, R. K., and P. M. Newberne. *Immunity and Infection—Mechanisms of Interactions.* Plenum, New York 1977.
3. Chandra, R. K. *Immunology of Nutritional Disorders.* Edward Arnold, London, 1980.
4. Beisel, W. R. Metabolic response to infection. *Ann. Rev. Med.* **26**:9, 1975.
5. Chandra, R. K. Nutritional deficiency and susceptibility to infection. *Bull. WHO* **57**:167, 1979.
6. Bwibo, N. O., and R. Owor. *Pneumocystis carinii* pneumonia in Ugandan African children. *West. Afr. Med. J.* **19**:184, 1970.
7. Basta, S. S., Soekirman, D. Karyadi, and N. S. Scrimshaw. Iron deficiency anemia and the productivity of adult males in Indonesia. *Am. J. Clin. Nutr.* **32**:916, 1979.
8. Chandra, R. K., B. Au, G. Woodford, and P. Hyam. Iron status, immunocompetence and susceptibility to infection. In: *Ciba Foundation Symposium on Iron Metabolism* 51 (New Series). Elsevier, Excerpta Medica, Amsterdam, 1977.
9. Suskind, R. M. (Ed.). *Malnutrition and the Immune Response.* Raven Press, New York, 1977.
10. Chandra, R. K. Rosette-forming T lymphocytes and cell-mediated immunity, in malnutrition. *Br. J. Med.* **3**:608, 1974.
11. Chandra, R. K. T and B lymphocyte sub-populations and leukocyte terminal deoxynucleotidyl transferase in malnutrition. *Acta Paediatr. Scand.* **68**:841, 1979.
12. Neumann, C. G., G. J. Lawlor, E. R. Stiehm, M. E. Swenseid, C. Newton, J. Herbert, A. J. Amman, and M. Jacob. Immunological responses in malnourished children. *Am. J. Clin. Nutr.* **28**:89, 1974.
13. Chandra, R. K. Reduced secretory antibody response to live attenuated measles and polio virus in malnourished children. *Br. Med. J.* **2**:583, 1975.
14. Sirisinha, S., R. Suskind, R. Edelman, C. Asvapaka, and R. E. Olsen. Secretory and serum IgA in children with protein-energy malnutrition. *Pediatrics* **55**:166, 1975.

15. Seth, V., and R. K. Chandra, Opsonic function, phagocytosis and bacterial killing capacity of polymorphs in undernutrition. *Arch Dis. Child.* **47**:282, 1972.

16. Selvaraj, R. J., and K. S. Bhat. Phagocytes and leukocyte enzymes in protein-calorie malnutrition. *Biochem. J.* **127**:255, 1972.

17. Chandra, R. K., S. K. Ali, K. M. Kutty, and S. Chandra. Thymus-dependent lymphocytes and delayed hypersensitivity in low birth-weight infants. *Biol. Neonat.* **31**:15, 1977.

18. Chandra, R. K., and K. M. Kutty. Immunocompetence in obesity. *Acta Paediatr. Scand.* **69**:25, 1980.

19. Chandra, R. K. Cell-mediated immune responses in genetically obese (C57B1 ob/ob) mice. *Am. J. Clin. Nutr.* **33**:13, 1980.

20. Chandra, R. K. Prospective studies on the effect of breast feeding on incidence of infection and allergy. *Acta Paediatr. Scand.* **68**:691, 1979.

Comment

GERALD KEUSCH

The interaction of nutrition and infection is, as Chandra points out, a complex, bidirectional influence of nutritional state upon immune function and, thereby, upon susceptibility and response to infection (1). At the same time, infection has a major impact on nutritional status (2). It is therefore highly appropriate to speak of this as a nutrition–infection complex (3), for we have now learned enough to know that efforts to improve nutrition are unlikely to reach the expected goals without attention to the problem of infectious disease in the population, particularly in young infants and children. In this context, what are the key issues that have relevance to policy and planning?

First, we can view the complex of immunological and nutritional status by defining the susceptibility of the host to an infectious agent, thus determining the response to this challenge. It may be diagrammed as follows:

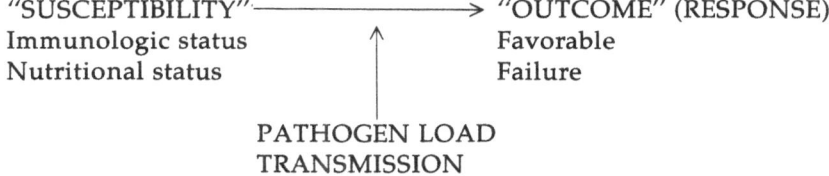

The classic elements of epidemiology—host, agent, and environment—thus combine to determine outcome (or response). This raises a very important issue concerning the range of deficit in either the immune or nutritional status and the extent to which specific levels of deprivation are reflected in altered functional responses. At which level of deficit is

GERALD KEUSCH • Division of Geographic Medicine, Tufts University Medical Center, Boston, Massachusetts.

function sufficiently affected to alter outcome? Is there a threshold for an effect to be seen?

This brings up the question of degree of malnutrition in a very important context, for, in fact, most of the studies that relate immunological and nutritional deficits have been performed in severely protein–calorie-malnourished subjects. In a sense this represents a state of gross functional failure; it is the far end of the scale of pathological changes. This group is also the tip of the iceberg in clinical malnutrition; most of the problem can be classified as mild to moderate. There are few studies, however, that attempt to define immunological abnormalities in the mildly to moderately malnourished. It is clearly important to do so, however, because this is a group at great risk of morbidity and mortality from infectious disease that can precipitate more severe malnutrition. They are at a borderline state of function that is not diagnosed by traditional anthropometric measures of nutritional status. Chandra's studies, and those in which I have participated at INCAP in Guatemala, suggest that certain immunological markers may be predictive of risk of diarrheal disease. Thus, immunological measures could perhaps be used for surveillance purposes and to guide policies and programs. This needs to be investigated.

It is also important to define the deficiencies, both nutritional and immunological, in order to target therapy. A schematic representation of this would be:

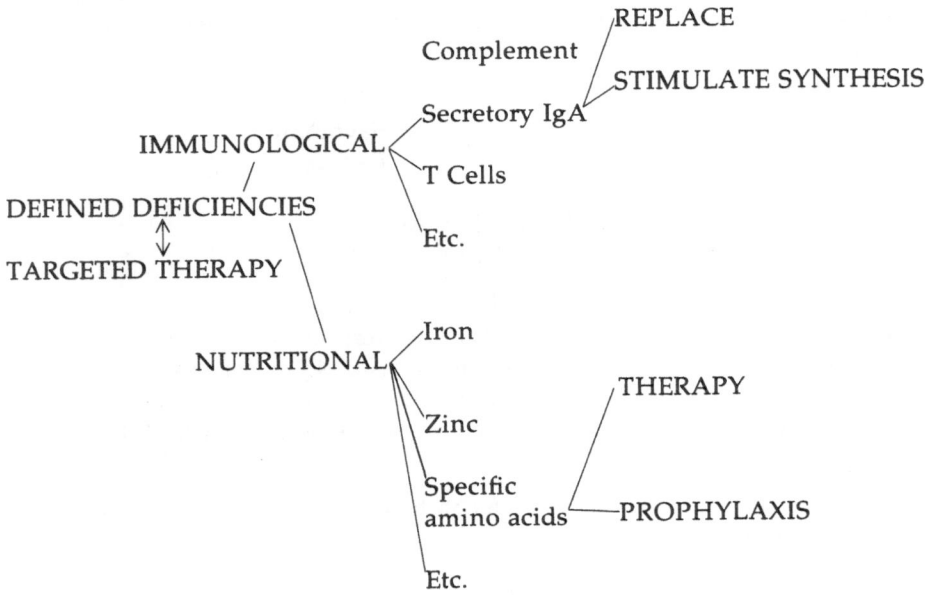

When immunological deficiencies are defined, three systems are found to be significantly affected by malnutrition: complement, secretory IgA, and T cells. Complement, for example, is very sensitive to nutritional insult and could well explain the propensity to Gram-negative bacteremia in malnourished hosts. It is possible to replace this component by plasma transfusion, and we are currently testing the ability of such therapy to reverse defects and reduce infection in the severely malnourished patient. It would be better, however, to find a way to stimulate the host to produce more complement under such conditions of stress, as occurs in the normal or mildly malnourished host. If a specific nutrient, or perhaps a specific amino acid, were rate-limiting, its replacement might permit such a desirable response. This is the reason that the study of the mechanisms of these host responses continues.

It is far better, however, to consider preventive measures that might be recommended now. Chandra has mentioned the most important ones, including prenatal surveillance (immunization and correction of nutritional deficits in the pregnant woman), breast-feeding, specific nutritional interventions in growth-faltering children, oral rehydration and early feeding in diarrheal disease, and immunization. Unfortunately, the last approach is limited because there are no vaccines for the most common infectious agents. More research is appropriate here, for it may be possible to increase the immune protective function of breast milk by immunizing the gut of the lactating woman to enteric organisms, since this route of antigen administration gives rise to mammary antibody-producing cells. What is needed are the vaccines with which to accomplish this goal.

In all of these interventions it is important to consider seasonality—seasonal prevalence of certain pathogens or the vectors that transmit them, seasonal malnutrition that increases susceptibility, and, of course, the influence of seasonal malnutrition on response to immunization. It may be necessary to provide nutritional supplements with vaccines or, alternatively, to vaccinate at a "nutritionally" better ttime of year. Programs to support family planning, to improve agricultural production and environmental sanitation, will have an impact as well and should be encouraged. As Chandra noted, multiple interventions are more likely to produce measurable effects than single options. Policies must be geared to these needs.

Discussion

Chandra's presentation included data showing that, in animals so zinc-deficient as to be near death, serum zinc levels do not change dramatically. Chandra was asked specifically whether this demonstrated a difference between people and experimental animals in terms of their ability to regulate zinc, or whether it represented some kind of artifact.

Chandra responded that there are cases in humans where zinc and immune function seem to be correlated. For example, acrodermatitis enteropathica is an inherited disorder of zinc absorption in which infants develop skin lesions, diarrhea, and many other infections. When zinc is administered, plasma zinc levels rise, cellular immunity increases, and susceptibility of these individuals to infection decreases. Similarly, a hereditary disorder of zinc absorption in sheep is responsive to zinc.

Some animal studies have shown that a low zinc intake causes decreased serum levels, while in others, a low intake of zinc had no effect on serum levels, although tissue levels decreased dramatically. More importantly, however, in all these situations the function of the thymus and other aspects of immunity are deranged. It is clear that zinc is important for cell-mediated immunity, but plasma zinc may be an unsatisfactory index of zinc nutrition. Perhaps measuring zinc content of hair and other available tissues may be used to supplement this information.

The second topic was of a broader nature. It questioned whether most work concerning immunity and malnutrition had been carried out in children, and whether people continuously exposed to unsanitary conditions tend to adapt, and therefore do not require public health measures. Chandra indicated that adults with mild to moderate malnutrition exhibit immunity deficits similar to those in undernourished children. For example, in famine situations, starving adults show increased susceptibility to infection.

Concerning adaptation, the important distinction between stunting and body wasting in children was emphasized. There are many biochemical changes that occur during wasting induced by nutritional deficiency not seen in stunting that occurs over a prolonged period. In the absence of conclusive data, the consensus was that the child who does not adapt well to acute nutritional stresses is more at risk of infectious disease and immunological deficiency than the child who is stunted in growth but well adapted.

It was also pointed out that the question of adaptation is a two-edged sword. The classic example is schistosomiasis, in which cell-mediated immune mechanisms cause the pathology. If the host did not develop a cell-mediated immune response, an individual could be infected and not have the severe pathological and physiological effects. In a circumstance where schistosomiasis is accompanied by malnutrition, the host is, to some extent, protected against that agent in its environment. Thus, it is important to consider the consequences of programs to rehabilitate malnourished individuals in an area where a disease like schistosomiasis is present. If cell-mediated immunity is improved in individuals who are already infected with the fluke, considerable additional damage may be caused that they are protected against while malnourished. The same kind of argument may apply to iron status. Low iron in the serum may be detrimental to the growth of microorganisms or their ability to produce specific virulent factors, such as toxins, that are the actual cause of the pathological manifestations of the particular diseases.

II

Food Fortification

For many years, it was argued that the most cost-effective means of combating malnutrition was to employ the technological capabilities of modern food science in order to enhance existing food staples with whatever nutrients were deficient in the diet of a given target group. There was, in fact, great enthusiasm during the 1960s and 1970s, as well as some early programmatic success, for such technological approaches to food and nutrition policy. It has become increasingly clear, however, that, whereas fortification interventions can play a useful role in dealing with micronutrient deficiencies of vitamins and minerals, they have limited applicability to the broader macronutrient deficiencies of protein–calorie malnutrition.

The issue paper contributed by Gershoff offers a candid and realistic assessment of the role that food fortification can play in current or future nutrition policy planning. Gershoff's properly restrained analysis is tempered by the country case studies on micronutrient fortification of sugar with vitamin A in Guatemala by Arroyave, and of staple foods with iron in South America by Layrisse. Additional case experiences and critiques are also offered by the workshop discussants and by the other participants.

Food Fortification

STANLEY N. GERSHOFF

Considering the theory of nutrient fortification and the successes that well-conceived fortification programs have achieved, it is shocking that probably no other type of nutrition intervention strategy has been more misused or abused. Possibly because nutrient fortification is relatively simple and inexpensive and provides a way in which to reach large numbers of people, it has been beset with problems ranging from poor science to charlatanism. To most of us, fortification of food or water is an attractive way to increase the nutrient intake of a population without the necessity of altering eating habits, and therefore without the need for elaborate, large-scale educational programs.

Fortification is of value under two different sets of circumstances. In one circumstance, it can be used to prevent or treat nutritional deficiency disease in a population subject to a nutritional disease with a sharply defined etiology. In the other, it can be used primarily by affluent societies to provide insurance against the occurrence of nutritional disease in segments of the population, often small and difficult to identify, who are at risk.

In a country such as the United States, fortification has been used for both purposes. It can be argued that the fortification of milk with vitamin D, of salt with iodine, and of water with fluoride have successfully treated and prevented nutritional disease. Furthermore, in the United States it has been common for about 35 years to add thiamin, riboflavin, niacin, and iron to cereal products; vitamin A to margarines and some dairy products; and other nutrients to food as a kind of insurance, with little evidence of the extent, if any, of their health impact.

There have been many statements and discussions about fortification through the years (1–5), and it can be concluded from these that a

STANLEY N. GERSHOFF • Tufts University School of Nutrition, Medford, Massachusetts.

successful fortification program in any particular society should have the following characteristics:

1. The intake of the nutrient(s) to be used as a fortificant is below a desirable level in the diets of a significant number of people. Both "desirable" and "significant" as used in this context are vague, and would of necessity be interpreted differently in different countries. In a wealthy nation the recognition that large numbers of people exhibited low or deficient biochemical indices related to nutrient intake, even though clinical deficiency signs were not a perceived problem, might be deemed sufficient reason to launch a fortification program. In a less affluent country or one with different priorities, the appearance of large numbers of people with clinical deficiency signs might be necessary before a fortification program would even be considered. Similarly, there would be differences from country to country in the percentage of the population expected to show undesirable biochemical indices or clinical signs before a significant number of people were judged to be in need of nutritional help. Furthermore, the number considered significant might vary with the nutrient in question.

2. A second characteristic of a successful fortification program would be that the carrier of the fortificants be consumed in relatively constant quantities by the population in need. Obviously, any carrier selected would have to be consumed by the majority of the population in need. If the quantities consumed varied over a wide range, the possibility might arise of not supplying sufficient amounts of nutrients to one group while exposing another to toxic levels. This kind of problem has come up in connection with vitamin A fortification programs in a number of developing countries. Concern about possible toxicity for a few people is a continuing problem for those advocating fortification programs. It provides a basic strategy for people who oppose fortification or many kinds of public health intervention programs. Consider the continuing fears spread about iron fortification and fluoridation. Questions about the possibility that fortification might create imbalances among essential nutrients have also been raised, although I am unaware of proposed fortification programs that might seriously pose such a risk.

3. In a successful fortification program the nutrients used must be stable and physiologically available under the prevailing conditions of storage and use to which they will be subjected. This presents a serious problem. Most developing countries are in tropical areas, and fortified foods or the fortificants of the premixes used

may have to be stored for long periods of time under conditions of high temperature and/or humidity, which may diminish the activity of unstable nutrients. The continued use of unavailable iron in iron fortification programs for decades is scientifically indefensible to the point of scandal.

Clearly, the choice of the proper fortificant carrier is of fundamental importance to the success of any fortification program. Berg and Levinson (2,3), as well as others, have written extensively on the characteristics of carriers and the problems that may occur in the implementation of fortification programs. As already mentioned, any carrier selected should be consumed by a sizeable portion of the public at risk. In developing countries this means that it should be cheap, palatable, and culturally acceptable. The carrier should be processed in amounts large enough to permit efficient, inexpensive control of the fortification. The fortification of grains milled in thousands of small village mills, as occurs in many developing countries, obviously presents a major problem. India, for example, has more than 500,000 rice mills. Nevertheless, even in India, if grain fortification were shown to be effective, a limited program might be in order. Too often impatient health workers have looked for supercomprehensive programs, while rejecting all others. As about 20% of Indians live in urban areas using large mills, a fortification program for these people might be feasible. Even though no benefits would be conferred on 80% of the population, over 100 million people might be served.

4. The fortification of a food should not alter its taste, odor, appearance, or cooking characteristics in such a way as to decrease consumer acceptance. There have been examples of problems related to the organoleptic properties of fortified food, including bad tastes caused by iodine, odors caused by thiamine, abnormal color imparted by riboflavin, and textural changes caused by the use of artificial rice fortification grains.

5. It is important that any fortified food requiring home processing not lose its nutritional value while being prepared for consumption. Fortified rice, which would retain nutrient activity when steamed as in Thailand, may lose this activity when boiled in excess water, as is often done in Bangladesh. Highly available ferrous salts, if added to flour, are converted to unavailable ferric salts by baking.

6. Finally, the carriers and fortificants used should not alter the economics of eating the fortified food in a way that will discourage its consumption. The economics of fortification has been a partic-

ular problem for planners who projected amino acid fortification programs. Because fortification programs affect all people in a population in order to get to a small at-risk segment, calculations of costs per person eating fortified food greatly underestimate the cost per person at risk. The latter cost may be so high that other types of intervention may become economically attractive.

Given a situation in which there is a scientifically sound basis for instituting a fortification program, in which a suitable carrier is available, and in which controlled field tests demonstrate that needed health benefits can be realized by fortification, a whole new series of questions arise.

Should the fortification be mandatory by government decree or should it be voluntary? If it is decided that it should be voluntary, how should the fortified food be distinguished from the nonfortified food? This would be a particularly important problem if the fortification did not change the color, taste, or odor of the food. Should the cost of fortification be passed on to the consumer, or should it be subsidized by the government? Should subsidies make fortified food cheaper than unfortified food? It is clear that many of the problems of implementing fortification or other nutrition programs are economic, particularly in the countries that need them the most because of the poverty of their people.

Decisions to develop fortification programs are often decisions to spend hard currency on imported nutrients and fortification equipment. Problems of setting and enforcing standards for the nutritional quality and purity of the fortificants are not restricted to developing countries; they are also present in industrialized countries. When the United States decided a few years ago to allow 30% texturized soy protein in the school lunch program as a substitute for other protein-containing foods many nutritionists became concerned. Not only was the biological value of the soy protein questionable, but the texturized protein did not contain the nonprotein nutrients in the foods being replaced.

This paper began with a strong caveat about the way in which fortification as a public health intervention technique has often been used, but also noted that fortification has also been highly successful. Let us look at a number of examples of fortification interventions and the special problems they have presented.

AMINO ACID FORTIFICATION OF GRAINS IN DEVELOPING COUNTRIES

About ten years ago, most of the scientists interested in protein–calorie malnutrition stressed the importance of protein. A conviction arose among some prominent and influential university and government scientists and administrators that the amino acid fortification of grains—the major source of calories for people living in developing countries—would be successful in solving many protein-related malnutrition problems. Others felt that it would not work. Still, the theory and prospects of helping large numbers of people were attractive, and U.S. AID decided to support several large-scale field trials of amino-acid fortification. Accordingly, three major studies of about four years duration were funded: the fortification of rice in Thailand, of wheat in Tunisia, and of corn in Guatemala (6,7). In each instance, the amino acid fortification was accompanied by appropriate micronutrient fortification and the studies were properly controlled. The results of all three studies became available about 4 or 5 years ago.

There was no effect on the anthropometric measurements made in any of the three countries, and with the exception of some dubious effects on morbidity and mortality in Guatemalan children, the interventions were without visible value for any of the parameters measured. These disappointing results did not appear to come from inability of the three separate groups of investigators to follow their protocols. The grains were fortified, and sufficient numbers of children who were markedly retarded in growth and development ate them; if the fortificants had addressed their primary nutritional needs, they should have responded significantly.

These studies raise two very disturbing questions. First: How is it possible that after 30 years of large numbers of nutritional studies in developing countries, including over 30 ICNND surveys, there is such a lack of understanding of the nutritional causes of retarded child growth and development in these countries? Second: Why, in the years since these studies were reported, has there not been a serious attempt to determine the reasons for their failure to produce positive effects?

IRON FORTIFICATION IN THE UNITED STATES

For more than 30 years, grain products in the United States have been fortified with iron compounds; in many the iron has little biological availability. Through these years there have been many concerns expressed about iron deficiency anemia in people throughout the world. Many countries, including the United States, have set nutritional standards for iron so high that women of child-bearing age cannot meet them by consuming ordinary diets. Even so, the conclusions of the American Ten-State Nutrition Survey (8) that iron deficiency anemia is a problem in American males and females of all ages shocked many public health scientists and administrators. Such a conclusion from the most comprehensive nutrition survey ever done in the United States understandably resulted in a variety of actions. The Center for Disease Control issued contracts for studies of the effects of iron fortification on anemic people of various ages. The Food and Drug Administration, at the urging of some of the most prominent American nutritionists, published a proposal to increase, by about three times, the amount of iron used to enrich bread (25 mg/lb) and flour (40 mg/lb).

Almost immediately a small, but very vocal, group appeared to oppose increased iron fortification, stressing the poor biological availability of the iron compounds used in fortification, while at the same time warning against possible iron toxicity. As often happens when public health intervention programs are proposed, an advocacy situation developed, with both sides spending their energies in attacking the opposing positions with words rather than data.

Unfortunately, it is difficult to characterize the anemias observed in the American Ten-State Nutrition Survey. We received a contract to study moderately anemic people over 60 years of age in Boston and concluded that they were not anemic as a result of iron deficiency (9). A similar conclusion was reached by the HANES survey (10). After 7 years of acrimony, the proposal to increase iron fortification of bread and grain products was withdrawn by the Food and Drug Administration. The reasons given in a sharply written statement (11) were that the proponents of increased iron fortification had not refuted the arguments of those opposing the proposal. One must conclude in this example that, once again, intelligent consideration of a fortification program was handicapped by a lack of scientific data.

The Fortification of Foods by Private Companies

People throughout the world have become increasingly aware of the need for good nutrition and recognize that this means the ingestion of a variety of nutrients. Unfortunately, most people have little understanding of the science of nutrition or are confused by it. For a number of reasons, many undesirable foods, which are fortified with all kinds of nutrients in varying combinations, are now being offered throughout the world, often with promises of extraordinary benefits. In the United States, it is now possible to buy breakfast foods containing 100% of the adult RDA for multiple nutrients in an amount of cereal representing about 5% of the adult RDA for calories. There is clearly a "vitamin race." The value of these foods has not been demonstrated, but they have resulted in a number of undesirable effects. They have provided false assurance of good nutrition to some. They have increased the price of food. They have confused people about the field of nutrition and the competence of nutritionists. They have provided arguments for those who distrust the food industry. Finally, their use and the claims made for them have misled legislators and government officials, both in developing and industrialized countries. It is increasingly difficult, for example, for American nutritionists working in developing countries to defend the proposition that the high amount of food fortification deemed useful in the United States is not suitable for people in poorer countries.

Whole Wheat (Atta) Fortification in Pakistan

Discussion of atta fortification is presented here because I have recently been asked to look at a proposed program in Pakistan. Approximately 9 years ago it was suggested to the government of Pakistan by the American government that a fortification program should be developed to reach 21 million urban poor, in which thiamin, riboflavin, niacin, and iron would be added to whole wheat. Over a period of time the Pakistani government was persuaded to make the atta fortification program a part of its national development plan. The agreement was that a 3-year program would be implemented, with the United States supplying over two million dollars and the government of Pakistan a lesser figure. Recently, there were conflicts between the United States and Pakistani governments concerning nuclear arms, and the United States suspended all aid to Pakistan. This left the government of Pakistan in the uncomfortable position of being committed to a public health program without the necessary funds. It is obvious from reading both American and Pakistani documents that marked health benefits were expected from this fortification program by both governments, and that once the program was implemented the public would be told about them.

A review of the information available to both the United States and Pakistani governments indicated that there were no published data showing significant public health problems in Pakistan owing to deficiencies of vitamins B_1, B_2, or niacin. While it is probable that considerable iron deficiency anemia exists in Pakistan, its causes have not been properly studied, and the effectiveness of an atta fortification program in alleviating it have not been demonstrated. Dietary surveys done in Pakistan do not reveal significant deficiencies of the nutrients of concern in Pakistani diets. Whole wheat, which provides the bulk of the calories for poor Pakistanis, is high in all of the nutrients that were to be added, although the availability of iron in the diet is questionable. Finally, the results of the grain fortification studies already discussed suggest that it is improbable that health benefits would accrue from the proposed atta fortification.

A variety of concerns have been raised by this program that now probably will not be implemented. This is not the proper place to discuss the withholding of promised health aid to a country with which there is a political problem, thus penalizing the most defenseless and needy people. However, it should be mentioned. The fact that this ill-advised program was developed by two governments over a period of years points out once more the inability of some planners to make use of the scientific information available to them. Frequently, it may be felt politically necessary to provide certain types of programs whether they are successful or not. However, the implementation of such a program raises the question of what would be the long-term effects on government officials and members of the public of failure to provide the major discernible benefits they had expected. Would such a failure have a harmful effect on the development, funding, and implementation of other more worthy projects?

Of interest are two other questions raised in Pakistan that apply to other countries. It was felt by some that the addition of nutrients to atta might concern some segments of the public that they were either being poisoned or treated with unwanted drugs for such things as population control. Even the millers, who were not concerned about the technology of wheat fortification—an uncomplicated process that has been used in other parts of the world—expressed minor concern that once the precedent was established, at some future time they might be asked to add other things that they might be opposed to for technological or other reasons. They were also worried about the possibility that if the fortification, which was to be directed to a restricted segment of the population, was accompanied by a massive public relations campaign, then a demand might be made by the rest of the public to have their atta fortified.

Vitamin A Fortification in Indonesia

For most, there are few consequences of nutritional deficiency more devastating than children becoming blind because of vitamin A deficiency. Vitamin A deficiency is a major public health problem in many parts of the world, resulting not only in blindness but also in impaired resistance to infectious disease, in retarded growth and development, and in death. Interventions to alleviate this problem have often been very disappointing, and vitamin A fortification programs are in various stages of development in a number of countries. Current estimates predict that, each year in Indonesia, 40,000–80,000 children develop corneal disease and become blind, and that 1–1.5 million develop conjunctival disease because of a deficiency of this vitamin.

The Indonesian government, unhappy with its vitamin A programs, is now considering vitamin A fortification. I have recently had the opportunity to work on this with Indonesian officials. Many of the basic conditions for a successful fortification program are now present. It is clear that the administration of adequate quantities of the vitamin to Indonesian children will protect them from blindness. Vitamin A is cheap and available. Thus, the problem has been to find a suitable carrier.

Initial studies of foods available for fortification indicated that only wheat flour, sugar, and monosodium glutamate (MSG) deserved consideration. Rough calculations of the cost of a program that would provide the target population with one-half the RDA for vitamin A indicated that an intervention using sugar as a carrier would cost $87 million per year, wheat $43 million, and MSG $4.5 million. Furthermore, because of the enormous individual differences in flour and sugar consumption in Indonesia, the use of either of these foods as carriers would provide a clear danger of vitamin A toxicity to large segments of the population. Thus, it has been concluded that only MSG meets the characteristics required of a suitable carrier.

Even so, the use of MSG presents several problems. Indonesian government officials are concerned that use of MSG might appear to be an endorsement by the government of a product produced by a commercial company. Representatives of consumer groups are concerned about MSG toxicity. There may also be resistance by the manufacturers of MSG who (1) foresee the disclosure of their production figures, which they often guard, (2) will have to stop advertising MSG as a pure white compound, (3) are reluctant to tamper with a successful merchandising operation, and (4) would need assurance that successful fortification with vitamin A would not be followed by further demands on them. There is also concern that the amount of unfortified MSG in current channels of distribution is so large that it will dilute the effects of fortified MSG for a considerable period of time.

The Indonesian example is interesting for another reason. Nutritionists, in representing programs, usually try to emphasize what these programs will do and how much they will cost. Rarely do they calculate the costs of *not* doing anything. Humanitarian and political considerations aside, the economic costs of not addressing health problems may be formidable. Carl R. Fritz of Helen Keller International has calculated what the economic cost of 40,000 Indonesian children going blind each year would be, with half of them dying by the age of four. His detailed, conservative estimate is that the costs to the families, communities, and nation add up to about $40 million per year, with the amount possibly tripled if the costs of an additional 10,000–40,000 children, who contract corneal disease but do not go blind, and an additional 1–1.5 million children, who contract noncorneal xerophthalmia each year, are included. It is obvious that if a vitamin A–MSG fortification program turns out to be only 10% effective, it would pay for itself.

CONCLUSION

This chapter has briefly described some of the major factors that must be considered in designing fortification interventions and has used various types of fortification programs, most of which I have had experience with, to illustrate some of the problems that arise. Fortification remains an attractive method for attacking certain types of well-defined malnutrition. However, to be successful the programs must be carefully designed and then evaluated once they are put into operation so that appropriate changes can be made if necessary.

REFERENCES

1. Austin, J. E. (Ed.). *Global Malnutrition and Cereal Fortification.* Ballinger, Cambridge, Massachusetts, 1979.
2. Berg, A. D., and F. J. Levinson. A new need: The nutrition programmer. *Am. J. Clin. Nutr.* **22**:893, 1969.
3. Berg, A. The Nutrition Factor. The Brookings Institution, Washington, D.C., 1973.
4. *Guidelines for Food Fortification in Latin America and the Caribbean.* Pan American Health Organization Scientific Publication No. 240, Washington, D.C., 1972.
5. Scrimshaw, N. S., and A. M. Altschul (Eds.), *Amino Acid Fortification of Protein Foods.* MIT Press, Cambridge, Massachusetts and London, England, 1971.
6. Gershoff, S. N., R. B. McGandy, D. Suttapreyasri, C. Promkutkao, A. Nondasuta, U. Pisolyabutra, P. Tantiwongse, and V. Viravaidhaya. Nutrition studies in Thailand, II. Effects of fortification of rice with lysine, threonine, thiamin, riboflavin, vitamin A and iron on preschool children. *Am. J. Clin. Nutr.* **30**:1185, 1977.
7. Gershoff, S. N. Evaluation of cereal grain enrichment programs. In: *Nutrition in Transition. Proceedings of the Western Hemisphere Nutrition Congress V.* P. L. White and N. Selvey (Eds.), American Medical Association, Chicago, Illinois, 1978.
8. *Ten-State Nutrition Survey 1968–1970.* DHEW Publication No. 72-8130–8134. Government Printing Office, Washington, D.C., 1972.

9. Gershoff, S. N., O. A. Brusis, H. V. Nino, and A. M. Huber. Studies of the elderly in Boston, 1: The effects of iron fortification on moderately anemic people. *Am. J. Clin. Nutr.* **30:**226, 1977.

10. *Preliminary Findings of the First Health and Nutrition Examination Survey, United States, 1971–72. Dietary Intake and Biochemical Findings.* DHEW Publication No. (HRA) 74-1219-1. U.S. Government Printing Office, Washington, D.C., 1974.

11. Kennedy, D. *Iron Fortification of Flour and Bread.* Federal Register Docket No. 77N-0356, November 7, 1977.

Comment

FERNANDO E. VITERI

I would initially like to comment on Gershoff's point that evaluation is lacking in the majority of iron fortification studies. To my knowledge, there are no adequate evaluation data to show that iron fortification in the adult population has any effect. Although some data indicate that iron-fortified milk and baby foods have had some positive effects on increasing the iron levels in children, data from the United States and England cast great doubt on the effectiveness of such efforts.

Before discussing my experiences in South America, some background information is necessary. First, it is important to recognize the existence of two simple measures to prevent iron deficiency in the child: The first is to delay ligature of the umbilical cord, thus allowing about one-third more iron to go into the infant at the time of delivery. The second is the promotion of breast-feeding because human milk contains a large amount of lactoferrin. It has been recently determined that the rate of iron absorption from breast milk is between 30 and 70%, which is extremely high in comparison to the approximately 4% absorbed from cow's milk.

Another point I would like to stress is that iron balance is a very delicate issue. Iron requirements are approximately 0.9–1 mg/day in children and adult males and about twice that in women of reproductive age. If we look at dietary components we see a trend toward decreasing amounts of iron as a result of the changing technology and consumption of purified foods. The trend is not only toward lower quantities, but also toward lower-quality iron. The reason for the lower quality is because there are generally only two sources of dietary iron: the nonheme iron in cereals and legumes, and the heme iron found in the blood and muscle

FERNANDO E. VITERI • Division of Human Nutrition and Biology, Institute of Nutrition of Central America and Panama (INCAP), Guatemala City, Guatemala.

of beef. Consumption of the latter products is decreasing among poor populations who rely almost totally on nonheme iron.

There are two other factors that must be considered in iron nutriture. One is that there are naturally occurring substances in the diet that depress iron absorption, e.g., phytates, phosphates, and fiber in cereals, and those that enhance iron absorption (among these the most important is ascorbic acid). For example, a diet containing nonheme iron plus some heme iron and adequate amounts of vitamin C would almost certainly ensure adequate iron absorption and fulfillment of iron balance. Therefore, the problems we face are both the low iron content in the diet and poor absorption owing to the types of iron available and interactions between iron and other dietary components.

Concerning the problem of iron deficiency in Central America, we found that anemia was present in about 22% of the population; the great majority of these anemias were caused by iron deficiency. Thereafter, we did a study on the effect of dietary supplementation. No difference was noted in the response of the population to iron or iron plus folate. With iron alone, or with iron plus folate, we could raise the hemoglobin levels to normal in 90–95% of the population. It was only after this research was complete that we started iron fortification.

To evaluate the success of this program, we are examining four levels of iron nutrition: iron reserves by measuring serum ferritin levels, iron transport, iron status of the bone marrow by measuring three erythrocyte protoporphyrins, and hemoglobin level. The question of what to expect from fortification trials in terms of these four measurements of iron status is unanswered. I can tell you that we have found a significant difference in the fortified communities versus the control community for all of the components examined.

The Program of Fortification of Sugar with Vitamin A in Guatemala

Some Factors Bearing on Its Implementation and Maintenance

GUILLERMO ARROYAVE

THE IDEA

In November 1968, a technical group was convened by the Pan American Health Organization (PAHO) to analyze the problem of hypovitaminosis-A in the Americas (1). Certain basic concepts derived from the analysis determined my path of research for the following eight years. The most important of these were:

> Results of many nutrition surveys show that a low dietary intake of vitamin A is widespread in sectors of the population in many parts of this hemisphere. Clinical and biochemical studies also indicate that hypovitaminosis-A exists in certain segments of the population. Cases of partial and total blindness resulting from severe vitamin A deficiency in association with protein–calorie malnutrition have been reported, often associated with high case-fatality rates. It may, therefore, be concluded that hypovitaminosis-A represents a public health problem in this hemisphere. . . .
>
> The milder forms of hypovitaminosis-A present even greater problems in assigning priorities in the context of public health. Obviously, consider-

GUILLERMO ARROYAVE • This is INCAP Publication I-1141. Division of Biology and Human Nutrition, Institute of Nutrition of Central America and Panama, Guatemala City, Guatemala.

ably larger numbers of the population are affected, and yet our present lack of knowledge of the effects of the lesser degrees of this deficiency makes it difficult to assign priorities realistically. From experiments in animals, however, it can be assumed that prolonged low intake of vitamin A and its precursors may have serious effects on growth and development and on resistance to infectious diseases.

Despite the apparent interest in this subject in scientific literature and the considerable epidemiological data available for this hemisphere, relatively little action has been taken to combat or control this disorder either in its severe or milder forms.

THE PROBLEM IN CENTRAL AMERICA, 1965–1967

During the years 1965–1967, a nutritional evaluation of the region revealed the dietary and blood serum data shown in Tables 1 and 2 (2). In addition, children with corneal lesions and blindness could be found, particularly in pediatric wards of public hospitals (3).

At the Institute of Nutrition of Central America and Panama (INCAP), I began research in 1969 to find an appropriate short-term intervention measure to eliminate or reduce this hypovitaminosis-A (4). In November 1975, sugar began being fortified with retinyl palmitate in Guatemala and Costa Rica. What follows is an account of certain important stages in the development of the program at the national level, from the birth of the idea to the day when the first measure of vitamin A premix was officially added to sugar at the factory level, a practice that continues today.

TABLE 1. Nutritional Survey in Central America and Panama (1965–1967)

Country	Number of families surveyed	Level of adequacy of vitamin A in the diet (percent of adequacy)				
		< 25	25–49	50–74	75–99	≥ 100
Guatemala	200	45[a]	22	10	6	17
El Salvador	278	69	19	7	3	2
Honduras	323	57	26	9	2	6
Nicaragua	331	45	23	13	8	11
Costa Rica	414	44	26	11	7	12
Panama	352	42	32	13	5	8

[a] All values expressed as percent of families at each level.

TABLE 2. Nutritional Survey in Central America and Panama (1965–1967). Prevalence of Hypovitaminosis-A in Children Younger than 15 Years (Determined According to Serum Levels)[a]

Country	0–4 Years		5–9 Years		10–14 Years		0–14 Years	
	Percent prevalence	Number of cases	Percent prevalence	Number of cases	Percent prevalence	Number of cases	Percent prevalence	Number of cases
Guatemala	26.2	219,100	16.2	108,300	11.1	62,700	18.8	390,100
El Salvador	43.5	241,200	43.5	190,700	22.4	82,300	37.8	514,200
Honduras	39.5	137,000	29.0	81,200	21.9	51,609	31.3	269,800
Nicaragua	19.8	56,900	18.5	50,500	6.4	14,400	15.5	121,800
Costa Rica	32.5	96,600	25.6	60,300	11.7	22,400	24.6	179,300
Panama	18.4	38,300	12.1	20,600	9.7	13,600	14.0	72,500
Total	31.2	789,100	24.7	511,600	14.3	247,000	24.4	1,547,700

[a] Values based on population estimates for July 1965.

PUBLIC PRESENTATION AND REACTIONS TO THE PROGRAM

RATIONALE OF THE CONCEPT

The concept that a fortification program may be justified on the basis of the existence of widespread dietary inadequacy and low biochemical indicators (nutritional basis) and the concept that it is not necessary and perhaps may even be unethical to wait until a high prevalence of incapacitating clinical lesions have occurred were difficult to explain. The interesting aspect of this was that the questioning and the opposition stemmed not only from non-nutritionally oriented groups, such as sugar manufacturers and ophthalmologists, but also, surprisingly, from some professionals working in the nutrition area, including some in specialized United Nations agencies.

Our argument, which eventually won favor, was that vitamin A deficiency affects important aspects of the organism before the "end of the straw" corneal lesions ensue. These are related to growth impairment, integrity of the epithelial tissues, resistance to infection, and night blindness, among others. All of these quantities are extremely difficult to assess as specific consequences of vitamin A deficiency in the complex situation of socially deprived populations, where the nature of most biological alterations is multicausal. The corneal damage is similar to kwashiorkor in the case of protein–energy malnutrition: it is the tip of the iceberg supported by an immense mass of a subclinically affected population.

TABLE 3. Distribution of Families by Percent Adequacy of Vitamin A Intake in Guatemala, 1975–1977

Survey period	No. of families surveyed	Level of adequacy of vitamin in diet (percent of adequacy)				
		< 25	25–49	50–74	75–99	> 100
Part A. Sugar without vitamin A						
Oct.–Nov. 1975 (basal)	358	60[a]	23	6	4	7
Apr.–May 1976	360	63	22	7	3	5
Oct.–Nov. 1976	360	54	27	10	4	5
Apr.–May 1977	360	43	25	14	7	11
Oct.–Nov. 1977	356	51	24	14	5	6
Part B. Sugar with vitamin A						
Oct.–Nov. 1975	358	—	—	—	—	—
Apr.–May 1976	360	13	15	22	15	35
Oct.–Nov. 1976	360	8	12	14	17	49
Apr.–May 1977	360	9	10	15	13	53
Oct.–Nov. 1977	356	8	9	15	13	55

[a] All values expressed as percentage of families at each level.

For that reason we stated the objective of the fortification program as follows:

> It is important to emphasize that the *main objective* of the program is to increase the adequacy of intake of vitamin A and, through this improved intake, to raise the body fluid and blood serum levels among the population at large, increasing thereby the supply of retinol to the tissues.

Our results were summarized in these words:

> It is concluded that the program of fortification of sugar with vitamin A has definitely contributed toward allowing the population of this country to ful-

TABLE 4. Daily Per Capita Intake of Retinol Equivalents[a] in Guatemala, 1975–1977

Survey period	From natural food sources	From fortified sugar[b]	Total
Oct.–Nov. 1975 (basal)	221	0	221
Apr.–May 1976	178	336	514
Oct.–Nov. 1976	198	425	623
Apr.–May 1977	251	419	670
Oct.–Nov. 1977	182	445	627

[a] All values expressed as μg.
[b] At a calculated level of fortification there are 10 μg retinol per gram of sugar.

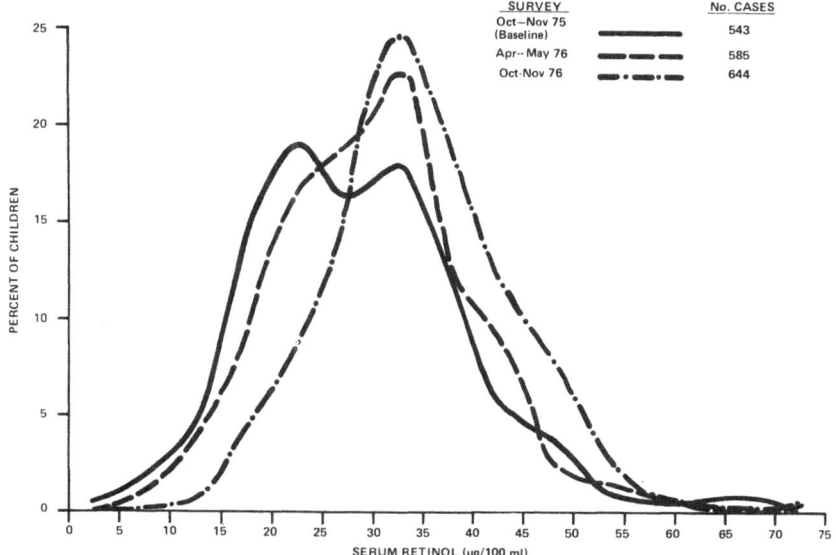

FIGURE 1. Effect of sugar fortification with vitamin A on the distribution of serum retinol levels of rural preschool children, 1975–1976.

fill its individual and social right to an intake of vitamin A in accordance with that considered necessary for maintaining adequate nutrition with respect to this essential nutrient.

The basis for these two statements are summarized in Tables 3 and 4 and in Fig. 1 (5).

OPPOSITION TO SUGAR AS THE DIETARY VEHICLE

The selection of white table sugar as the dietary carrier was made after a thorough analysis of many possible foods in accordance with certain criteria. A vehicle suitable for this purpose should have the following characteristics: (1) the vehicle must be consumed by essentially all of the population; (2) the vehicle must show little variation in its day-to-day per capita consumption; (3) fortification should result in unappreciable change in the organoleptic characteristics and acceptability of the vehicle; and (4) the cost and nature of the vehicle must be such as to allow for an economically feasible industrial process.

In a previous publication (6) I pointed out that in developed countries, the number of possible vehicles is large because of the equally large number of components in the daily diet. The following foods have been used as vehicles for fortification:

Food	Coverage
Prepared infant formula	Infants
Instant breakfast	Principally children
Ready breakfast	Principally children
Margarine	All age groups
Milk	All age groups

The inapplicability of these to less developed countries is obvious. These foods, for all practical purposes, are not consumed by the population sectors in need of vitamin A in these countries. For some countries, like Guatemala, even wheat or rice are not universally available, and their consumption is significant only in the higher socioeconomic strata. Corn is most commonly eaten, but it is home-processed with no possibility of a central point in its food chain where the nutrient could be added. In addition, the corn is drastically cooked and the cooking water is discarded.

From the start, the nutritional risk attached to excessive sucrose intakes was considered. The Guatemalan population at large (particularly rural) consumes sugar although not in excess (about 30–40 g/day average). Nevertheless, measures were taken to avoid any promotion of higher sugar consumption as a source of the vitamin. Any reference to vitamin A content in the labeling was legally prohibited, as well as any advertisement. Presidential Decree SP-G-105-74 (7) translated reads:

> All promotion that attributes therapeutic properties to fortified sugar is prohibited, as is any presentation of this product as a unique source of this nutrient (vitamin A). The products that are formulated with fortified sugar cannot indicate it as a quality of the product. Those who fail to comply with, or violate, this law will be subject to the sanction stipulated in the law. (7)

In spite of this, strong criticism and opposition developed from some groups and even from some individuals belonging to scientific and technical organizations, such as WHO and PAHO. The battle was hard, but we succeeded. A typical, not unique, case is illustrated by the two letters that follow.

Vermont, November 5, 1972

Dear Dr. Arroyave,
   It was reported by the New York Times Service that you plan to fortify sucrose with vitamin A in order to combat dietary shortages of this vitamin.

One of our biggest world problems is correcting one problem by a method that produces another less obvious, although just as serious a dietary predicament.

I direct your attention to research done in England on the effects of "pure" sucrose sugar on the body.

Dr. John Yudkin has written a book geared to lay people on the subject of sucrose sugar called, *Sweet and Dangerous.* His research papers, however, are more convincing for the professional and would no doubt still be available from Queen Elizabeth Hospital, London, England.

Dr. Emmanuel Cheraskin of the University of Alabama, Birmingham, Alabama, also has data available. They, too, have researched this area for thirty years. No one in government here listens because of the powerful pharmaceutical lobby in Washington. With hard work on our parts, we are hoping to correct this dreadful situation.

In the meantime, I do hope that you will not continue to support such a program to your people, but will instead find an alternate solution.

Sincerely,

A. J. H.

Guatemala, November 21, 1972

Dear A. J. H.:

Your letter disturbed me a great deal, as it made me realize how poorly informed you are about the nutrition problems of our third world and how little you care about them.

The fact that excessive sugar consumption is undesirable is well documented. I do know the literature on that subject. But it is also true that sugar *per se* in amounts that are not excessive is not harmful. This is also true for many foods such as fats, and even several minerals and vitamins. For those populations already consuming too large an amount of sugar there is room for efforts to try to decrease it. Those same privileged populations are also enjoying an abundance of practically every food and everything else. But that is your problem. Ours is the opposite. Our people consume sugar (not excessively) and badly need vitamin A. We do not see how we could make them stop eating sugar, even if we wanted to. Therefore, we think we can use it as a vehicle for a needed nutrient. No one is thinking of promoting a higher consumption of sugar because it will be fortified, nor would anyone promote a higher consumption of table salt, for example, because it is iodized. We have done a lot of research and thinking about this and find no better solution for the vitamin A deficiency problem in our areas. If you can think of some alternate solutions, let me know. But *please* don't try to suggest fortifying milk or margarine until you have a chance to know the socio-economic and socio-cultural patterns of the populations of our concern.

In the meantime, we will continue to support the program. Let me add that, as undesirable as dental caries are, I still prefer to see a child with poor teeth to seeing him *blind.*

I will welcome further comments.

Sincerely yours,

Dr. Guillermo Arroyave

THE PROS AND CONS OF THE PROFESSIONAL GROUPS

When the laboratory and pilot research was in progress, but well advanced at INCAP, the news about the program filtered out and became a subject of public debate. The first reaction—and indeed a violent one—came from the president of the Association of Chemical Engineers of Guatemala, who argued a number of technological objections that, in his opinion, made it impossible to mix vitamin A with sugar. He carried with him the whole official opinion of this association. The main objections were: (1) the danger of toxicity, and (2) the technological impossibility of mixing vitamin A with sugar, in view of the fat-soluble character of one and water solubility of the other. This public debate was carried out through meetings, letters, and even the mass media (newspapers, television, radio). The professional in question even consulted with technical persons of the U.S. Food and Drug Administration, but asking the questions in such a way as to receive the answer that he needed, for example: Is vitamin A toxic? The answers, usually recommending caution in its use, were put to use to frighten lay sectors about the proposed program.

In fact, the president of this society had business and family ties with one of the most powerful sugar manufacturers in Guatemala. With carefully presented scientific and technical arguments, and with the support of health and social science professional sectors, the opposition was defeated after three years. Among the strongest supporters of fortification were the Guatemalan Medical Association, the Pediatric Association, the Association of Chemists and Pharmacists, the School of Medicine and the School of Pharmacy of the University of San Carlos, and the National Committee for the Blind and Deaf.

THE REACTION OF THE GOVERNMENT

When the process was fully developed and tested, the time came to propose it to the government through the Ministry of Health. The idea was officially received well and a green light was given to INCAP to continue with the work. Liaison professionals from the Maternal and Child Care Division of the Ministry of Health were appointed to work with INCAP and with representatives of the sugar manufacturing sector in the elaboration of the law. When the law was finally drawn up, it included an article making the sugar manufacturing sector responsible for covering the cost of fortification, including the purchase of the vitamin A product. The law went through the offices of executive power with "normal" sluggishness. The trouble began in Congress. The lobbying by the sugar manufacturers was hidden but powerful, and the law was defeated on September 12, 1973. Later, we learned that the sugar manufacturing sector was divided in its opinion, a large and powerful majority being against fortification of sugar. One particular man in this private sector deserves special mention because of his support and cooperation for the project. He is Mr. Roberto Dorión, then President of Ingenio El Salto, S.A., Guatemala. To the others he was a black sheep among the flock.

Then the mass media began to play a role, with overwhelming support in the form of editorials and news releases emphasizing the need of the "poor" for such a program. Literally hundreds of articles were published criticizing the decision of Congress. As the election day for congressional representatives approached, we began a second offensive. At this stage, the Committee for the Blind and Deaf played an instrumental role in generating very strong social pressure, and the law was formally approved on June 11, 1974 (8). The political circumstances at that particular moment had added the necessary political appeal and value to the program.

The First Three Years of the Program on a National Scale

Identifying the Main Constraint: The Economic Factor

Sugar is produced in Guatemala during a certain period of the year called "zafra." This sugar production season normally begins at the end of November and extends through June or the beginning of July. During these seven months, sugar cane is converted into either crude sugar for export or centrifuged white sugar for internal use. It is estimated roughly that about 75% of the latter goes for direct table use. The rest is used for industrial purposes, mainly sweet drinks and processed foods. It is that 75% of table sugar that has the highest priority in terms of vitamin A fortification, as processed foods and beverages are very infrequent dietary items for the poor sectors, particularly in the case of the rural population, where vitamin A intakes are most inadequate.

At the time this paper is being written, the sugar from four "zafras" has been fortified: 1975–1976; 1976–1977; 1977–1978, and 1978–1979. The evaluation has been completed and published (5). The publication includes: (1) the efficiency of the delivery system for fortified sugar to the population, (2) the nutritional effectiveness, and (3) estimates of the cost.

This evaluation allowed us to determine that 75% of the total white sugar production for local consumption was fortified in 1976–1977, and 72% was fortified in 1977–1978. Without going into a detailed analysis of this situation, this was considered quite satisfactory, and indeed, resulted in dramatic positive effects on the indicators of vitamin A nutritional status of the population (5).

The results of 1978–1979 were somewhat disappointing. Data on the efficiency of fortification are now emerging that show that during this third sugar production season, only 52% of white sugar for local consumption was fortified.

In this section I shall try to describe the economic–financial factors that, directly or indirectly, have become constraints threatening the maintenance of the fortification program and that, in my view, specifically explain the low efficiency during the 1978–1979 "zafra."

There are several ways in which the economic aspects of the program on a national scale can be analyzed in order to identify the positive as well as the negative factors that affected its implementation and maintenance. This is discussed in the following two sections.

THE CONSUMER'S POCKET

The national laws of fortification of sugar with vitamin A in Guatemala, as well as in three other countries of the Central American region, specify that the cost of the fortification process must be absorbed by the sugar manufacturers and that the price of sugar to the consumer cannot be increased on the basis of the costs of the program. The facts behind the rationale supporting that decision are explained thus:

In 1974, at the time the Guatemalan law was approved by Congress, the cost of the water-dispersible retinyl palmitate specified by the technology was U.S. $10/kg. Then the purchase of the product was calculated as representing about 90% of the total cost of the fortification program, the remaining 10% being the costs of the operation at the factory level, plus supervision and control. On that basis, the cost of fortification was 11 U.S. cents per qq,* or 0.11 cents (about one-tenth of a cent per pound).

At that time, the retail price of sugar was 8 cents per pound and the smallest fractional coin in Guatemala is 1 cent (U.S. $1 = 1 quetzal). Obviously, it was impossible to put into practice an exact increase in price per pound to compensate for the actual fortification costs. In addition, 0.11 cents is only 1.3% of 8 cents, which was considered by Government economists to be a light "load."

*qq is the Spanish measure of weight equal to 100 lb, or 46,000 g.

Although the figures changed somewhat in 1979, the relative "load" essentially has not. Repeating the calculations with the present cost of the vitamin product (U.S. $19.50 per kg)* gives a total of 21 cents per qq, or 0.21 cents per pound. At present, for various reasons obviously unrelated to the cost of fortification, sugar is selling at 15 cents per pound, and 0.21/15 is equivalent to a 1.4% overcost.

THE SUGAR MANUFACTURERS' SIDE

In dealing with this aspect we shall consider again the total cost (90% for the product and 10% for other costs), although we realize that this method overestimates slightly the costs absorbed by the manufacturers, because they are responsible for only part of the supervision and control.

According to the figures shown previously, the fortification of each qq of sugar costs 21 cents (U.S.). The wholesale cost of the qq (at the factory), where money goes directly to the manufacturers, is U.S. $13.50. Therefore, the ratio shows a 1.6% increase (0.21/13.50). To all concerned outside of the sugar business, this looks like a very favorable price to pay for "some" nutrition.

But how do the manufacturers look at it? Exact figures are not easy to obtain, but I do not think they are necessary for the purpose of this argument. We will assume, in addition, that the total production of white sugar subject to vitamin A fortification is now (1979) the same as it was in 1975, which is a harmless assumption. The value could be rounded to 3.6 million qq sacks. Multiplying this figure by U.S. 11 cents per qq gives a total investment of U.S. $396,000 for 1975, while in 1979, the same 3.6 million × U.S. 21 cents was U.S. $756,000.

The previous analysis and the relationships derived therefrom, are only a partial view. To it I would like to add what I call "the impact of the New Economic Order on a nutritional intervention in an underdeveloped country."

The facts and figures to be considered in the discussion are as follows: From 1975 through 1979, the sugar manufacturers in Guatemala produced about 50% of the total white sugar for local consumption, and the other approximately 50% crude sugar for export markets. This, according to their economists—and it seems to make sense—means that to a large extent their financial stability depends on international sugar prices. Any drop in this international price cannot be easily compensated by an increase in the price of local sugar because sugar, which is consid-

*In May 1979, the price of retinyl palmitate 250 CWS was U.S. $25/kg.

ered as a basic food in Guatemala, has a top price control placed on it by the Government and, for political reasons, it is extremely difficult to adjust the price frequently and repeatedly.

In connection with this, it is appropriate to analyze the data in Table 5. This table shows the changes undergone by the international market prices for export sugar and for retinyl palmitate imported for the fortification of sugar. Note that in 1974, the year that fortification was approved and that the sugar industry adopted responsibility for its financing, the ratio "price of export sugar/price of vitamin A" was 1.3; the ratio was only 0.4 in 1978, with a tendency to drop even lower by the end of 1979. This type of phenomenon, of questionable ethical basis, has been perhaps the most important negative factor affecting the maintenance of the program. With local sugar prices under government control, the "slight" gain obtained at the local level through a strenuous political struggle is claimed not to compensate the loss resulting from the deterioration of the international sugar market. Not being in a position to analyze this particular relationship in more technical detail, I present it only as the main complaint from the sugar manufacturing sector. Panama has, in fact, interrupted the program on this basis and has accused the vitamin manufacturers of monopoly and price abuse.

DISCUSSION

The question to consider is: *Should a private industrial sector pay for a nutrition–public health intervention?*

The answer from the private-enterprise economic expert: "They never will. They will find a way to charge it to the consumer. If they cannot, because of strong government price control on the commodity, they will not cooperate, laws or no laws."

The answer from the consumer: "They should; they are making enough money as it is; they are all millionaires" [in general, they are!]; "they have an obligation to do it." The government says the same thing. That is, it accepts in theory the same premise, an attitude that is politically *wise* (votes!).

The opinion of INCAP at present: The view of the consumer seems logical and INCAP favored the inclusion in the law of the specific article charging the sugar manufacturers with the responsibility to absorb the costs. This position appeared, at the time, to be supported by precedents in developed countries, where literally hundreds of manufactured food products are enriched with nutrients at the expense of the producer, and

TABLE 5. Market Prices of Export Sugar and of Retinyl Palmitate 250 CWS in U.S. Dollars

Year	Sugar[a] (100 lb)	Retinyl palmitate (1 kg)
1972	9.00	7.00
1974[b]	29.50	10.00
1975	22.48	11.00
1976	13.32	13.00
1977	11.00	15.00
1978	7.82	19.50
1979 (latest)	8.86	25.00

[a] Farrman & Co., New York.
[b] Year that the fortification law was approved in Guatemala.

even in developing countries, in some instances, such as in the case of salt iodization in Central America.

In regard to this crucial point, our recent analysis of the situation leads to the following conclusions: (1) When there is no government control on the price of a food, such a premise is a fallacy, because in the long run, the price tag is manipulated so that the consumers finally do pay the bill. (2) When there is price control by the government because the food is considered a basic item (such as sugar, corn, and salt) and the manufacturer sees that it is impossible, or very difficult, to apply the mechanisms described in (1), resistance against compliance develops among manufacturers; a number of imaginary faults are attributed to the process and program, ending in partial (Guatemala) or total (Panama) boycott and failure.

CONCLUSION

In my opinion, as a "scientist–biochemist, self-made public health nutrition worker–dreamer," a nutrition intervention program of this type should be structured in such a way that it constitutes an integral part of the Food and Nutrition National Plan. In this context, its cost must be borne by the public sector (government), which should obtain and allocate appropriate funds for such purposes, perhaps within a programmatic policy of "short-term measures to improve the dietary adequacy of the population at large."

Finally, I believe that, of all of the possible aspects and constraints discussed with regard to the fortification of sugar with vitamin A, the conceptual, technological, political, and operational aspects have feasible and relatively easy solutions. The key to success is the wisdom to design the most appropriate and politically acceptable policy to ensure financial support on a long-standing, sound economic basis.

REFERENCES

1. Pan American Health Organization. *Hypovitaminosis-A in the Americas. Report of a PAHO Technical Group Meeting, Washington, D.C., November 28–30, 1968.* PAHO Scientific Publication No. 198, PAHO, Washington, D.C., 1970.
2. Institute of Nutrition of Central America and Panama. *Nutritional Evaluation of the Population of Central America and Panama: A Regional Summary.* DHEW Publication No. [HSM] 72-8120, U.S. Department of Health, Education and Welfare, Washington, D.C., 1972.
3. Oomen, H. A. P. C., D. S. McLaren, and H. Escapini. Epidemiology and public health aspects of hypovitaminosis-A: A global survey on xerophthalmia. *Trop. Geogr. Med.* **16:** 271–315, 1964.
4. Institute of Nutrition of Central America and Panama. *Fortification of Sugar with Vitamin A in Central America and Panama.* U.S. Department of Agriculture, Economic Research Service, Washington, D.C., 1975.
5. Arroyave, G., J. R. Aguilar, M. Flores, and M. A. Guzmán. *Evaluation of Sugar Fortification with Vitamin A at the National Level.* Pan American Health Organization Scientific Publication No. 384, PAHO, Washington, D.C., 1979.
6. Arroyave, G. Distribution of vitamin A to population groups. In: *Proceedings of Western Hemisphere Nutrition Congress III, August 30–September 2, 1971,* P. L. White (Ed.), pp. 68–79. Futura, New York, 1972.
7. Government of Guatemala. *Reglamento para el Enriquecimiento del Azúcar con Vitamina A.* Acuerdo Gubernativo SP-G-105-74, Guatemala, 1975.
8. Government of Guatemala. *Decreto No. 56-74,* Guatemala, June 11, 1974.

Prevention of Iron Deficiency

MIGUEL LAYRISSE

It is well known that lack of iron is the most common nutritional deficiency in the world, especially in developing countries. Its highest prevalence is observed in women during their reproductive life, and also in infants, children, and even in adolescents. The deficiency is produced when there is an imbalance between the iron absorbed from food and that eliminated in the shedding of epithelium, the formation of new tissue, the loss in menstrual blood, and the fetus's need for iron during gestation. Additional iron loss is caused in developing countries by hookworm, trichuris, and *Schistosoma haematobium* infections. Consequently, the frequency and severity of iron deficiency are more evident in populations where those infections prevail.

Physiological iron requirements vary with age and sex: 1.5 mg for children less than 2 years old; 1 mg for children between 2 and 14 years of age, and 1.2–2 mg for women during their reproductive years (1).

It was generally taken for granted until very recently that 12–20 mg of iron per day ingested with food could fill these requirements, assuming that approximately 10% of food iron is absorbed daily from the diet and utilized by the organism. However, this assumption has been completely discarded during the last 12 years as the result of studies on food iron absorption, in which foods were tagged with radioactive iron before ingestion, permitting more accurate measurement of absorption. These studies have provided increasing knowledge on the mechanisms that regulate the different patterns of iron absorption.

The first phase of these studies was the determination of iron absorption from a single food (2–4). It showed in general that iron absorption from animal food products, especially meat, is three to four

MIGUEL LAYRISSE • Universidad Central de Venezuela and Instituto Venezolano de Investigaciones Científicas, Caracas, Venezuela.

times greater than absorption of iron in vegetables. However, iron absorption from eggs, milk, and milk products is close to the percentage absorbed from vegetable foods (5–9). Studies with animal foods such as meat, fish, and liver have shown that the amount of iron absorbed depends on the proportion in which heme, ferritin, and hemosiderin are present. Iron absorption from purified heme is poor—about 4%—but increases about three times when it is ingested as hemoglobin, and even more when it is consumed in the form of hemoglobin and myoglobin from meat (2,10–12). Iron from purified ferritin and hemosiderin is also poorly absorbed—about 2%—but absorption increases several-fold when iron is provided by liver and other meats (13,14).

The second phase of these studies dealt with the effect of mixed-diet food interactions on iron absorption at the lumen of the gut; this provided a better insight into dietary iron absorption than that obtained from a single food. Studies using foods biosynthetically labeled with different radioactive iron isotopes and fed first separately and then together at 15-day intervals to the same individual have shown that iron absorption from vegetable foods is very similar when they are fed together (4), and a similar absorption pattern is found when one vegetable food is mixed with an iron salt either as a ferric or ferrous compound (8,16,17). Iron absorption from vegetable food is about double when the vegetable(s) is combined with meat, liver, or fish (11,18,19). Iron absorption from vegetables is also increased when either ascorbic acid or fruit is added (20,21).

The effect of vegetables and chelating agents on the absorption of iron from animal tissue depends on the proportion in which heme, ferritin and hemosiderin are present in the food. Absorption of heme iron is not affected by vegetables and chelating agents (12), but absorption of ferritin and hemosiderin is affected (13,14). This explains why vegetable foods do not affect iron absorption from most meat, but do reduce iron absorption from liver.

The results obtained from these studies on the effect of mixed diets on iron absorption provided fundamental knowledge for establishment of the concept of two iron pools: heme and nonheme iron. Iron compounds belonging to the same iron pool show the same percentage of absorption when they are administered together. The heme iron pool is formed by hemoglobin and myoglobin and the nonheme pool by vegetables, eggs, iron salts, and possibly milk and dairy products (22). It was also demonstrated that these pools can be measured by mixing a radioactive iron compound belonging to either the heme or nonheme pool into foods (Fig. 1). By this means, a small amount of labeled ferric or ferrous iron salt can indicate the percentage of absorption from the non-

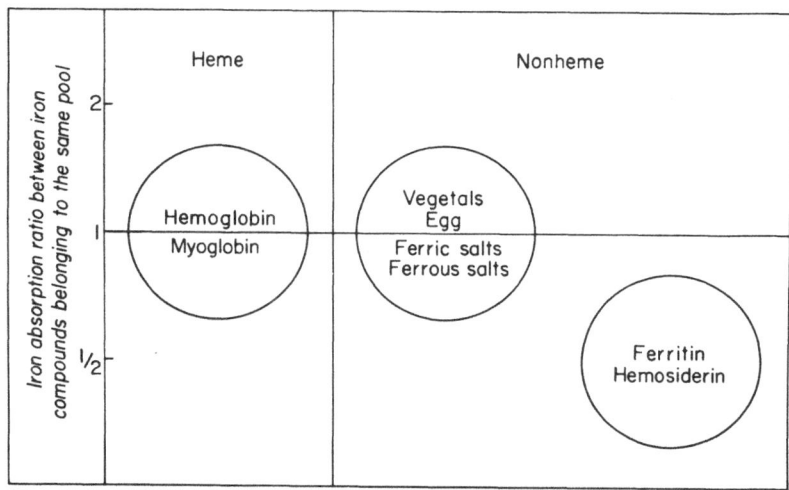

FIGURE 1. Iron compounds pertaining to heme and nonheme iron pools. Purified ferritin and hemosiderin showed distinctly lower absorption when they were administered with vegetables.

heme pool (8,16,17), while a small amount of labeled rabbit hemoglobin can measure that from the heme pool (16). It is also possible to measure accurately the iron absorption from ferritin and hemosiderin using a small amount of purified rabbit ferritin (14). These new techniques, called "extrinsic tag methods," have replaced the tedious work associated with biosynthetic incorporation of radioactive iron into foodstuffs, especially vegetables.

The third phase of iron absorption studies was the determination of the total iron absorbed from a meal and from a daily diet, and also involved the determination of iron absorption from the different pools, as described in the above studies. The total iron absorption from standard diets consumed in different countries has already been determined by this new methodology, demonstrating that the total iron intake does not reflect the amount of iron absorbed, and that the composition of each meal is of paramount importance for the absorption of nonheme iron (20,23–29). Thus, foods, such as animal tissue and fruits, are helpful in obtaining adequate iron absorption from a meal, and beverages, such as tea (30) or coffee (31), reduce iron absorption from a meal. These studies also show that the total iron utilized from some of these diets is very low, and undoubtedly does not permit a physiological iron balance, at least in the vulnerable segments of the population.

The fourth and most recent of these investigations, also based on the "extrinsic tag method," has been concerned with several kinds of iron fortification of various foods to prevent iron deficiency. It was shown that not all iron salts are suitable for fortification. While ferrous sulfate, reduced iron, iron glycerophosphate, ferric ammonium citrate, and ferric chloride (9,28,31–37) are absorbed in amounts that parallel absorption of intrinsic iron in the food vehicle, ferric orthophosphate and sodium iron pyrophosphate are less well absorbed. It was also demonstrated that certain food vehicles, such as maize, contain excess chelating substances that inhibit absorption even when doses of up to 60 mg of iron are given (32), and that other vehicles, such as refined sugar, are devoid of inhibitors (31).

We have already tested six potential food vehicles that could be put to use depending on the food consumption patterns and industrial facilities in each region. The absorption ratio for 3 mg of ferrous sulfate mixed with each vehicle was the same as that for iron salt given alone, which showed that neither refined sugar nor sugar cane syrup contains detectable absorption-inhibiting substances. The other absorption ratios were 0.35 for sweet manioc, 0.25 for milk, 0.16 for wheat, and 0.08 for maize. It is assumed that iron absorption from rice and beans is the same as that from maize.

Even though iron absorption from the majority of iron salts already tested is almost the same when they are administered with the same food vehicle, we have recently reported the peculiar characteristics of Fe(III)-EDTA (38,39) compared with those observed when ferrous sulfate is administered with the same vehicle (Table 1). The results indicated that

TABLE 1. Iron Absorption from Fe(III)-EDTA Complex and Ferrous Sulfate Mixed with Various Foods and Calibrated According to the Absorption from the Reference Dose

	Iron absorption (%)		
Food enriched	Fe(III)-EDTA (3 or 5 mg Fe)	Ferrous sulfate (3 or 5 mg Fe)	Composite mean absorption from reference dose (3 mg Fe)
Refined sugar	8.4	30.0	
Sugar-cane syrup	8.4	25.8	
Milk	13.1	7.9	31.5
Sweet manioc	12.8	11.8	
Wheat	11.5	4.9	
Maize	8.2	2.0	

when ferrous sulfate is the fortification agent iron absorption is inhibited by the chelating substances present in foods, whereas absorption from the Fe(III)-EDTA complex is only slightly affected by such substances. In addition, this iron complex exchanges completely with vegetable iron in the lumen of the gut, and the absorption of both extrinsic and intrinsic food iron is equally good, but the amount absorbed is twice as high than would be expected from other iron salts used under the same experimental conditions. Accordingly, wheat and maize are not satisfactory food vehicles for fortification with ferrous sulfate or other iron salts, but they can be made adequate by enrichment with Fe(III)-EDTA. A small amount of this salt, about 10 mg per day, would be sufficient in most instances to cover the physiological needs for dietary iron.

The amount of information on iron absorption from food and on iron fortification and the new methodology derived from these studies permit accurate assessment of the daily availability of iron from the usual diet of any population, and reveal the amount of iron fortification required to prevent iron deficiency in most subjects. We began recently to coordinate a collaborative study, sponsored by the United Nations University and the Instituto Venezolano de Investigaciones Científicas, to determine the local iron availability from the most common Central and South American diets and to establish a base line for iron fortification in each region. This collaborative study includes a training program at the Reference Center in Caracas for those investigators who are not familiar with the techniques developed for this kind of study. Further collaboration will begin when local research is under way. Four investigators from different countries are already participating in the program, and it is expected that this number will be increased in 1980. Preliminary information from two countries indicates that standard diets consumed by people in the low-socioeconomic groups do not provide the amount of iron necessary to meet the normal requirements of these populations.

SUMMARY

The high prevalence of iron deficiency in the world urgently requires public health actions to prevent it, especially in developing countries where parasitic infections and inadequate diets significantly increase iron losses and where dietary factors interfere with the absorption of the iron. It is an illusion to think that changes in eating habits that might take place in the near future would resolve this situation. The only preventive measure that seems truly feasible is iron fortification of food. The extrinsic tag method introduced in the medical literature within the last decade permits accurate measurement of not only the total iron absorbed and utilized from a daily diet, but also the absorption of iron added to food. Refined sugar is by far the best food vehicle for iron fortification because it is devoid of chelating factors that inhibit iron absorption, while wheat and maize contain inhibitors that markedly reduce absorption of most iron salts. Fe(III)-EDTA is the only iron salt tested that is only slightly affected by foods like wheat and maize. A small amount of this salt, about 10 mg per day, would be sufficient in most instances to cover the physiological requirements for iron.

ACKNOWLEDGMENTS. This work was initially supported by WHO and the Williams Waterman Foundation. In recent years it has been supported by the Consejo Nacional de Investigaciones Científicas y Technologicas, Caracas, and by the United Nations University.

REFERENCES

1. World Health Organization. Nutritional Anaemias, Technical Report No. 503. WHO, Geneva, 1972.
2. Layrisse, M., J. D. Cook, C. Martínez-Torres, M. Roche, I. N. Kuhn, and C. A. Finch. Food iron absorption: A comparison of vegetable and animal foods. *Blood* 33:430–443, 1969.
3. Layrisse, M., and C. Martínez-Torres. Food iron absorption: Iron supplementation of food. *Prog. Hematol.* 7:137–160, 1971.
4. Martínez-Torres, C., and M. Layrisse. Nutritional factors in iron deficiency: Food iron absorption. *Clinics Haematol.* 2:339–352, 1973.
5. Chodos, R. B., J. F. Ross, L. Apt, M. Pollycove, and J. A. E. Halkett. The absorption of radioiron-labelled foods and iron salts in normal and iron-deficient subjects and in idiopathic hemochromatosis. *J. Clin. Invest.* 36:314–326, 1957.
6. Moore, C. V. Iron nutrition. In: *Iron Metabolism*, pp. 241–265. F. Gross (Ed.), Ciba International Symposium, Springer-Verlag, Berlin, 1964.
7. Callender, S. T., S. R. Marney, and G. T. Warner. Eggs and iron absorption. *Br. J. Haematol.* 19:657–665, 1970.
8. Bjorn-Rasmussen, E., L. Hallberg, and R. B. Walker. Food iron absorption in man. I. Isotopic exchange between food iron and inorganic iron salt added to food: Studies on maize, wheat and eggs. *Am. J. Clin. Nutr.* 25:317–323, 1972.
9. Layrisse, M., C. Martínez-Torres, M. Ruphael-Divo, W. Jaffe, and J. E. Torres-Suarez. Iron absorption from skim milk enriched with iron glycerophosphate. *Arch. Latinoam. Nutr.* 23:145–150, 1973.
10. Turnbull, A. L., F. Cleton, and C. A. Finch. Iron absorption. IV. The absorption of hemoglobin iron. *J. Clin. Invest.* 41:1897–1907, 1962.
11. Conrad, M. E., S. Cortell, H. L. Williams, and A. L. Foy. Polymerization and intraluminal factors in the absorption of hemoglobin-iron. *J. Lab. Clin. Med.* 68:659–668, 1968.

12. Martínez-Torres, C., and M. Layrisse. Iron absorption from veal muscle. *Am. J. Clin. Nutr.* **24:**521–540, 1971.
13. Layrisse, M., C. Martínez-Torres, M. Renzi, and I. Leets. Ferritin iron absorption in man. *Blood* **45:**689–698, 1975.
14. Martinez-Torres, C., M. Renzi, and M. Layrisse. Iron absorption by humans from ferritin and hemosiderin. *J. Nutr.* **106:**128–135, 1976.
15. Layrisse, M., C. Martínez-Torres, and M. Roche. The effect of interaction of various foods on iron absorption. *Am. J. Clin. Nutr.* **21:**1175–1183, 1968.
16. Layrisse, M., and C. Martínez-Torres. Model for measuring dietary absorption of heme iron: Test with a complete meal. *Am. J. Clin. Nutr.* **25:**401–411, 1972.
17. Cook, J., M. Layrisse, C. Martínez-Torres, R. Walker, E. Monsen, and C. A. Finch. Food iron absorption measured by an extrinsic tag. *J. Clin. Invest.* **51:**805–815, 1972.
18. Martínez-Torres, C., I. Leets, M. Renzi, and M. Layrisse. Iron absorption from veal liver. *J. Nutr.* **104:**983–993, 1974.
19. Martínez-Torres, C., I. Leets, and M. Layrisse. Iron absorption from fish. *Arch. Latinoam. Nutr.* **25:**199–210, 1975.
20. Layrisse, M., C. Martínez-Torres, and M. González. Measurement of the total daily dietary iron absorption by the extrinsic tag model. *Am. J. Clin. Nutr.* **27:**152–162, 1974.
21. Sayers, M. H., S. R. Lynch, R. W. Charlton, T. H. Bothwell, R. B. Walker, and F. Mayet. The fortification of common salt with ascorbic acid and iron. *Br. J. Haematol.* **28:**483–495, 1974.
22. Layrisse, M. Dietary iron absorption. In: *Iron Metabolism and Its Disorders, Excerpta Medica* Series 366, pp. 20–33, 1975.
23. Bjorn-Rasmussen, E., L. Hallberg, B. Isaksson, and B. Arvidsson. Food iron absorption in man. Application of the two-pool extrinsic tag method to measure heme and non-heme iron absorption from the whole diet. *J. Clin. Invest.* **53:**247–255, 1974.
24. Cook, J. D., and E. R. Monsen. Food iron absorption I. Use of a semi-synthetic diet to study absorption of non-heme iron. *Am. J. Clin. Nutr.* **28:**1289.–1295, 1975.
25. Monsen, E. R., and J. D. Cook. Food iron absorption in human subjects IV. The effects of calcium and phosphate salts on the absorption of nonheme iron. *Am. J. Clin. Nutr.* **29:**1142–1148, 1976.
26. Hallberg, L., E. Bjorn-Rasmussen, L. Rossander, and R. Suwanik. Iron absorption from Southeast Asian diets. II. Role of various factors that might explain low absorption. *Am. J. Clin. Nutr.* **30:**539–548, 1977.
27. Bjorn-Rasmussen, E., L. Hallberg, and L. Rossander. Absorption of fortification iron. Bioavailability in man of different samples of reduced iron and prediction of the effects of Fe fortification. *Br. J. Nutr.* **37:**375–388, 1977.
28. Hallberg, L., E. Bjorn-Rasmussen, L. Garby, R. Pleehachinda, and R. Suwanik. Iron absorption from South-East Asian diets and the effect of iron fortification. *Am. J. Clin. Nutr.* **31:**1403–1408, 1978.
29. Monsen, E. R., and J. D. Cook. Food iron absorption in human subjects V. Effects of the major dietary constituents of a semisynthetic meal. *Am. J. Clin. Nutr.* **32:**804–808, 1979.
30. Disler, P. B., S. R. Lynch, R. W. Charlton, and T. Bothwell. The effect of tea on iron absorption. *Gut* **16:**193–200, 1975.
31. Layrisse, M., C. Martínez-Torres, M. Renzi, F. Velez, and M. González. Sugar as a vehicle for iron fortification. *Am. J. Clin. Nutr.* **29:**8–18, 1976.
32. Layrisse, M., C. Martínez-Torres, J. D. Cook, R. Walker, and C. A. Finch. Iron fortification of food. Its measurement by the extrinsic tag method. *Blood* **41:**333–352, 1973.

33. Cook, J., V. Minnich, C. V. Moore, R. Rasmussen, W. B. Bradley, and C. A. Finch. Absorption of fortification iron in bread. *Am. J. Clin. Nutr.* **26**:861–872, 1973.
34. Garby, L. Iron fortification from fish sauce in Thailand. *Am. J. Trop. Med. Hyg.* **68**:467–476, 1974.
35. Disler, P. B., S. R. Lynch, R. W. Charlton, and T. H. Bothwell. Studies on the fortification of cane sugar with iron and ascorbic acid. *Br. J. Nutr.* **34**:141–143, 1975.
36. Grebe, G., C. Martínez-Torres, and M. Latrusse. Effect of meals and ascorbic acid on the absorption of a therapeutic dose of iron as ferrous and ferric salts. *Cur. Therap. Res.* **17**:382–397, 1975.
37. Layrisse, M., C. Martínez-Torres, and M. Renzi. Sugar as a vehicle for iron fortification: Further studies. *Am. J. Clin. Nutr.* **26**:274–279, 1976.
38. Layrisse, M., and C. Martínez-Torres. Fe(III)-EDTA Complex as iron fortification. *Am. J. Clin. Nutr.* **30**:1166–1174, 1977.
39. Martínez-Torres, C., E. L. Romano, M. Renzi, and M. Layrisse. Fe(III)-EDTA Complex as iron fortification: Further studies. *Am. J. Clin. Nutr.* **32**:809–816, 1979.

Discussion

Discussion focused first on the choice between using scarce resources for a fortification program or for a more broadly based "development" effort, such as income generation or employment. The question arises, therefore, whether to use resources to eliminate nutrient deficiencies in the short run or to work toward longer-term problems. While some may argue that these trade-offs do not necessarily exist in many countries, such as India, it is difficult for some to carry the financial burden of a large-scale fortification project. In other instances, such as the Indonesian example, the fundamental problem with vitamin A fortification is not the cost (considering the income received from the sale of oil), but the difficulties introduced by technical constraints and lack of political will.

In reference to the technical problems, there was concern that food science professionals have not been paragons of certainty; the provision of demonstrable benefit from fortification programs has been problematic. This led to discussion of the necessity of having conclusive proof before initiating fortification programs. There is an obligation to present evidence to governments of the potential returns from their investment. It is inexcusable not to have a clear understanding of the nutrient deficiencies present in a country and of the specific fortification schemes available to address the problems identified. If both prerequisites are met, fortification efforts should be strongly recommended, and it is then up to governments to determine their priorities.

Although it was agreed that questions such as whether or not to prevent blindness through vitamin A fortification are fundamentally ethical dilemmas, the need for understanding opportunity costs was stressed. The limitations on resources must be considered. It may be more fruitful, for example, to concentrate on the infection–malnutrition complex through a variety of interventions.

It was also suggested that, if the opportunity cost of a nationwide fortification program (for a nutrient like iron) is too great, designing intervention policies specifically for vulnerable groups is an alternative. However, the difficulty in determining vulnerability in many populations and the subsequent need for targeting detract from this consideration.

In conclusion, it was noted that single intervention schemes such as fortification efforts are not the optimal answer to improve health and nutrition. Few would deny that multifactorial efforts are more fruitful, e.g., the evidence presented by Arroyave that the infection–vitamin A deficiency problem is inextricably bound. However, there is a need to initiate efforts, even if they do not represent final solutions, with the understanding that demonstration of benefits may be contingent upon addressing related problems extant in a community. Similarly, fortification programs must be responsive to local conditions; continual evaluation and redesign are required.

III

Supplementary Feeding and Formulated Foods

No nutrition programs have been more beset with problems of implementation and doubts as to their nutritional impact than those concerned with supplementary feeding. Supplementary feeding programs are appealing because a logical solution to malnutrition would seem to be the provision of food to those who need it. However, experience has demonstrated the difficulty of ensuring that supplementary food actually reaches those most in need. It is of interest that arguments in defense of feeding programs often have little to do with their success in correcting nutritional deficiencies.

The issue paper, case studies, and discussion explore and analyze the problems encountered with attempts to implement various kinds of feeding programs. The difficulties of achieving the stated goals of such programs in actual practice are also addressed. It is clear that studies must be carried out on unintentional, as well as intentional, consequences of feeding programs.

The issue paper by Scrimshaw emphasizes many of the problems and difficulties encountered in attempts to implement supplementary feeding programs and to introduce formulated foods. At the same time, it emphasizes the importance of implementing programs to make appropriate weaning foods available to all populations. Case studies by Koval and Allen in Egypt, by Ropes in the Philippines, and by Tandon in India represent three quite different intervention programs, all falling far short of their goals, but still making valuable contributions.

The editors wish to acknowledge the contribution of Carol Meredith, who served as rapporteur for this workshop.

Programs of Supplemental Feeding and Weaning Food Development

Nevin S. Scrimshaw

The principal issues related to programs of supplementary feeding concern: (1) the desirability, timing, and nature of weaning foods to complement breast milk; (2) the usefulness, or lack of it, of supplementary feeding programs for older preschool children and for school children; (3) the value of supplementary feeding programs for pregnant and lactating women; (4) the role of supplementary feeding programs for adult workers; and (5) the identification of methods of supplementary feeding that will reach target groups however they are designated. This paper will concentrate mainly on the issues involved in supplementary feeding of the preschool child during and following the weaning period.

For that great majority of children in developing countries who are still breast-fed for an extended period, the timely complementation of breast milk with foods that supply additional protein, energy, iron, and other nutrients is essential for normal growth and development, for resistance to infection, and for the prevention of increased morbidity and mortality. This critical transition period commences with the need to introduce food to complement breast milk and ends when the child is consuming fully the family diet. The mother must be encouraged to complement breast milk properly during this period and to understand when to do so. She must have available to her explicit options for doing this that are practical, effective, and suited to existing resources and her total family responsibilities.

Nevin S. Scrimshaw • International Nutrition Program, Massachusetts Institute of Technology, Cambridge, Massachusetts, and World Hunger Programme, United Nations University, Tokyo, Japan.

Even for infants of healthy, well-nourished mothers under favorable conditions of environmental sanitation and personal hygiene, some complementation of breast milk is desirable by 4–6 months, depending on the individuals. It is generally needed earlier if the mother is poorly nourished and/or environmental conditions are less favorable. Data from developing country populations suggest 3–4 months as more usual (1), and under highly unfavorable circumstances, even earlier (2).

The first consequence of failure to complement breast milk is a falling off of growth and development. The second is a lowering of resistance to infection that is soon reflected in episodes of diarrheal, respiratory, and other infectious diseases, including pyoderma, pharyngitis, and conjunctivitis. Because of the diarrheal disease so commonly seen at this time, it has been argued that complementary food should be avoided because of the risk of enteric infection owing to its contamination. In other words, growth faltering should be tolerated as the lesser evil.

The assumption that the increase in enteric infection is largely due to contaminated food is erroneous. Field studies suggest that diarrheal disease in this age group is caused primarily by contact spread from heavily contaminated hands and an unsanitary environment (3). Moreover, weaning foods need not add significantly to this risk and can prevent the drop in resistance to infection that is associated with the malnutrition responsible for the weight faltering. The fact that nonenteric infections also increase when weight begins to falter argues against the withholding of weaning foods on the grounds of their possible contamination. However, bottles can represent a source of massive infection; they are quite unnecessary and should be entirely avoided as a vehicle for providing foods to complement breast milk.

In the latter part of the first year and during the second year of life, weaning foods must provide an increasing proportion of the child's nutrition. Even in the second year, however, a small amount of high-quality breast milk protein can contribute significantly to the nutrition of children receiving predominantly vegetable protein. The weaning period, which by definition begins when the first foods are given to supplement breast milk, ends when the child is no longer receiving breast milk and is consuming the regular family diet. During this period government interventions to help ensure the availability of suitable complementary foods are needed in most developing countries.

The period immediately subsequent to weaning, whether it occurs early in the first year or some time in the third, represents a period of special risk to the child. Without breast milk protein, the diet is often too low in calories relative to protein for recovery and catch-up growth following frequent infectious episodes, and the clinical protein deficiency syndrome of kwashiorkor develops, usually superimposed on some degree of marasmus owing to chronic undernutrition during and subsequent to the weaning period.

If breast-feeding during at least the first year is the norm, intervention programs will have their greatest value in the second and third years of life. If, as in Chile and some urban populations, breast-feeding terminates much earlier, intervention is required correspondingly earlier. To the extent that such intervention is unsuccessful in prolonging breast feeding, there may be no immediate alternative to concentrating on adequate substitutes for breast milk, be they home-prepared, commercial, or distributed by governments or nongovernmental agencies.

Accordingly, if supplementary feeding programs are to benefit the group at highest nutritional risk and need, they must somehow reach the child from 6 to 36 months of age; yet programs for the preschool child, for the most part, miss this target group and reach only the older preschool children who have survived the period of maximum nutritional hazard and who usually have attained normal weight for height, even though they are grossly retarded in weight and height for age.

Use of the Gomez classification of malnutrition, which is based on weight for age, is very useful for younger preschool children, but it has led to much misuse and misjudgment of supplementary feeding and nutritional rehabilitation programs involving older preschool children (4). Children 3 or 4 years of age may be classified as II degree (25–40% below standard weight) or even III degree (40% below standard weight) malnutrition when their weight for height is normal. In that case, attempts to improve weight for age by supplementary feeding can only lead to obesity.

The value of supplementary feeding is thus dubious for most older preschool children and even more so for school children. Study after study has shown that even children entering school 3 or 4 years retarded in weight for age nevertheless grow at rates paralleling those of well-nourished children, and that supplementary feeding of school children can seldom be shown to result in any objective signs of nutritional improvement (5). Other arguments are advanced for school feeding programs, particularly their educational value and beneficial effect on school attendance. In fact, they often utilize foods not available except in the school feeding program and rarely involve any significant educational component. It may be that they improve school attendance in some situations. Such benefits are often claimed, but are almost wholly undocumented. They may, however, function as a useful income supplement for poor families.

When mothers breast-feed for at least the first 6 months, as is still the case for the majority of mothers in most developing countries, the principal issues are: (1) the timing for the introduction of suitable weaning foods as growth begins to falter with exclusive breast-feeding; (2) the concern for an adequate diet in the period immediately following weaning; and (3) the limited nutritional value of any supplementary feeding once the period of maximum risk has passed, i.e., after the second year in most countries. If the mother terminates lactation before weaning foods can be appropriately introduced without the use of a bottle, whole different sets of problems are associated with substitutes for breast milk that are beyond the scope of the present topic.

It is sometimes argued that milk should not be given to populations known to lose lactase activity in childhood, a characteristic of most children in all of the developing countries. Without this intestinal enzyme, the principal sugar of milk, lactose, passes undigested into the large intestine where, if the quantities of milk are large, its bacterial fermentation causes gas and sometimes abdominal pain and diarrhea. Experience has shown, however, that in practice, even if intestinal lactase activity is low, school-age children have, or develop, sufficient tolerance to lactose that problems are not encountered with supplementary feeding programs utilizing moderate amounts of cow's milk (6). For younger preschool children, an age group that still has lactase activity almost undiminished, the problem does not arise.

NATURE OF WEANING FOODS

Weaning foods to complement breast milk can be divided into several categories:

Milks. In industrialized countries and among the affluent populations of developing countries, the most convenient and nutritious weaning foods are animal milks. Unfortunately, these are rarely available to the majority of the families in developing countries because supplies are limited and costly. Therefore, acceptable substitutes must be provided for these groups. It is possible to produce a vegetable milk with soy protein that has physical and nutritional properties similar to cow's milk, but the sophisticated processing and packaging required results in a product that is still too costly as a weaning food for the very poor.

Lower-Cost Mixtures. To help fill the role of milk in most industrialized countries, there is a need in every developing country for a weaning food that is based on locally available ingredients and that is as low in cost as possible. Fortunately, the combination of approximately two-thirds of any ground cereal and one-third of any well-processed oilseed meal will produce such a mixture, and both components are available in most developing countries. Although the proportions differ, legumes, such as chick peas (Bengal gram, garbanzos), mung beans (green gram), and pigeon peas, cow peas, and common beans *(Phaseolus vulgaris)*, can also be used effectively in combination with cereal or root staples.

Solid Foods. Many components in the family diet can be fed directly as weaning foods if broken into small pieces, mashed, or strained. Bread, tortillas, or chapaties are commonly given, depending on the culture. Eggs and bits of meat would be nutritionally better but are usually too costly. Legume dahls in India, refried beans in Mexico and Central America, and tempeh in Indonesia are good protein sources. Home-made multimixes can also be excellent as weaning foods and cheaper than those that are commercially processed.

Processed weaning foods that must be sold cannot benefit families that lack the necessary minimum purchasing power and therefore cannot be expected to solve the problem of malnourished preschool children in a country. It has become popular in some nutrition and development circles to criticize the processed weaning foods for this reason and to overlook their important positive aspects. These include:

Nutritional Value. It is possible to improve the protein–calorie quality and density of traditional cereal or root staples by the addition of legumes or oilseed meals at relatively low cost compared with products of animal origin of similar nutritional value.

Convenience. Time is a limiting factor in the efforts of overburdened, low-income mothers, many of whom are involved in food production or in earning money. In their struggle for the survival of their families, there is much evidence that they eagerly accept any labor-saving step that is economically feasible. The monetary cost appears justified to them, for example, in the machine grinding rather than hand grinding of corn for tortillas, in the machine milling of rice, or in the purchase of spaghetti. Given a true choice between home preparation of multimixes as weaning foods and the convenience of an already-mixed, processed weaning food, most low-income mothers would choose the latter. Even when they cannot afford to purchase processed foods they are unlikely to have the time and knowledge necessary for preparing comparable mixtures at home and instead use nutritionally inadequate traditional weaning foods.

Cost Advantage Compared with Foods of Animal Origin. Processed weaning foods will range in price from those that are precooked and packaged in relatively sophisticated ways to those that are simple powdered mixtures dispensed in bulk or in plastic bags. The latter can make available weaning foods to a significant segment of the population that is too poor to buy sufficient foods of animal origin for the purpose. The size and significance of the market for processed weaning foods will vary with local cost, purchasing power, and other circumstances.

Potential Savings to Governments and Private Agencies Conducting Feeding and Welfare Programs. For a government or private agency depending on their own resources in the purchase of food for hospitals, day-care centers, and the like, and for the relief of families unable to obtain sufficient food by either home production or purchase, relatively unsophisticated and low-cost mixtures, such as Bal Ahar in India or Incaparina in Guatemala, have important advantages compared with the purchase of milk for this purpose. The latter usually must be imported with scarce foreign exchange, fails to utilize locally available agricultural products, and introduces dietary habits that cannot be sustained without continued subsidy.

The issue has been distorted by the provision of dried skim milk (DSM) by a number of industrialized countries to developing countries at greatly subsidized costs or even without charge. Since the DSM was usually surplus that the industrialized countries were obligated to buy from farmers because of their own farm support legislation, and had to be disposed of in some fashion, neither the normal economic considerations nor the economic and agricultural impact on the recipient developing country entered significantly into consideration. However, these programs had political appeal in donor and recipient countries alike. When the United States began to run short of surplus DSM in the 1960s, the same mechanism was used to dispose of other agricultural products. Corn–soy milk (CSM), beginning in 1966, and later wheat–soy blend (WSB) were shipped in amounts totaling many millions of tons under PL 480 Title II. These huge shipments of foreign-produced processed weaning foods, both convenient and nutritious, have been a major factor in many countries inhibiting the success of similar indigenous developments. Why should a government spend its limited resources to purchase a locally produced weaning food for use in its institutions and welfare programs when it is offered, at no cost, a quantity that is more than it can use effectively?

Too often individuals promoting this massive distribution of weaning foods through foreign assistance channels have discounted local efforts for the production of similar products. In India, however, where the government produced and distributed Bal Ahar without charge, this mixture has played a major role in government feeding programs, and millions of tons have been distributed since 1966. In Guatemala, now that the government has begun to purchase Incaparina for use in some of its programs, the modern factory producing it is operating on a 24-hr basis and is unable to meet the demand.

Although all efforts to develop local processed weaning foods at relatively low cost have tended to be considered failures, and most such efforts have failed, there is nevertheless a steady demand from developing countries for technical assistance for the development of such foods. This is evident in the inquiries received from every region by The United Nations University World Hunger Programme requesting advanced training that will facilitate the local development of such weaning foods.

Fortunately, INCAP,* which pioneered the development of Incaparina and a family of other similar weaning mixtures, and CFTRI,† which developed Bal Ahar along comparable lines shortly afterwards, are associated institutions of The United Nations University World Hunger Programme for research and training in this area. They have long experience in the development of such products and have also done much research on suitable combinations of local staples for home-prepared mixtures.

Some nutritionists in industrialized countries have tended to emphasize only the *disadvantages* of processed weaning foods and only the *advantages* of home-prepared ones. Such a position does not take into sufficient account the constraints on lower-income mothers. Finding the extra time required to follow some of the directions for preparation of home weaning foods may simply be impossible for them. It is true that, without external assistance, the only way the diet of children of mothers with little or no additional purchasing power can be improved is through better use of foods already available for the family, but the difficulties should not be underestimated. Unfortunately, nutrition education programs have not proved effective in this regard. A program of periodic weighing, with weight charts kept by the mother, can provide the motivation and guidance for mothers to take advantage of local foods (7, Chapter 13, this volume) and is the best way to do so. The problem here is that major national efforts are required to organize such programs on a significant scale, and not many countries are either economically or logistically able to make such an effort, or are unwilling to make the political decision to do so, or both.

COMPLEMENTARY AND SUPPLEMENTARY FOODS FOR INFANTS AND YOUNG CHILDREN

The WHO/UNICEF Conference on Infant Feeding addressed the issue of how foods complementary to breast milk should be fed and agreed that for normally breast-fed infants the bottle should not be used. Weaning foods should be given by cup, spoon, or suitable traditional

*Institute of Nutrition of Central America and Panama, Guatemala City, Guatemala.
†Central Food Technological Research Institute, Mysore, India.

implement or utensil, or even clean fingers rather than risk the contamination of improperly sterilized bottles and bacterial growth in them.

The physical form of the weaning foods must obviously be adapted to the method of feeding. It is particularly important that complementary foods be offered after the infant has suckled and not before. If this practice is not followed, the quantity and duration of lactation may be adversely affected. If given after nursing, the child's appetite is a good indication of the amount of supplement needed, provided it is of suitable protein-energy density.

Five Interventions Involving Complementary or Supplementary Feeding

Nutrition Education in Extension

Nutrition education programs designed to improve infant and child-feeding practices among the low-income populations of developing countries have had only limited success when confined to such conventional techniques as lecture demonstrations, posters, and other forms of printed material. The use of mass media is not sufficient either. Most successful have been programs for the weighing of infants and young children at the community level, with weight records actually kept by the mother in the home. In this manner, the mother is able to see when the growth of her child begins to drop below normal, she can compare her child's performance with that of other children in the community, and she can come to recognize when the postweaning diet of the child is inadequate. In those cases where the family is simply too poor to obtain the food, some means of providing it is essential, whether through local community initiative or government initiative. In general, these programs have functioned thus far mainly on a pilot scale, but efforts to extend them on a nationwide basis are only beginning. Some success in this regard is being registered by the nutrition programs in Java and the Philippines (Chapters 13 and 16, this volume).

Provision of Weaning Foods without Cost to Mothers

Although these programs have been widely popular and heavily supported by international, bilateral, and voluntary agencies, they are of questionable value for the specific purpose of preventing malnutrition in infancy once breast milk is no longer sufficient as the sole source of food. The programs may reach a certain proportion of older preschool children who are having nutritional problems in the postweaning period, but they rarely affect a significant number of children during the critical weaning period. Efforts to ensure that the target children receive the intended food by having them brought daily to a central point for supervised feeding is wholly impractical for countries where the ordinary health delivery system reaches only a small proportion of the target population, where mothers are simply too busy to bring their children regularly to such a center, and where the costs of extending such a program on a national scale are prohibitive.

The alternative of providing mothers with food weekly, biweekly, or monthly to take home for their weanling child may benefit the family without having any significant effect on the target child. This is because the food is generally shared among other siblings or with the entire family and withdrawn from the child for whom it was intended when diarrhea or other illness occurs, which happens with relatively high frequency. However, where weighing programs can be instituted, or where mothers bring undernourished children to clinics or day care centers, then free or subsidized distribution of acceptable nutritious foods suitable for the weaning period can help the specific families involved. Whether the food available is an externally donated powdered skim milk, a processed mixture, such as CSM or WSB, a locally purchased milk, or a locally processed, predominantly vegetable mixture may be of economic and political importance to the country, but irrelevant to the improved nutrition of the child.

SCHOOL FEEDING

The practical way of disposing of large quantities of donated food, or of introducing politically attractive feeding programs, is through the schools. As indicated earlier, there is little evidence that this is a measure of importance for either the nutritional status of the child or nutrition education. Whether school feeding contributes to school attendance and to the concentration of children who come to school is uncertain, but it is considered by economists to be an effective way of targeting income redistribution efforts, and is generally popular with parents and school teachers. For these reasons, strict cost-benefit considerations seldom influence decisions regarding school feeding programs.

MATERNAL FEEDING

There is no doubt that cycles of pregnancy and lactation deplete the low-income mother nutritionally and result in a high proportion of low-birth-weight babies and in quantities of breast milk considerably below those of well nourished mothers in more privileged circumstances. Low-birth-weight babies show poorer growth and higher morbidity and mortality during the first year of life, and the combination of low nutrient reserves at birth and reduced quantity of breast milk means a need to introduce complementary feeding at an earlier age. This, in turn, adds to the risk of infection with enteric organisms and increases the likelihood of malnutrition beginning relatively early in the first year. Presumably, this adverse sequence of events could be prevented by improving the nutritional status of the mother.

Clearly, much more attention needs to be given to programs to do so, especially during pregnancy and lactation, and for low-income mothers, some kind of subsidized food supplementation may well be necessary. How this can be achieved without the food's being so distributed among the family members as to be ineffective for the intended purpose is not clear. To place unacceptable demands on the time of the mother to come regularly to a central distribution point is impractical.

SUPPLEMENTARY FEEDING PROGRAMS FOR WORKERS

A large proportion of low-income adults in developing countries are consuming diets providing considerably fewer calories than FAO/WHO estimated for average requirements. To survive on these diets, they must restrict their total physical activity. Work capacity is reduced, and unnecessary nonwork physical activity is almost eliminated for many populations. Under these circumstances, any measures that will increase the food available for consumption will result in a higher level of physical activity. Employers may well find it worthwhile to provide such supplementary food to their workers in some form, because an increase in work capacity is likely if there is need and incentive for it.

SUMMARY

While feeding programs may appear to be a simple direct way of correcting the malnutrition of such vulnerable target groups as infants, preschool children, and pregnant and nursing mothers, there are serious logistic, economic, and cultural obstacles to their effectiveness on a national scale. School feeding programs are easier to implement, are politically popular, and may be economically feasible with the assistance of donated foods through bilateral or international assistance, but they are of limited benefit because this is not the population group for whom malnutrition is a widespread or significant problem. Supplementary feeding of undernourished workers will increase their level of physical activity and potential work output.

Every developing country should have available relatively low-cost, processed weaning foods utilizing locally produced components of vegetable (or predominantly vegetable) origin that can be purchased by a spectrum of the population able to buy some processed foods, but not otherwise able to afford sufficient foods of animal origin for weaning purposes. Such foods also represent a more economical and rational way of providing food for hospitals, day care centers, and other institutions, and a way of providing for supplementary feeding programs that purchase milk products, especially if they must be imported.

REFERENCES

1. Scrimshaw, N. S., and B. A. Underwood. Timely and appropriate complementary feeding of the breast-fed infant—an overview. In: *Food and Nutrition Bulletin*, Vol. 2, No. 2, pp. 19–22. The United Nations University World Hunger Programme, April 1980.
2. Whitehead, R. G. The infant food industry. *Lancet* ii:1192–1194, 1976.
3. Bruch, H. A., W. Ascoli, N. S. Scrimshaw, and J. E. Gordon. Studies of diarrheal disease in Central America. V. Environmental factors in the origin and transmission of acute diarrheal disease in four Guatemalan villages. *Am. J. Trop. Med. Hyg.* 12 (4):567–569, 1963.
4. Beaton, G. H., and J. M. Bengoa (Eds.). *Nutrition in Preventive Medicine*, World Health Organization Monograph Series No. 62. WHO, Geneva, 1976.
5. Beaton, G. H., and H. Ghassemi. Supplementary feeding and nutrition of the young child. *Am. J. Clin. Nutr.*, 35 (4) Supplement, April, 1982.
6. Protein Advisory Group (PAG). A statement on low lactase activity and milk intake, No. 17. In: *PAG Compendium, Worldmark International Documentation*, Vol. E-1, p. 349. John Wiley, New York, 1975.
7. Rohde, J. E., D. Ismail, and R. Sutrisno. Mothers as weight watchers: The road to child health in the village. *Environ. Child Hlth.* 21:295–297, 1975.

Comment

ALBERTO CARVALHO DA SILVA

Where sanitary conditions are very precarious and the prevalence of infectious disease is high, I wonder whether supplementing breast-feeding infants before the age of 6 months is as important as compensating for higher risks of infection. Two examples illustrate the reasons for my concern:

1. In a rural area of the State of São Paulo, Brazil, a maternal–child health program sponsored by a medical school has succeeded in extending breast-feeding to the age of 6 months in several cases, with good child development and a low prevalence of infection. But when these children were weaned at 6 months of age, the incidence of infection and malnutrition rose markedly.
2. In a poor section of the city of Salvador, Bahia, a group of 500 children were followed from birth to the age of 6 months, weaning being almost complete by the third month. Morbidity was so high that, on average, each child spent 28% of its first 6 months of life with infection (8% respiratory and 20% gastrointestinal); 80 children died during the 6-month period, most of them in the first months.

These two examples clearly illustrate situations in which risk of infection was so high that it might have been safer to postpone risk of contamination, since with breast-feeding, it was possible for infants to reach the age of 6 months with normal nutrition and without exposure to infection.

Should food supplementation prove necessary, then the best way to do it may be through the mother during pregnancy. A recent evaluation

ALBERTO CARVALHO DA SILVA • Programa Multidisciplinar de Nutrigao, The Ford Foundation, Rio de Janeiro, Brazil.

of the PRONAN program in Bahia has indicated better child growth when the mother received food supplements while pregnant than when they were given to the child after birth.

School lunch programs should be evaluated as delivery systems for food supplementation and social stimulation for preschool children. In some schools dropout rates are as high as 50% in the first grade-school year; correcting this low school performance may be viewed as the first priority for nutrition policy in a developing country. Should school lunch programs prove to be effective in reversing this trend, they should be maintained, ultimately considering the preschool component as the main target and the grade-school age component as a marginal effort.

Food Aid for Supplementary Feeding
A Case Study from Egypt

STEPHEN R. ALLEN AND ANDREW J. KOVAL

INTRODUCTION

This chapter details the experience of one voluntary agency in handling a moderately large supplementary feeding program for preschool children in Egypt, using foods supplied by the U.S. Government under the PL 480 plan.

A nationwide feeding project such as the one about to be described poses conflicts, not so much between the donor and the recipient ministry, as between the central planner in government and the health care personnel at grass-roots level. The ministry goal of 700,000 recipients in a preschool age population of 5.6 million is laudable enough, but the distribution rush for the physicians or their assistants may be overwhelming and appear to be an infringement on more pressing problems. The central planner is anxious to increase the coverage to more than 12% of the eligible population and to have greater precision in the allocation of resources, but the physician at the health unit is already burdened by the logistics of distributing this quantity of food with some sense of dignity if not purpose. If told that the target population must be increased five-fold, the physician must of necessity be resigned to forsaking the practice of medicine for the role of a glorified inventory clerk.

We have chosen to focus our attention on a few key problem areas in the practical administration of such a large program. If supplementary

STEPHEN R. ALLEN AND ANDREW J. KOVAL • Catholic Relief Services, Cairo, Egypt. The views expressed in this paper are those of the authors alone.

feeding programs have a role to play in the future, some attention must be given to these difficulties, and if we were to select just one recommendation, it would be the repackaging of blended foods into convenient sized packages. This would facilitate a dignified and hygienic distribution procedure and enhance the value of the weaning food in the eyes of the mother.

THE STATE OF HEALTH AND NUTRITION IN EGYPT

Egypt is a large but mainly arid country with a population that is estimated at 40 million. Although the population growth rate (2.6%) and the gross national product per capita (GNP U.S. $320) (1) do not put Egypt among the poorest of the developing countries, the Food and Agricultural Organization of the United Nations (FAO) has classified Egypt as a most seriously affected developing market economy because of the quantity of food it must import to feed the population and the size of the balance of payments deficit.

The Physical Quality of Life Index (PQLI) developed by Morris David Morris and modified for the Egyptian Governorates by John Field (2) shows that this country is in the bottom one-third of nations when ranked internationally but its performance in promoting popular well-being is quite creditable, especially when comparison is made with some of its oil-rich neighbors (Table 1). The PQLI scales infant mortality, life expectancy at the age of one year, and the literacy rate on an index of 0–100, and, although there are serious doubts about the reliability of official estimates of the infant mortality rate, measures that focus on the

TABLE 1. Egypt and Six Other Countries with PQLI
Scores Close to 43 Compared in Terms of Per Capita
Income[a]

Country	PQLI	Average per capita income (U.S.)
United Arab Emirates	34	14,368
Libya	45	4,402
Iraq	45	999
Iran	43	1,260
Bolivia	43	332
Egypt	43	245
India	43	133

[a] Data presented from Reference 2.

TABLE 2. Main Causes of Infant Mortality According to Season[a,b]

Season	Diarrhea and gastroenteritis	Congenital abnormality	Respiratory problems	Others	Total
January–April	8.9	3.6	3.5	2.4	18.4
May–June	24.9	9.9	9.4	6.7	50.9
September–December	14.8	5.9	5.6	3.9	30.2

[a] Data presented from Reference 4.
[b] Percentages expressed as percent of total deaths.

social impact of overall development could be useful to food program planners if the index can be shown to predict the magnitude of nutritional need in various areas of the country.

When the Catholic Relief Services (CRS) supplementary feeding program was begun in 1975 there were no reliable data on which to base a judgment about the type, quantity, and location of Title II food assistance. The FAO food balance sheet that indicated the average per capita calorie intake was 2634 kcal not only gave Egypt a head start over most of its neighbors with respect to food availability, but also led to speculation about how a country with an overall surfeit of food and with such an apparently low level of frank malnutrition could have an officially quoted infant mortality rate of 106 per thousand and a second-year mortality rate of 50 per thousand live births. The controversy is still unresolved and further data have added more confusion.

There is evidence accumulating from the rural health delivery project[*] that the true infant mortality rate is well in excess of 106, yet the recent national nutrition survey (3) suggests that only 2.3% of Egyptian preschool children are suffering from undernutrition, defined as less than 85% of reference median weight for height. However, when the data from the national nutrition survey are classified according to Gomez, 0.8% of the sample was suffering from third degree malnutrition and a further 8% of the sample had second degree malnutrition, a much less comforting picture. Moreover, the nutrition survey was conducted in the winter, when it is widely felt that disease transmission is reduced and when the synergistic effects of disease and undernutrition are moderated. Table 2 presents the results of one investigation into the cause of death in infancy by season (4).

There has been speculation about the validity of the results of the national nutrition survey, mainly because they contradict all previous work undertaken to measure the extent of malnutrition in Egypt. Among

[*] Strengthening Rural Health Delivery Project (SRHD), funded by USAID, Egypt.

the questions raised is the biological significance of the type of classification of undernutrition employed by the U.S. Center for Disease Control (CDC). Although differentiating between the acute and chronic processes in the way that the CDC recommends has certain advantages, particularly when one wishes to distinguish the tall, thin child from the small, well-proportioned child, it seems likely that most children in Egypt suffer from acute malnutrition superimposed on chronic malnutrition, or from the latter alone. There has also been doubt expressed about the sensitivity of the sampling method for revealing the full extent of the problem of acute malnutrition, but the answers to these questions may be forthcoming if the CDC has an opportunity to repeat the survey during the summer months.

So we are left with a dilemma. On the one hand, we have an accumulation of work that is methodologically unsound, but, on the other hand, the nutrition survey has produced results that strain credibility, given what is already documented and, especially, given the alarmingly high infant and young child mortality rate in the country. It seems that there is a good deal of underreporting of deaths in infants, and true infant mortality rates in the country as a whole may exceed 150 per thousand live births. How much malnutrition one might expect in a country where the mortality rate in the second year of life is 70 per thousand is not clear; although the methodology, sampling, and coverage of the National Nutrition Survey was more scientifically thorough than other studies were, it would probably be premature to reject the other work and accept uncritically the fairly positive findings of the survey.

THE ORIGINS OF A CRS FOOD PROGRAM

When CRS was invited by the government of Egypt to expand the PL 480 Maternal Child Health (MCH) program from a pilot scheme in one governorate to a nationwide program, the data, surveys, and studies about the nutritional status of the preschool population were sparse, outdated, and often contradictory. While they showed a very high infant mortality rate, they also recorded disturbingly high rates of mild to moderate protein–calorie malnutrition. (A UNICEF assessment classified over 55% of the child population in this category, while a Nutrition Institute study, published in 1967, reported that 70% of the children were less than 90% of the Harvard reference standard at the end of the second year.) Instances of severe malnutrition were, however, found to be as low as in the most recent findings. It was on the basis of these data that CRS and the Ministry of Health sat down to decide jointly on a year-by-year

TABLE 3. Distribution by Commodity in Each Program Year[a,b]

Commodity	1975	1976	1977	1978	1979	1980
Bulgur	3,474	3,474	6,434	8,002	9,568	11,137
Wheat–soy blend	3,960	7,641	9,436	11,760	14,064	16,368
Vegetable oil	2,398	1,737	2,145	2,667	3,160	3,712
Wheat flour	7,920	1,737	—	—	—	—

[a] Data presented from Catholic Relief Services, Ministry of Health Program Statistics, Egypt, 1979 (unpublished).
[b] Units are metric tons.

target for a program of providing supplementary food (Table 3). Of course, considerations about the cost and availability of storage space and transportation facilities imposed severe constraints on the targets set.

It is frequently difficult to decide on a suitable strategy for the distribution of large quantities of supplementary food. If on-site preparation of food is impossible, the problem is likely to be greater; but in Egypt the Ministry of Health has an extensive health care delivery system based upon some 2100 rural health units (each staffed with at least one physician), and close to 300 MCH centers in the urban areas that are logical sites for food distribution. The level of health care in the country is not what one might expect of such an extensive infrastructure, and probably the single biggest problem—although the identification of the root causes of this problem has not been undertaken—is the underutilization of the Health Service and the failure of the service to reach out to a significant proportion of the population for whom it exists.

Also, although the difficulty is of lesser importance, the rapid growth of population has left centers, especially in the urban areas, with the impossible task of trying to provide health care for many more people than originally intended. In Cairo, there are 38 MCH centers for a population that is conservatively estimated to be 8 million. The opportunities for the staff of these centers to impact positively on the health status of more than a handful of the 100,000 mothers and preschool children they serve are clearly limited.

Nor is the situation too different in the rural areas where the unit/population ratio may be more favorable and often as low as one unit per 5000 persons. One study in Kalubeya showed that more than 90% of mothers never consulted the health service either in the pre- or postnatal period despite the fact that the service is available at no cost and within easy travelling distance. The traditional midwife (daya), who has no official status in the country, is present at almost all deliveries. The attitude of the health ministry to the daya has varied considerably in recent times, but currently she is seen as an unwelcome and unsanitary birth attendant.

Despite its inefficiencies, the delivery system of the Ministry of Health seemed the logical route for channeling supplies of supplementary food as well as offering an opportunity for passing on nutrition information to mothers. The advantages and disadvantages of this will be examined later in this paper.

The provision of food aid to combat undernutrition in Egypt has also to be seen in the context of the extensive food subsidy system that has operated in this country for more than 20 years. The price of "baladi" bread has remained unaltered for almost 40 years, and it is possible for an adult Egyptian to meet his daily calorie requirement at an expenditure of 7 U.S. cents. The official minimum wage in the country is approximately U.S. $25/month, and it is fortunate that food can be purchased so cheaply when it has been calculated that U.S. $250 is needed as a minimal annual sum to provide a least-cost diet if the purchaser chooses food according to seasonal availability and optimizes the nutrients from each unit weight of food (5).

The situation with respect to food prices and subsidies appears extremely unstable. Uncontrolled food prices have escalated rapidly in recent years (1958–1959, 100; 1974–1975, 269*), and the cost to the government of maintaining the prices of basic foodstuffs (such as flour, sugar, oil, and tea) at a level that can be afforded by the bulk of the population has increasingly strained the already overburdened economy. The cost of the subsidy system has risen from LE 9M in 1960 to LE 622M in 1975, and to LE 650 M in 1978. A heavily constrained agricultural sector, defense budgets, and spiraling world food prices of cereal grains have all added to the difficulty; but the importance of stable food prices can be assessed on the basis of the public reaction following a government suggestion to partially decontrol food prices in 1977. The decision was reversed within the week following the so-called food riots, and the International Monetary Fund no longer seems so anxious to press Egypt to relieve itself of this balance of payments burden as a prerequisite to further loans.

The income-saving effect of food aid can be significant for poor families, but in general, with food prices at such a low level, many items provided free of charge for nutritional purposes are not considered valuable. One indirect beneficial effect of a cheap food price policy in a country is that people are less inclined to cash in the food in the mar-

---

*This indicates one problem for the analyst of the Egyptian scene. Aside from the unreliability of the data, these figures are considerably out of date.

ketplace. This cheap food price policy does have other less desirable consequences; it has probably resulted in reduction in domestic food production and, consequently, the costs to the Egyptian economy of importing food are now enormous. In 1979, it was anticipated that more than four million tons of wheat alone would be imported. This is more than 80% of the total domestic requirement and makes Egypt the largest food grain importer outside the Communist bloc countries.

THE ORIGINAL FIVE-YEAR PLAN

USAID planning requires a voluntary agency to submit a five-year projection of requirements for individual commodities as well as an annual estimate of requirements for the projected target group in each program category. Accordingly, the Ministry of Health worked out a 1975 base-year figure of 220,000 recipients and a projected annual increase of 100,000 until achieving its goal of over 700,000 in 1980 (Table 4). The MCH's plan was initially premised on the basis of one-third of the target group being pregnant or lactating mothers and two-thirds children under 6 years of age. Field observations during the first two years confirmed that, in actual practice, over three-quarters of the recipients were pregnant and lactating mothers. In 1977, the MCH and CRS narrowed the focus to children 6 months to 3 years of age. At no point was

TABLE 4. Number of Recipients by Year of Program Operation plus Estimated Cost of Operation According to the Ministry of Health's Project Plan[a]

Calendar year	Number of recipients	Value of program[b] (U.S. $)
1975	228,039	8,900,000
1976	321,814	8,450,000
1977	417,814	10,650,000
1978	513,814	12,700,000
1979	609,814	14,800,000
1980	705,814	17,000,000

[a] Data presented from Catholic Relief Services, Ministry of Health Program Statistics, Egypt, 1979 (unpublished).
[b] This sum is calculated as the value of the food, plus the cost of shipping to Egypt, together with the Egyptian Government's contribution to storage and inland transportation. Figures are recalculated to 1979 values.

the projected target group linked to any estimate of children suffering from malnutrition. However, it has always been emphasized that food and education should be directed to those children who, in the opinion of the physician at the health unit, are suffering from undernutrition and hence, those for whom food aid will be a positive benefit. Furthermore, we strongly recommend that, once a child has been identified as undernourished, he be given food for a minimum of one year. The roots of malnutrition may well be in early childhood, and the disease may gradually develop from an initial faltering of growth to a clinically recognizable disease state, and the treatment of the problem may require considerable time.

The goals of the CRS project were as follows:

1. To improve nutritional status, especially of the vulnerable groups 6–36 months old, through supplemental feeding, especially of high-protein blended foods.
2. To provide the "at-risk" children with a more balanced diet and to improve eating habits through nutrition education for mothers of vulnerable children.
3. To improve weaning practices, especially the introduction of an appropriate supplement at an early age, through awareness and training sessions with mothers.
4. To stimulate the formulation of a national food and nutrition policy.
5. To stimulate the National Nutrition Institute of the Ministry of Health to play a more dynamic and fruitful role in the improvement of the nutritional status of the population.
6. To increase the amount of in-service training, especially in nutrition education of personnel working in health centers.

The Evaluation of the Program

One of the most significant weaknesses of any program of this size is the failure to evaluate properly the impact of the assistance, hence the difficulty in making recommendations for the alteration and revision of a program that would bring about a more efficient use of scant resources. There are fundamental problems associated with measuring the impact of supplementary feeding programs. The outcomes are generally long run and thus difficult to measure because of the intervening time lag. The longer the time between the intervention and the measurement of its outcome, the harder it is to link the program to the hypothetical impact. In the interim period other environmental, behavioral, or natural changes may take place to affect the outcome.

Notwithstanding the problems, our evaluations have tended to be scanty in coverage, biased, and conducted on an ad hoc basis. No good baseline data exist on the children who enter the program, so it is not possible to unravel the effects of the supplementary feeding from a multitude of other changes that have taken place in these last 5 years.

The most important and fruitful efforts to collect information on the impact of the supplementary feeding program were through a research project conducted by the International Islamic Centre for Population Studies and Research of the University of Al Azhar, under the guidance of Professor M. R. Barakat (7). The most severe limitation of this approach is the applicability of an in-depth study (the research project has many more components than the impact of supplementary feeding) to the wider context. There is almost certainly some observer bias, particularly in terms of the usage and acceptability of blended foodstuffs. Our experience in other situations has indicated that wheat–soy blend (WSB) has serious acceptability problems even when time and effort are given to nutrition education sessions to demonstrate the usefulness of a bland food mixture.

Table 5 summarizes the nutritional status of children in the most vulnerable age group (6–36 months) in the study villages. For the purposes of the study, all the families in the area are classified as recipients.

TABLE 5. Percentage of Children in Each Weight for Age Category[a,b]

Age (in months)	Weight as a percentage of reference					
	60	60–70	70–80	80–90	90–100	100
3–5	1.0	0.5	1.5	3.0	3.0	1.0
6–8	0.5	1.5	2.0	3.0	6.0	2.5
9–11	—	0.5	2.0	2.5	5.0	4.0
12–17	1.0	2.0	8.0	7.5	2.5	4.0
18–23	—	0.5	0.5	3.0	3.0	3.0
24–35	1.0	1.0	6.0	6.0	8.0	4.0
Total	3.5	6.0	20.0	25.0	27.5	18.5

Number of children with third-degree malnutrition = 14 (3.5%)
Number of children with second-degree malnutrition = 51 (16%)

[a] Weight for age is expressed as a percentage of the Ministry of Health and Center for Disease Control reference population.
[b] N is 510.

Our goal in this project has been to ensure that each recipient family receives food at regular intervals together with appropriate nutrition education for the preparation of preweaning foods, and an appreciation of the need for hygienic precautions in the preparation of such foods. It is too early to state whether or not the project has had a positive impact on the nutritional status of the preschool child population. Preliminary indications suggest that this has been the case, but it is difficult to isolate the feeding program as the sole contributory factor. Communications in the area have improved vastly in the past year, and the socioeconomic circumstances of a good proportion of our participating sample has been altered. We have also made major efforts to improve nutrition awareness in the area with an outreach program, and it is, therefore, likely that our final analysis will present an equivocal opinion about the impact of the food alone.

When we look at the operation of the program at the national level, the picture is much less encouraging. The distribution of more than 30,000 metric tons of food per year inevitably brings with it difficulties associated with central storage and distribution to the periphery. At the health unit, most physicians claim that having an overall responsibility for food aid interferes with their main work as medical practitioners. It is acknowledged that a poor understanding of the nutritional needs of children being weaned, resulting in inadequate quantities of the wrong type of food being given at a later age, is an underlying factor in most of the diseases that they encounter in the clinic. They further claim that the usefulness of food supplements is undermined by packaging in 25-kg bags. These bags are more convenient for the shipper and for inland transportation, and the cost of repackaging in-country is thought to be prohibitively high. In our judgment, serious attention should be given to this problem and the possibility examined of packaging in small (e.g., 2-kg) containers in the United States.

Blended high-protein weaning foods are expensive commodities (average cost U.S. $310/ton, plus an average of U.S. $80/ton transportation) (Table 6), and the additional costs of packaging may be recouped by better utilization of the food. Repackaging would improve the convenience of the food, the image to the mother and the family, and perhaps result in a greater utilization at the time when these foods can probably be of greatest value—from 4 months through to completion of weaning.

With the problem of distribution taken away from them, the physicians could take more time to discuss the health of the child and explain the use of a preweaning food for infant feeding. This activity could complement present efforts to introduce nonformal nutrition education as a

TABLE 6. The Quantities and Value of PL 480 Food
Commodities Shipped to Egypt Since 1954[a]

Category	Quantity ($\times 10^3$ pounds)	Value ($\times 10^3$ U.S. $)
Voluntary agencies	1,850,362	182,114
Bilateral agreements[b]	409,864	20,748
World Food Programme	114,120	10,898
Total	2,374,346	213,760

[a] Data presented from Reference 6.
[b] Bilateral agreements for the supply of food commodities under Title II of PL 480 are no longer in existence. The significance of these amounts can be seen when compared to the total quantity of PL 480 commodities shipped to Egypt under Title II (i.e., grant) through voluntary agencies, bilateral agreements, and the World Food Programme.

part of the activity of the health unit (CRS and the Ministry of Health have a grant for such a project that foresees the introduction of nutrition education as part of the work of 150 health centers). The early introduction of an appropriate food to the diet of an infant is often viewed skeptically because it is imagined that this will lead to a decline in breast-feeding. We believe this problem has been inadequately studied, and group educational techniques that advocate nutritional supplements but otherwise do not have a detrimental effect on breast-feeding are improperly understood.

The idea of a bland food supplement that can be adapted to local dishes has had little general success in Egypt. The skill and imagination needed to incorporate WSB into recipes is considerable, and may, in any case, be counterproductive by encouraging consumption by the whole family. Our predominant problem is that for long periods in infancy there is little or no food to complement breast milk.

As an infant pap, WSB has been quite well accepted because it is precooked and easily digested. From a nutritional standpoint WSB is very adequate, although it is difficult to feed a child sufficient quantities of WBS alone to satisfy energy needs. It also appears that iron, though present in sufficient quantities (208 mg/100 g) and in an absorbable form, is nevertheless not absorbed by the body (Dr. James Cook, personal communication).

The integration of WSB into a local foodstuff requires considerable skill and patience, and it is doubtful whether people are prepared to invest this time when their appreciation of the intrinsic nutritional value, despite education efforts, may be low. In an effort to combat this, our own program stresses the benefits of WSB for the young infant (upward from 4 months) and the ease of preparation when it is simply mixed with water.

We should now like to reexamine the original goals of our project with the benefit of our five years of experience:

1. *Improvement of the nutritional status of the vulnerable groups.* It is not possible to assess this priority goal with certainty for the entire target group. There is some evidence to suggest that supplemental feeding of vulnerable preschool children under careful conditions can be beneficial. This requires careful follow-up by the health team, continuous education, and enrollment in the program for at least one year. To what extent food alone is a positive contributing factor is not possible to elucidate. It may well be that the investment in education for the preparation of preweaning foods at home would be of equal benefit. This absolutely critical question has remained unanswered in all but a handful of studies of rather limited scale, and a careful, prolonged analysis is overdue. Some clarification is needed in our program of the potential nutritional pay-offs we are likely to obtain if we direct food aid to pregnant women.

2. and 3. *Improvement of weaning habits through education.* A nutrition-education program has been begun recently by the Ministry of Health in cooperation with CRS. More effort and money could, and should, be spent in this direction and nutrition should become an integral part of medical education. Without some substantial improvements in the method for identifying, monitoring, and distributing the food to the target group, nutrition efforts, in their present format, are likely to meet with limited success.

4. *A national food and nutrition policy.* This has not been implemented. In 1978, the then Minister of Health convened an *ad hoc* nutrition committee, but to date no policy paper has emerged. The situation is little changed from the time of the U.S. National Academy of Sciences Institute of Medicine report (8). A recently held nutrition workshop recommended that this committee be charged with identifying and setting in motion projects that will positively impact on Egyptian mothers and preschool children, although it is too early to see how this will be put into operation. Even such economically important interventions as the bread subsidy have never been analyzed for nutritional benefits.

5. and 6. *The role of the nutrition institute and increased in-service train-*

ing. In part, at least, this has improved. Largely as a result of the National Nutrition Survey, for which the Institute received much praise (and rightly so), the atmosphere in the Institute seems improved. The CRS-supported nutrition education project is going ahead with their assistance at the training course stage and this, too, will have beneficial consequences. It is less certain that the Institute is the body that should be assigned the task of planning and executing nutrition interventions, although they would be expected to play a role in this.

THE NEED FOR A PREWEANING FOOD IN EGYPT

No issue of human nutrition has aroused more controversy and misunderstanding than the relative importance of protein and energy deficits in the causation of malnutrition. Because of the need to provide protein for growth, the requirements of young children, when related to body weight, are higher than for adults and, although there appears to be less controversy about the protein needs of small infants, uncertainty still exists about the recommendations made by FAO/WHO in 1973 (9) for older children and adults. During the course of the 1970s, the emphasis on the importance of protein deficiencies was dropped and nutrition planning was frequently formulated with the aim of meeting calorie needs, whereupon it was assumed that protein needs would, in the great majority of country situations, be satisfied. Inevitably, projects that aimed to provide supplementary foodstuffs came in for criticism, although the basis of this criticism was not always the high-protein content of the food blend (10).

There is now an increasing and impressive body of evidence to suggest that the concern with the satisfaction of calorie needs to the exclusion of examining protein requirements was inappropriate, and the effects of this evidence should eventually lead to a modification in nutrition policy. The consequences of such changes of heart are confusing, especially for the nonspecialist policy maker who, it seems, must now rethink his long-range food planning. It is especially difficult in developing countries where specialists and nonspecialists alike may have made considerable efforts to secure funds for tackling the protein problem only to be told that they could have achieved the same result with a totally different approach. Fortunately, it is now possible to examine critically the need for high-protein preweaning foods without facing a barrage of critics claiming the question to be irrelevant.

It is quite possible that young infants in the developing world require a specially manufactured supplementary food in addition to breast milk, although efforts to introduce such a food should not counteract existing traditions for prolonged breast-feeding, but rather should be supportive of this. There is evidence to suggest that the malnutrition that may be seen in most severe form beyond 12 months of age may come about following growth retardation beginning as early as the third month (11). We know from our data in Egypt that growth begins to falter around the sixth month of life, although, unfortunately, the most comprehensive survey of child growth in this country excluded children under 6 months of age from the sample.

Dietary insufficiency, however caused, is almost always an important reason for growth impairment, and if this is beginning so early in life, then we have a responsibility to investigate the need for appropriate (in terms of price, acceptability, and nutritional composition) preweaning foods. We know practically nothing about the present use of traditional preweaning foods in Egypt, and especially lacking are the quantitative data that would enable us to estimate dietary deficiency in the first few months of life. This information is an essential prerequisite for those who will be involved in trying to provide such foods.

More data are available about the growth of young children, and these have been examined elsewhere in this paper. The deficit in height for age reaches a peak in the 12- to 35-month age, and while there is a high percentage (10.2% of the sample with a height for age less than 89.9% of the reference median) of children with a height deficit in the 6- to 12-month age group, there were no data collected on children under this age. From this we conclude that children from 1 to 3 years of age are at greatest risk, and they form the target group for our supplementary feeding program.

The experience with Superamine (a UN-supported, locally produced, nutritious preweaning food) has not been encouraging for those who would suggest that local production should make up the gap in the need for supplementary food. The quantity of Superamine manufactured has always been small and has never come close to the latest targets of 1000 metric tons/year. Difficulties have been encountered with formulation, but most seriously, the blend has been a complete commercial failure, resulting in the elimination of a scheme to fund distribution through profits obtained from sales. This is discouraging, but the time (and money) invested in the scheme has been relatively short, and experience with other foods of this kind indicate that it takes several years before a successful product with a suitable image in the marketplace can be manufactured. More work is needed on the factors that impede the development of local weaning foods; especially lacking are the vigorous marketing skills that give commercial brands such heavy sales despite price barriers.

Using the nutrition survey estimate of 10% of preschool children with either second or third degree malnutrition, then at least 30,000 metric tons of food supplement would be required annually. This production capability does not now exist in Egypt, and it is unlikely that a major donor would be in a position to make this kind of investment unless it could be convincingly demonstrated that the percentage of children who are in greatest need could be identified and appropriately followed. It seems, however, that this requirement will not be met by the Ministry of Health. Furthermore, such a program takes no account of the prevention of malnutrition in the sizeable proportion of the population who are at risk, although not in the second or third degree category. Hence, the preventive side of the program is limited to those children who are already undernourished.

CONCLUSIONS

Supplementary feeding programs are difficult to design, organize, and evaluate, especially when conducted on a national scale. The identification of children "at-risk" and follow-up to ensure improvement in health status is a prerequisite, yet all too difficult to find in the health services of many developing countries.

There are problems with specially formulated preweaning foods that interrupt the smooth running of a feeding program. It is strongly recommended that careful thought be given to the repackaging of weaning foods, both to facilitate the work of the health staff and to improve the image of the preweaning food. Distributions to the mothers of children at risk should be frequent to avoid long periods when the supplement is not available for the child, and mothers should be integrated into a program of basic health education. The systematic weighing of all children in heavily utilized health centers is probably beyond the capacity of the staff, although if it can be organized and the information is used by the staff, it is invaluable.

There is an urgent need for a careful, systematic evaluation of a large-scale country program to assess the benefits of providing supplementary foods, and to indicate where improvements can be made in program operation.

REFERENCES

1. Food and Agriculture Organization. Food Balance Sheets, 1972/1974, FAO, Rome, 1976.
2. Field, J. O. and G. Ropes. Development in the Egyptian Governorates. *L'Egypte Contemporaine*, May, 1979.
3. Egypt National Nutrition Status Survey. Nutrition Institute, Cairo, and the Center for Disease Control, Atlanta, Georgia, April, 1979.
4. Gabr, M. Malnutrition and diarrheal disease. In: *Practical Approaches to Combat Malnutrition with Special Reference to Mothers and Children* (Proceedings of an IUNS Conference, Cairo, Egypt, May 25–29, 1977), N. Scrimshaw and M. Gabr (Eds.). Arab World Printing House, Cairo, Egypt, 1979.
5. Central Agency for Public Mobilisation and Statistics. Family Budget Survey, 1974/1975, Cairo, 1977.
6. Food for Peace. *1977 Annual Report on Public Law 480*, Agency for International Development, Washington, D.C., 1979.
7. Allen, S. R. Report of Joint Activities and Recommendations for Future Work. CRS and University of Al-Azhar, April, 1979.
8. Institute of Medicine, National Academy of Sciences. Health in Egypt: Recommendations for U.S. Assistance. NAS, Washington, D.C., 1979.
9. *Energy and Protein Requirements*, Report of a joint FAO/WHO ad hoc expert committee, WHO Report Series No. 522. World Health Organization, Geneva, Switzerland, 1973.
10. Simon, M. Food aid for supplementary feeding programmes—An analysis. *Food Policy*, November, 1978.
11. Waterlow, J. C. and A. M. Thomson. Observations on the adequacy of breast feeding. *The Lancet*, August 4, 1979.

The Nutri-Pak

Experience with an Indigenous Supplementary Feeding Intervention in the Philippines

GEORGE H. ROPES

The subject of this paper is the Philippine nutrition intervention known as Nutri-Pak, but it is impossible to discuss Nutri-Pak without describing the context within which it was developed. I shall therefore preface my discussion of Nutri-Pak with some comments on the Philippine Nutrition Program (PNP), which is the programmatic expression of two entities: the National Nutrition Council (NNC), and the Nutrition Center of the Philippines (NCP). The former is a public body composed of the heads of more than a dozen ministries and professional organizations, responsible for formulating nutrition policy and coordinating implementation of all government nutrition activity. The latter, a private sector counterpart of the NNC, plays a supporting role. Both bodies were established in mid-1974, the NNC by President Ferdinand E. Marcos, the NCP by the First Lady, Mrs. Imelda Marcos. Such high-level political support for nutrition makes the Philippines something of a rarity.

Three imperatives faced the nascent PNP: to create an organizational infrastructure, to increase popular awareness of malnutrition, and to articulate a coherent nutrition program. The first task, that of building an organization, was accomplished by replicating the NNC at the regional, provincial, municipal, and village levels. A hierarchy of nutrition committees was thus formed that reached down to the lowest administrative level. The nutrition committee of each barangay, as vil-

GEORGE H. ROPES • International Nutrition Program, Massachusetts Institute of Technology, Cambridge, Massachusetts.

lages are called in the Philippines, spawned a barangay network that had one unit leader for every 20 families. At each level, the nutrition committee was composed of representatives from all the public agencies involved in nutrition-related activities and was headed by the appropriate executive official. The organizational effort was diligently pursued and highly successful. Within two years, committees had been formed in all 12 regions of the Philippines, in all but one of 76 provinces, in almost 75% of the 1500 municipalities, and in about 40% of the 42,000 barangays (1).

The second task facing the NNC/NCP, which was to make the populace aware of the extent and seriousness of malnutrition, was undertaken concurrently with the organizational drive. Principally, it was accomplished via the massive Operation Timbang, or OPT, in which more than four million preschoolers (about half of the 0- to 6-year-old population) were weighed and classified according to the Gomez scale. This mass mobilization itself alerted the public to malnutrition as much as did the aggregate results: over 30% of these children were suffering from second- and third-degree malnutrition. OPT also served to locate and identify the malnourished.

The third task—that of articulating a national nutrition program— also proceeded quickly. The plan drawn up by the NNC/NCP called for interventions in five broad areas: food assistance, health protection, food production, family planning/nutrition information, and education. These schemes were aimed particularly at the following priority groups: infants and preschool children, pregnant women, nursing mothers, and school children.

Other tasks, only slightly less pressing, also occupied the NNC/NCP in its formative stages. These included training personnel, setting up a monitoring and reporting system, generating publicity, and doing research on food and nutrition. This is not the place to elaborate on these aspects of the PNP, but they bear mention to underscore how active it was in its youth.

Having provided, albeit briefly, the context into which the Nutri-Pak fits, I propose next to address the intervention itself, presenting in some detail its origin, evolution, and current status. Following that review, I will raise what I consider the most interesting questions emerging from the Filipino experience with Nutri-Pak. The genesis of what later became the Nutri-Pak concept occurred early in 1974 in the province of Laguna, southeast of Manila. The staff of the Laguna Provincial Nutrition Program set up a production system for converting inexpensive, locally available protein sources—small shrimp and fish—into finely ground protein powder and sealing it in small plastic packets.

About a dozen women were organized to do the necessary cooking, grinding, packing, and sealing. Each packet contained one level teaspoon of protein powder, which provided about 9 g of protein or roughly one-third of the RDA for a weanling. The protein packets were sold through well-baby clinics, feeding centers, and schools of Laguna. Directions instructed mothers to add the powder to the traditional weaning foods; other suggested uses were as seasoning or as a nutritious condiment. The project leaders saw it as a way to increase local food self-sufficiency, and as such, a model suitable for other provinces to follow. They also recognized the employment- and income-generating potential of the project (2).

The Philippine Food and Nutrition Program (PFNP), then responsible for coordinating all nutrition activities in the country, did little to promote the innovative Laguna Project (3). However, PFNP'S successors, NNC and NCP, proved more receptive to the concept, incorporating the project, albeit after substantial modification, into the nascent PNP. The NCP, who were assigned responsibility for developing the intervention, gave the name of Nutri-Pak to the modified concept early in 1975 (4).*

The most significant modification made by the NCP was the addition of rice and oil, also individually packaged in sealed plastic packets, to the protein powder of the Laguna intervention. These changes improved the nutritional pay-off (and balance) of the Nutri-Pak to about 12 g of protein (roughly one-half of the RDA for an infant) and about 400 cal (approximately one-third of the RDA).

Another aspect altered by the NCP was the intended target group of the intervention, namely, from infants 0–6 months old to children 6–60 months old. This shift reflected the NCP's recognition that, given prevailing hygienic conditions, breast milk is clearly the feeding method of choice during the first 6 months of life for the majority of Filipinos. Because the NCP wanted to encourage, not discourage, breast-feeding for newborns, it stressed Nutri-Pak as a supplement to breast milk after the age of 6 months.

This shift in the age of the intended beneficiaries prompted the development of three sizes of Nutri-Pak, to meet the nutritional needs of an expanded range of recipients. Type I was intended for infants, Type II for toddlers, and Type III for children 4–5 years old. Also, NCP developed additional protein sources, adding anchovy and mung bean varieties to the minishrimp. Some formulations included skim milk to boost

*The first use of the term "Nutri-Pak" was in a draft memo dated March 5, 1975, which later appeared in slightly modified form (4). This pamphlet is the principal source for the information that follows on Nutri-Pak.

protein quantity and quality. The nonfat dry milk, supplied by USAID through PL 480 Title II, was the only nonindigenous part of Nutri-Pak.

Several alternatives for production of Nutri-Pak were put forward, although it seems clear that NCP preferred the Laguna model, in which municipalities established simple processing plants in accordance with their needs and resources. Because a grinder, either manual or electric, was about all the machinery required to process locally available foodstuffs, a municipal-level Nutri-Pak processing plant could produce enough low-cost rations to rehabilitate the municipality's third-degree malnourished children. Thus, such plants could promote self-reliance—one of the main themes of the PNP—at both local and national levels. A community would provide for its own target population, while dependence on uncertain supplies of donated foods from abroad would be reduced. These features made this option very attractive politically.

Alternatively, the NPC offered to sell high-protein powder to municipalities unwilling or unable to process their own. Municipalities could also order complete Nutri-Paks from NCP at cost. Early promotional literature stressed that home preparation of Nutri-Pak rations was both possible and desirable.

With respect to distribution, whereas the Laguna protein packets had been sold, NCP initially conceived of the Nutri-Pak as being provided free of charge to all children identified by Operation Timbang as suffering from third-degree malnutrition. The distribution channel was envisioned as being from the municipal nutrition committees through the barangay networks to the families of those children. Although not explicitly stated in the Nutri-Pak literature, there is little reason to doubt that the NCP was aware that Nutri-Pak could provide tangible, ongoing functions for the municipal nutrition committees and barangay networks—functions that could sustain commitment after the initial enthusiasm of forming a committee and participating in the OPT campaign had waned. In the beginning Nutri-Pak was seen as an integral, indeed vital, component of the PNP. Such were the features and functions of the Nutri-Pak as originally conceived and promoted by NCP in 1975.

Given the concerns of this conference, two questions are in order: *What* has been the experience with Nutri-Pak in the interim? *Why* has Nutri-Pak evolved as it has? The answer to the first question is fascinating, and I will sketch the broad outlines of that experience. The second question is difficult, perhaps even impossible, for someone who did not participate personally, to answer. Therefore, I will do no more than speculate regarding the reasons for Nutri-Pak's evolution.

In discussing the Nutri-Pak experience, the first point to make is that there are really two Nutri-Paks: the first is the official, brand name Nutri-Pak developed and produced by the NCP; the second is a generic term covering a variety of locally produced Nutri-Pak-type interventions over which the NCP had little control and, until recently, about which it has had little information.* That this situation could exist illustrates the strengths and weaknesses of the Philippine approach to nutrition programming. Policy directives from Manila extolling Nutri-Pak and exhorting municipalities to establish processing plants did generate considerable activity on the periphery, but much of that activity remained beyond the effective supervision or even the knowledge of the NCP. Given the limited manpower of NNC and NCP at the national level, the ambitious scope of the endeavors incorporated within the PNP, and the formidable obstacles to communication in the Philippines, it is not altogether surprising that much Nutri-Pak activity went on unobserved.

The result, however, has been that the Nutri-Pak experience has not been cumulative; local initiatives have benefited little from central guidance and support, nor has the NCP fully capitalized on the lessons learned in the field. Fortunately, this problem has been recognized by the NNC and NCP, and steps have been taken recently to address it.

Late in 1978, the NNC commissioned a study to learn what had really been happening to Nutri-Pak in the field (5). By combining reports from several sources, the investigators found that 133 Nutri-Pak processing plants had been established throughout the country since 1975. The vast majority of these plants were set up by municipalities in response to early PNP publicity stressing that option. The exact classifications by intended level of coverage were:

National	1
Regional	2
Provincial	16
City	6
Municipal	106
Barangay	2
Total	133

Of these plants, 107 were equipped with manual grinders, 25 had electric grinders, and one plant had both. According to the reports, 108 plants (81%) were operational. The accuracy of this last statistic was challenged when the researchers visited 41 of the plants and discovered that the status of more than a third was not as reported.

What else did the research team learn from its survey of field experience? First, they found a system that was functioning—one could almost say flourishing—despite years of scant attention from the national level. Basing their calculations on the production figures of 21

*Reference 5 is the principal source for information on generic Nutri-Pak.

of the 41 plants visited, the evaluators estimated that these plants met 32% of the yearly feeding requirements for the areas served. Extrapolating this production rate to all areas with reported Nutri-Pak facilities, and then to the country as a whole, they calculated that 13 and 7%, respectively, of the feeding requirements were being met by the intervention. Although speculative, these figures are the best available on Nutri-Pak's outreach. It is worth noting that the term "yearly feeding requirement" denotes the number of OPT-identified cases of third-degree malnutrition in an area multiplied by 42 (1 Nutri-Pak per day for 6 weeks). This means that the estimated total annual production nationwide is over three-quarters of a million Nutri-Paks. Even if this estimation procedure overstates actual production by 50%, about one-half million infant rations a year are being produced with only minimal assistance or direction from the center.

A second thing the survey team found was a diverse, heterogeneous system. Twenty-eight of the 41 plants produced Nutri-Paks similar in composition to the "official" Nutri-Pak. Most of the rest produced packets that omitted the oil or skim milk components, or both. Four plants added other ingredients, such as sugar, boullion cubes, and banana powder. The researchers identified three distribution schemes that were used with roughly equal frequency by the plants that were operating. These schemes were: to distribute directly to households; to use the feeding center approach; and to distribute at designated outlets, such as health centers or the plant itself. About half the plants followed no set feeding program; the rest dispensed Nutri-Pak to recipients for varying lengths of time. Plants that designated only children with third-degree malnutrition as their target recipients matched those that targeted both second- and third-degree malnutrition cases; four plants in the survey did not discriminate on the basis of nutritional status at all. The investigators could not determine whether or not the actual recipients were the ones targeted. However, their survey indicated that few recipients consumed the recommended number of packets because of flagging maternal interest and intrafamilial sharing.

Within all this diversity, the evaluation team did discern some common features. The first of these was underutilization. No plant ran at more than one-third capacity, and on average, the plants operated only 3 hr per day. The evaluators' concern for efficiency seems misplaced, however, since they recognized that the number of target recipients at any given time largely determined the volume of production. Cost effectiveness criteria are inappropriate when capital cost is so low (approximately U.S. $1200 for a municipal plant) and distribution costs are ignored.

Another feature common to many Nutri-Pak processing plants was insufficient planning. Too little attention, the evaluators felt, was paid to citing, capitalization, and marketing considerations. Rarely did decisions regarding whether to establish a Nutri-Pak plant, and where to locate it, hinge on either nutritional or logistical criteria. Lack of funds was the most commonly cited reason for a plant's being inoperative. Most plants organized at the provincial level, in practice, distributed Nutri-Paks to only a few nearby municipalities.

A third common characteristic was inadequate management. Only two plants of those surveyed had full-time supervisors. In the others, the person in charge was a provincial or municipal action officer, or a government agency worker who devoted only a limited time to managing the Nutri-Pak plant. That part-time person had to perform multiple functions, supervising the production, distribution, and financial aspects of the operation, as well as serving as overall project manager.

A final common feature was deficient record-keeping. Only 10 of the 41 plants surveyed kept detailed production records, 16 others maintained records of varying completeness and utility, and 15 kept no records at all.

Experience with the "official" Nutri-Pak has differed considerably from that of its generic counterparts. Since 1975, the Research and Development Section of the NCP has been engaged continuously in activities to improve Nutri-Pak. These product development activities, which include acceptability, shelf life, utilization tests, marketing strategy studies, and the evaluation of delivery schemes, have benefited from the active involvement of the Coca-Cola Company, which has lent its expertise in food technology and communications to a pilot project that is centered around the regional Nutri-Pak plant in Tolosa, Leyte.

From this cooperative venture have come several improvements in the production and marketing systems of the Nutri-Pak. On the production side, minishrimp and anchovy were dropped as protein sources because of stability problems; replacements were developed from donated commodities and textured vegetable protein. For simplicity, the three types (sizes) of Nutri-Pak were reduced to one. These innovations, however, were disseminated only to those few Nutri-Pak plants that had established contact with NCP. Regarding the marketing, three promotional approaches were tested: face-to-face communication, comic books, and video cassettes. The last method showed sufficient promise that, in a program administered by the Communications Section of NCP, vans called "Nutri-buses" now visit villages regularly to present televised "lessons" dramatizing the nutritional needs of infants and Nutri-Pak's role in meeting them. Nutri-Pak's separately packaged ingredients make it a valuable educational tool for teaching mothers the importance of each one.

It is worth noting that, unlike all the other Nutri-Pak plants surveyed except for another in close contact with NCP, the Nutri-Paks produced in the Tolosa plant are sold. Although the cost to the consumer is subsidized by NNC and NCP in an attempt to reconcile the conflicting objectives of rehabilitation and self-reliance, the overall approach pursued by NCP at Tolosa is at some odds with the original concept of Nutri-Pak. The "official" Nutri-Pak embodies a centralized, top-down, high-technology, "expert" way of doing things that contrasts sharply with initial intentions and with actual field experience. Most fundamentally, the meaning of self-reliance has been subtly altered; where it once referred to the national and community levels, it now applies largely to the family.

I shall return now to the question I raised earlier as to *why* the Nutri-Pak has experienced this rather unusual course of development. Why, after such heavy initial emphasis and such high expectations, was Nutri-Pak so downplayed and largely ignored? Why has the "official" Nutri-Pak project at Tolosa taken directions so at variance with earlier conceptions of the scheme? No definitive answer is yet forthcoming, but I will suggest two possible explanations. The first is technical. It hypothesizes that some early problems with Nutri-Pak led to a reevaluation and deemphasis of the intervention. The plethora of program initiatives that claimed the attention of those directing the PNP during its first years crowded Nutri-Pak out of the limelight. Data from many sources inundated the monitoring and reporting system; low priority programs did not receive much scrutiny. Personnel from Manila, too busy for more than sporadic contact with the field, did not learn until recently that Nutri-Pak is alive, if suffering somewhat from neglect.

The second possible explanation is political. It proceeds from the premise that at the level of populations and of societies, the causes and cures of malnutrition are primarily political in nature. In the absence of a disaster, either natural or man-made, widespread hunger usually can be taken as *prima facie* evidence of systematic inequity. Questions of allocation (i.e., who gets what?) are inherently political, none more so than who has access to affordable food sufficient in quantity and quality to avoid hunger and starvation, to sustain normal growth and development, and to reach one's biological potential. A government's food and nutrition policies and programs will therefore reflect political realities. Thus, examination of the political context in which such policies and programs are embedded is necessary to understand why some policies are adopted but not others, and why some programs are prosecuted vigourously while others languish.

The Philippines has been under martial law since September 1972. One need not question the presumably humanitarian motives of the present regime to observe that by establishing the NNC and the NCP they simultaneously preempted a potentially volatile issue as their own and gained much political capital both at home and abroad. Nor need one know why the government empowered the NNC to coordinate only activities *directly related* to nutrition to note that, broad as this mandate seems, it constrains the NNC to seek technical solutions to a fundamentally political problem.

A political interpretation of the Nutri-Pak experience in no way impugns the competence or dedication of anyone associated with the PNP. It merely suggests that the architects of the PNP, although quick to appreciate and exploit the benefits of political support, in time came to apprehend the constraints imposed on the program both by its benefactors and by the wider political environment. The PNP increasingly adopted a problem definition that stressed ignorance, not poverty or powerlessness, as the proximate cause of malnutrition. Its programmatic solutions came more and more to reflect a technocratic orientation; decentralized, community-based, largely autonomous approaches like that of Nutri-Pak as originally conceived evolved into more centralized, individual-oriented, controlled concepts like the "official" Nutri-Pak. In short, this explanation suggests that politics—the macropolitical context—is very much a factor in determining why certain policies find programmatic expression, and how those programs are implemented.

The recent discovery of significant Nutri-Pak activity in the countryside has renewed the PNP's interest in, and support for, the intervention. It will be interesting to observe how Nutri-Pak develops over the next few years. Time should tell whether the technical or the political explanation has greater power to account for the Philippine experience with Nutri-Pak.

REFERENCES

1. The Malnutrition Problem in the Philippines. Processed working paper prepared for the International Study Symposium on Policy Making and Planning to Reduce Malnutrition, Berkeley, California, 29 March–1 April, 1977.
2. *Philippine Food and Nutrition Program News*, p. 3, March 1974.
3. *Philippine Food and Nutrition Program Annual Report*, p. viii, 1 July 1973 to 30 June 1974.
4. Annex 3 of *The Philippine Nutrition Program, 1975–1976* (a pamphlet).
5. Alfonso, M., E. Bañez, L. Pineda, R. Florentino, D. Adorna, and R. Guirriec. Organization, Production, Distribution, and Utilization of Nutri-Pak—An Evaluation. (This unpublished report is the principal source for information on the generic Nutri-Paks.)

Supplementary Nutrition
A Case Study from India

BADRI TANDON

Supplementary nutrition is an important approach for prevention and treatment of malnutrition among children, pregnant women, and lactating mothers. It is being implemented in India through a number of government and nonofficial programs. We are aware of the limitations and shortcomings of this approach, yet for health and nutrition, educational and social welfare, economic and political reasons, supplementary nutrition programs in India have continued to increase the coverage of the target population during the last two decades.

India has a population of about 548 million (1971 census); of this total, 225 million are children under 12 years old, 132 million are preschool age, and 62 million are below the age of 3 years. There are 38 million pregnant and nursing women. The projected figures for 1983 are: total population, 697 million; 264 million children, of whom 151 million will be preschool age; and 49 million pregnant and nursing women. Forty-six percent of the population in India is living below the poverty line, with a per capita expenditure of Rs. 66.5 (equivalent to U.S. $8.00) per month, which is too little to provide adequate food. Based on the 1976–1977 food prices, monthly per capita expenditure for food is less than Rs. 61.8 in the rural areas and Rs. 71.3 in the urban areas.

Several dietary surveys have indicated that the diet of preschool children is deficient in calories, protein, vitamin A, riboflavin, vitamin C, and calcium. Nearly 90% of the children receive 300–600 kcal below the recommended daily allowance, and one-third consume less than the

BADRI TANDON • Department of Gastroenterology and Human Nutrition Unit, All-India Institute of Medical Sciences New Delhi, India recommended daily allowance of protein. This deficiency of dietary nutrients combined with recurrent infections results in varying degrees of malnutrition. A multicentric study reported by the Indian Council of Medical Research (ICMR) showed that the weight of Indian children averages at 60–70% of the American standard. A recent study from the National Institute of Nutrition in Hyderabad, and a nationwide Integrated Child Development Services (ICDS) survey indicated a high prevalence of grade II and grade III malnutrition. Eighteen to 21% of the preschool children had 3rd degree malnutrition (greater than 40% weight deficit); 35–65% had a 25–40% weight deficit (Grade II), and 14% were 10–25% underweight.

Dietary deficiencies in pregnant and lactating women and low-birth-weight infants further aggravate the high prevalence of malnutrition among preschool children.

India is divided into 30 states, including union territories. Health and nutrition are state responsibilities, but considering the importance of nutrition for health, a major effort for prevention and treatment of malnutrition has been initiated by the central government. Since independence (1947), the Indian government has organized its activities through five-year plans. The first five-year plan began in 1951, and at present the sixth five-year plan is in effect. Unfortunately, nutrition programs did not receive any attention in the first two five-year plans, some efforts were made during the third and fourth five-year plans, but real action began only in the fifth five-year plan, which has been further intensified in the current plan.

Table 1 shows the different major nutrition schemes being enacted today in India. The list does not include the small and medium size pro-

TABLE 1. Major Centrally Sponsored Supplementary Nutrition Programs in India (Sixth Five-Year Plan)

Name of project	Year of study	Financial outlay (crores)	Target population
Midday meal	1962–1963	57.4	Children 6–11 years of age: 18 million in 13 states
Balwadi	1970–1971	8.0[a]	Children 3–5 years of age: 250,000
SNP	1970–1971	70.5 (WFP,[a] CARE[a])	Children 0–6 years of age: 10 million
ICDS	1975–1976	40.0	Children 0–6 years of age: 1.6 million

[a] Through voluntary agencies.

TABLE 2. Per Capita per Day Requirements of Different Food Groups for a Balanced Diet in India, and Their Estimated Availability during the Years 1973–1976

Food group	Grams required for a balanced diet	Estimated per capita per day availability[a] for 1976 (g)
Cereals	366.0	404.9
Pulses	64.1	51.8
Vegetables (leafy)	116.4 ⎱	38.0
Vegetables (others)	61.3 ⎰	
Roots and tubers	68.9	60.0
Fruits	39.6	54.0
Milk and milk products	189.4	111.5
Fats and oils	39.3	13.9
Flesh foods	37.6	14.5
Sugar and jaggery	41.5	55.6
Total number of calories available	2362	2136
Total protein available	57.8	52.0

[a]Estimated quantities of available food supplies are not necessarily the quantities of food actually consumed.

grams organized by state sectors and voluntary organizations. *At present, roughly six million preschool children are being covered by supplementary nutrition programs, and in the next five-year period it is hoped that this figure will double.* It is estimated that there will be about 150 million preschool children by 1983, among whom about 61 million will need significant nutritional supplementation, yet at best, only 20%, or about 12 million of them, can hope to get nutritional help through government programs. Of the 49 million pregnant and nursing women anticipated in 1983, seven million are targeted to receive supplementary food, but probably only about two million will actually be reached.

What is the state of food availability within the country in reference to requirements? Table 2 provides this information, obtained from the Ministry of Agriculture. In general, there is a chronic marginal shortage of calorie and protein sources that has become worse owing to a recent countrywide drought.

In an effort to alleviate the problem of malnutrition, the Ministry of Agriculture, the government of India, and smaller establishments at the state level have been engaged in the production of nutritious food for supplementary nutrition programs. Balahar, Balamul, and Miltone are some of the foods manufactured on a large scale.

Balahar. This foodstuff was developed by the Central Food and Technological Research Institute (CFTRI) in Mysore, and first used on a large scale during the Bihar famine in 1966–1967. Its production has been increasing continuously during the last decade (Table 3). The constituents and specifications of Balahar are given in Tables 4 and 5.

Balamul and Ready-to-Eat. These foodstuffs are two important weaning products. Their formulation is shown in Tables 6 and 7. Approxi-

TABLE 3. Production of Balahar ($\times$ 10^6)

Fourth five-year plan	49,062 metric tons
Fifth five-year plan	142,146 metric tons
Target for sixth five-year plan	250,000 metric tons

TABLE 4. Formulations of Balahar

	Formula A (21%)	Formula B (16%)	
A. Soy-fortified bulgar Wheat	85%	75%	85%
Groundnut flour	15%	5%	3%
Wheat flour	—	20%	12%
B. Maize flour	70%	85%	—
Groundnut flour	15%	7.5%	—
Soy flour	15%	7.5%	—

TABLE 5. Specification of Balahar[a]

	Formula A (21%)	Formula B (16%)
Protein ($N \times 6.25$) (dry basis)	Min. 21%	Min. 16%
Free fatty acid	Max. 5.0%	Max. 30 μg/kg
Acid-insoluble ash (dry basis)	Max. 0.2%	Max. 30 μg/kg
Total ash (dry basis)	Max. 3.0%	Max. 30 μg/kg
Moisture	Max. 10.0%	Max. 30 μg/kg
Crude fiber (dry basis)	Max. 3.5%	Max. 30 μg/kg
Aflatoxin	Max. 30 μg/kg	Max. 30 μg/kg

[a] Quantity of vitamins and minerals added to 1 kg of Balahar: vitamin A, 4 mg; vitamin B_1, 9 mg; vitamin B_2, 13 mg; vitamin B_{12}, 15 mg; folic acid, 1 mg; calcium, 4 g; ferrous sulfate, 750 mg.

TABLE 6. Formulation of Weaning Food
Products

	Balamul	Ready-to-eat
Protein	22%	15%
Fat	7%	10%
Carbohydrate	60%	65%
Calories	391	410

TABLE 7. Proximate Composition of
Balamul[a]

Full fat soya	25%
Moong	12.5%
Bengal gram	7.5%
Skimmed milk powder	10.0%
Rice	17.5%
Wheat	7.5%
Sugar	10.5%
Iodized salt	2.5%
Calcium phosphate	2.5%

[a] Vitamins A, B_1, B_2, C, iron, and methionine are also
added.

TABLE 8. Nutrient Composition of Miltone[a]

Protein	4.0 g
Fat	2.0 g
Solid nonfat	9.5 g
Lactose	5.0 g
Calories	54
Vitamin A	150 IU
Vitamin C	6.0 g
Vitamin D	16.0 IU
Thiamine	0.15 mg
Folic acid	20 g
Vitamin B_{12}	0.27 μg
Vitamin E	0.8 mg

[a] Composition per 100 g.

TABLE 9. Production of Miltone

Year	Lakh (liters)
1973–1974	10.51
1974–1975	9.62
1975–1976	5.20
1976–1977	8.80
1977–1978	25.00

mately 1750 million tons of weaning food were produced during the year 1977–1978.

Miltone. CFTRI developed this milk substitute from groundnut flour. Its composition and production levels are shown in Tables 8 and 9.

ORGANIZATIONAL STRUCTURE FOR SUPPLEMENTARY NUTRITION PROGRAMS

Organizational structure has gradually evolved during the last 10 years and has reached an optimum level in the ICDS program. The Special Nutrition Programme (SNP), the largest, is organized very simply. One SNP center provides supplementary nutrition for 100 beneficiaries in tribal areas and 200 beneficiaries in urban slums. Each center is manned by one organizer and one helper, who are paid a small honorarium. Twenty-five paise (about U.S. 4 cents) per child are provided to cover the costs of food and transportation. Children are provided 200 cal and 8 to 12 g of protein, and mothers receive 500 cal and 25 g of protein daily for 300 days a year from this nutritious food. It is supposed to be a spot feeding program.

The ICDS is a more comprehensive program that provides supplementary nutrition as a part of a package of health, nutrition, and education for the beneficiaries. The package includes supplementary food, immunization, health check-ups, primary medical care, and education (informal nutrition and health). Supplementary nutrition is restricted to a spot feeding program every day of the year. While SNP is primarily supervised by the Social Welfare Department, the ICDS is a joint program of the Social Welfare and Health Departments. Balwadis provide informal education and supplementary food through voluntary agencies.

TABLE 10. Nutritional Benefits of the Integrated Child Development Services Project

Type of project area	Baseline survey					Second survey					Third survey				
	Number	Normal and I[a]	II	III and IV	No record	Number	Normal and I	II	III and IV	No record	Number	Normal and I	II	III and IV	No record
Rural	17,904	46[b]	28	22	4	16,920	52	27	15	5	15,572	59	28	11	2
Tribal		46	23	22	9		54	21	11	14		59	18	6	17
Urban		43	34	22	1		54	33	12	0.6		73	20	6	2
All		45	28	22	5		53	26	13	7		63	23	8	6

[a] I, II, III: Gomez classification of grade of malnutrition based on weight for age.
[b] All values given as percentages.

Impact of Supplementary Nutrition on the Nutritional Status of the Beneficiaries

The main objective of supplementary food is to improve the nutritional status of children and to prevent undernutrition. What have been the results of different supplementary nutrition programs in India? A midday meal program has been in effect for children from 6 to 11 years of age. No systematic study on its nutritional benefits is available. The Ministry of Education has data suggesting that the school dropout rate and absenteeism have decreased and registration of new pupils has increased. SNP, the largest of the supplementary feeding programs, has also not been subjected to planned scientific study. Recently, the Interagency Evaluation Group (World Food Programme) has prepared a general evaluation report on this project. A few studies have been carried out at Hyderabad, Delhi, Rajasthan, and Pondicherry. In summary, nutritional benefits to the recipients cannot be projected through hard data, but soft data suggest that children receiving supplementary nutrition were in better nutritional status than were those who did not.

The ICDS has better data to measure the nutritional benefits of its supplementary nutrition program. A longitudinal study carried out during a two-year period shows a significant decrease in the prevalence of severe malnutrition and a shift toward a Grade I status and normal status (Table 10). The time interval between the baseline survey and the second survey was 10–12 months, with 8–11 months between the second and third surveys. ICDS data clearly demonstrate the value of supplementary food in improving the nutritional status of preschool children. It must be qualified, however, that in the ICDS program, supplementary food has been provided by spot feeding as a part of a package of health services.

Major Difficulties of Supplementary Nutrition Programs

The Indian experience with supplementary nutrition programs presents the following limitations and difficulties:

1. Programs have very limited outreach to the children under 3 years of age for these reasons: (a) Children of this age group are unable to come to the "feeding centers" without an accompanying family member. (b) A nutritious food like Balahar is not acceptable to very young children, and weaning foods are more

costly for the program. (c) The carry-home system results in too much sharing of food within the family, so young children do not receive enough of the supplement to benefit.

2. The social structure of the villages and urban slums does not permit selection of beneficiaries among the preschool-age children by either nutritional or economic criteria. Failure to restrict supplementary food for the most needy children thus limits the best utilization of meager resources. I have already indicated that about 60 million children at present need supplementary nutrition, and at best 20% of them will receive it in the current five-year plan. If selection of the most needy group were possible, the resources could be diverted to them. All efforts for selection of beneficiaries from within the families in the rural and urban communities have been unsuccessful in large-scale, national programs.

3. The spot-feeding program, which seems to be the only effective approach to get nutritional benefits to needy children, is relatively costly and limits the coverage of the target population. The carry-home system, which is less costly, is of little nutritional benefit to the target group as has been demonstrated by the All-India Institute of Medical Sciences and the National Institute of Nutrition studies in the India Population Projects.

4. Centralized production of nutritious foods like Balahar for distribution to the feeding centers is quite an unsatisfactory policy for the following reasons: (a) The administrative system of procurement and the logistics of supply are such that, by the time Balahar reaches the farthest point of distribution, it is unfit for human consumption. Most of the time the beneficiaries have fed it to their animals. (b) There are frequent breaks in supplies because of local weather and communication difficulties. Irregular supplies in feeding programs lead to poor cooperation from the communities. (c) Centralized production of food means that often the products are not suited to local tastes, and hence the food is rejected by the children.

Some of these difficulties have been solved by partial decentralization of nutritious-food production by setting up regional units. In order to suit local tastes, cereal ingredients are often changed. These modifications are useful but do not solve all of the problems. *Nutritious food production must be done at the most peripheral point, and if possible, at the village level.*

5. Most of the nutrition programs do not develop a proper organizational structure from apex to base. The projects are not moni-

tored. Such programs fail to demonstrate measurable nutritional benefits.

6. Minimal health inputs, such as immunization, primary medical care, safe drinking water, and sanitation, often do not receive attention simultaneously in supplementary nutrition programs.

Nutritional benefits *are* noted if supplementary food is provided as part of a package of services for health, nutrition, and education, as has been done in the program of the Integrated Child Development Services in India.

Supplementary Feeding and Formulated Foods
Some Comments

RICARDO BRESSANI

By definition, programs of supplementary feeding and use of formulated food aim to improve the nutritional status of populations by upgrading the quality of the diet. This may be accomplished either through the introduction of a single nutrient, if this is what is needed, or through the introduction of a mixture of nutrients for a more balanced food. Formulated foods may have other functions as well, such as, helping to bring about a transition to consumption of better diets, serving as an adjunct to breast milk during weaning, serving as ingredients for extending present dietary components, complementing food intakes, and replacing food items that, for one reason or another, are not consumed by the target population.

Therefore, to be able to understand how dietary improvement can be achieved with supplementary feeding and formulated foods, the information listed in Table 1 is needed. Table 1 includes the kinds of answers to the questions generally asked in dietary surveys, such as food habits, actual food intake, kinds of foods consumed, amounts of food consumed, time of introduction, frequency with which foods are consumed, mode of preparation, and forms in which food is consumed by all members of the family. Once such information is available, specific activities may be undertaken. For purposes of this discussion, the possible activities for nutrition planning and implementation for improving the protein quality of the diet, and thus the nutrition of the family, have been classified into those actions that could be derived from agriculture, from

RICARDO BRESSANI • Institute of Nutrition of Central America and Panama (INCAP), Guatemala City, Guatemala.

TABLE 1. Desirable Information for Dietary
Improvement

Food habits
Actual food intake
Kinds
Amounts
Patterns of intake
Frequency
Age of consumer when a food is introduced
Mode of preparation
Forms of consumption

food technology development, and from nutrition education and home economics.

For such a discussion, the kind of background information shown in Table 2 is necessary. These data were obtained on small weanling pigs fed the two main foods consumed by rural populations in many areas of Latin America. The small animals, in individual pens, were fed *ad libitum* for 12 weeks. Therefore, there was no competition among animals, and food was constantly available. The main results were (1) shifting the corn to bean ratio in the diet improved weight gain; (2) addition of single groups of nutrients, such as vitamins, minerals, energy, and two essential amino acids, improved growth to varying extents; and (3) when these nutrients were all added, weight gain was still greater, but not to the extent observed in the control group. The main conclusion is that for such a diet all the nutrients are needed, as opposed to just one, which is not surprising.

An additional point that is highly significant but seldom recognized is the effect of improved dietary quality on food intake. Figure 1 shows

TABLE 2. Weight Gain of Young Pigs Fed Corn–Bean
Diets with Various Supplements Alone or Combined

Supplement	Corn–bean diet 87/13 kg	Corn–bean diet 70/30 kg
None		
+ Amino acids	2.35	10.88
+ Vitamins	14.75	13.63
+ Minerals	8.50	15.88
+ Calories	6.00	8.63
All nutrients	35.00	37.00
Control	54.88	54.88

the food intakes of small animals consuming different experimental diets. Food intake on an unsupplemented maize/bean diet decreased over a 12-week period, while that of animals consuming the same basic diet supplemented with all necessary nutrients stimulated appetite and increased food consumption. These results make the problem of energy intake easier to solve. The results are relevant to the topic under consideration because they show that a change in food composition, quantity, and quality, e.g., from milk to dried foods, is comparable to what takes place in children during the weaning process.

Figure 2 presents additional background information. It shows the protein-complementary effect of a cereal grain (maize in this case) combined with legume foods (common beans and soybeans). With the maize–bean diet, a peak nutritive value is obtained when both foods are consumed in a 7 : 3 ratio. The protein quality decreases when the ratio is changed above or below this level. In the case of an opaque-2 maize–bean system, an identical peak appears in nutritive value, but on the bean side of the peak the quality drops, although it does not with opaque-2 corn. The same response takes place for the maize–soybean system, except that quality decreases on the maize side and remains constant and high on the soybean side.

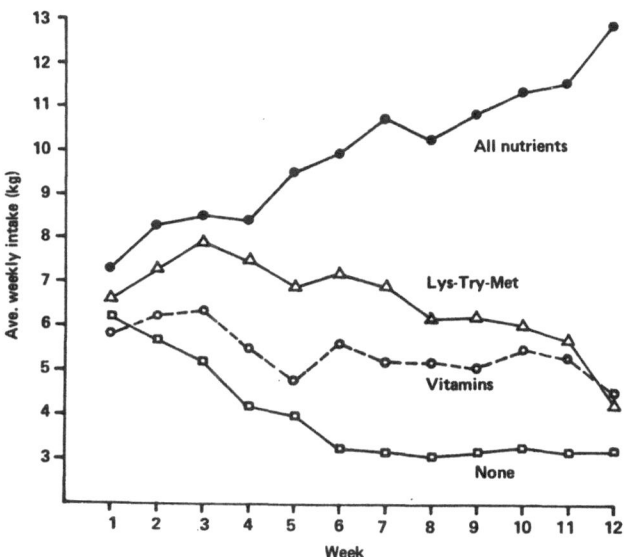

FIGURE 1. Feed intake of young pigs (5 weeks) fed an 89/13 corn/bean diet with various supplements.

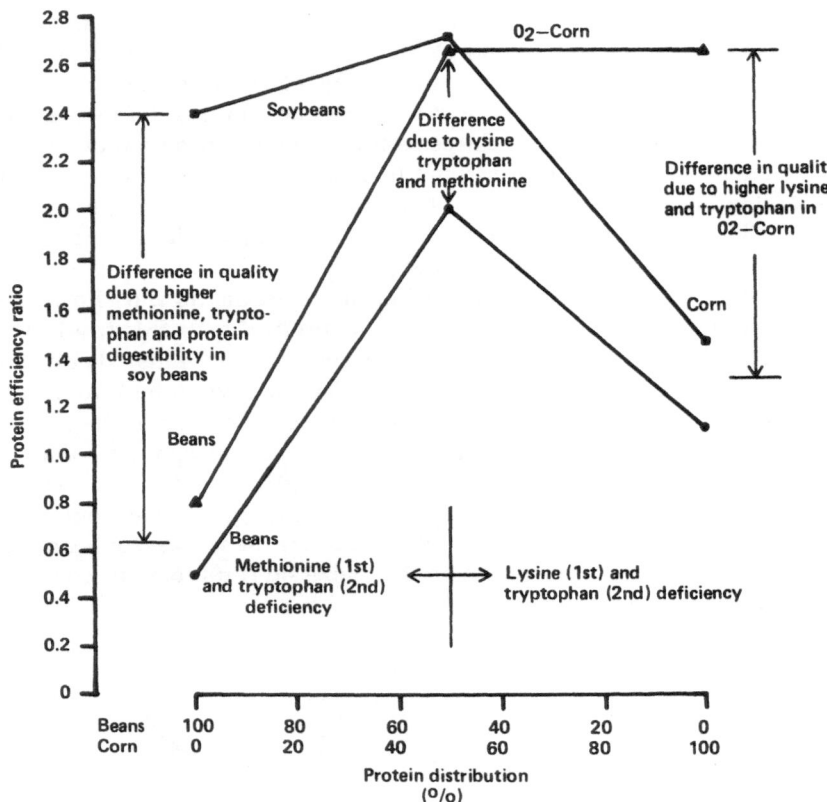

FIGURE 2. Protein quality of mixtures of corn and beans.

This information provides a background for nutrition policy implementation for improvement of dietary quality. The role of agricultural production is shown in Fig. 3. This figure shows the optimum protein quality value (A), the quality of the average diet consumed by the population (B), the quality of the mixture usually given to four- to five-year-old children (C), and the quality of maize alone (D), which is used extensively as the main weaning food. The upper line represents the opaque-2 maize–bean system. There are various possibilities for improving the diet. One method is to increase production, distribution, and consumption of beans in order to move the protein quality level from B, C, and D to A.

Much attention is being given to increasing the bean yield, but so far yields have not improved, and on a per capita basis they are actually

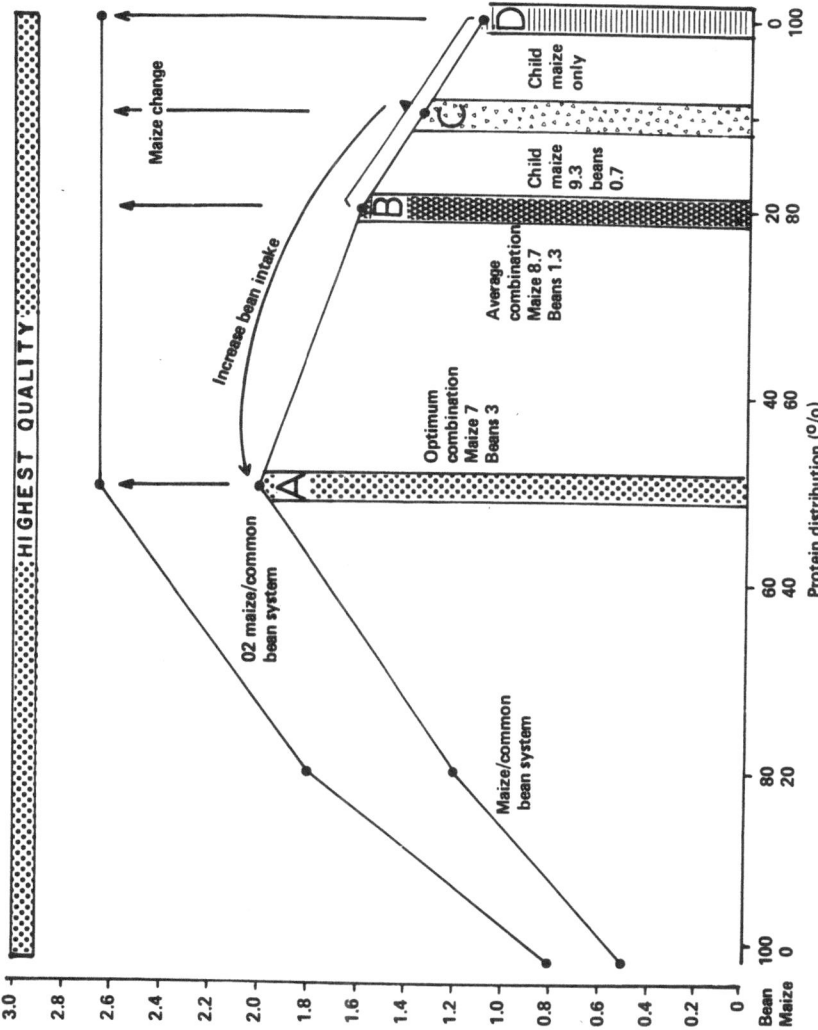

FIGURE 3. The role of an increased agricultural bean and corn production and availability on the nutritional quality of rural diets.

decreasing. The alternative is to produce opaque-2 maize and keep the present dietary maize/bean ratio. However, opaque-2 maize production is not yet a reality, even though much research is being done on the modified types. A better quality bean is also a possibility; however, if yield improvement has yet to be accomplished, the possibility of combining high quality with high yield is even more remote. This kind of agricultural information has not been disseminated, and it is therefore not used as extensively as it should be. Furthermore, it cannot be expected that those generating the research will also be responsible for its implementation, which should be the function of people trained in transferring such information to the producers and policy makers. National food and nutrition policy should thus promote this activity.

Another possibility for increasing dietary protein quality for children is to provide supplementary feeding with animal protein sources. A diet consisting of the present maize/bean ratio, or even maize alone, can be improved with relatively small amounts of animal proteins. Various results have shown, as summarized in Table 3, that 50 cc of liquid milk, 30 g of poultry meat, or 14 g of fish per 100 g of maize diet, consumed daily, will induce significant improvement in protein quality. The nutritional value of animal proteins is well recognized, but the main point is that the amounts needed are so small. Food and nutrition policy should, therefore, consider this when planning agricultural production programs as well as when deciding on how much animal protein to import and export. The amount of animal protein could be even lower if the diet consisted of the optimum ratio of maize and beans, as shown in Fig. 4. It should also be noted that with the increase in protein quality there is also an increase in protein quantity in addition to other nutrient factors, including energy.

Food technology offers at least two possibilities for improving dietary protein quality. One is the development of fortified foods and the other is to develop formulated foods. As indicated in Fig. 4, the qual-

TABLE 3. Minimum Amounts of Some Animal Proteins Necessary, if Consumed Daily, to Improve Maize–Bean Diets

Animal Protein	Amount found effective (g/ 100 g maize)	Protein equivalent (g)	Food weight equivalent (daily)
Milk	5	1.75	50 cc
Fish	4	3.60	14 g
Chicken	8	5.50	30 g

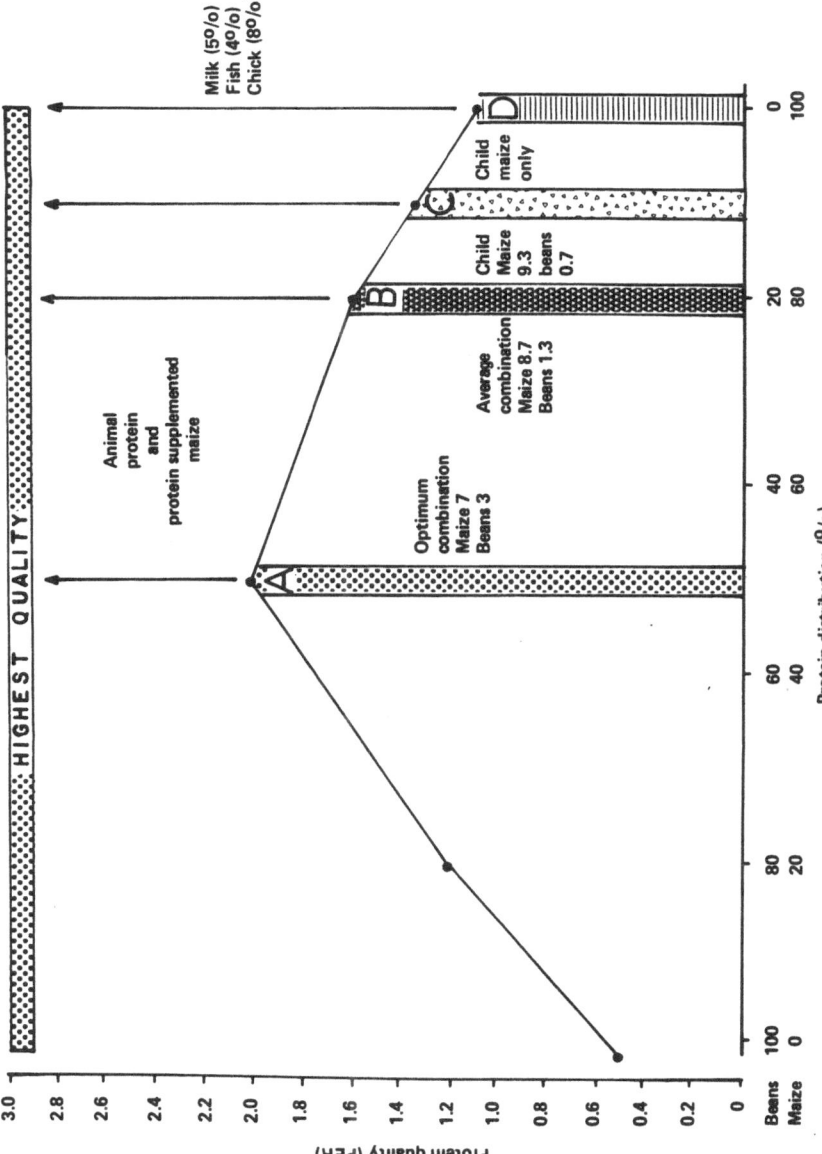

FIGURE 4. The role of small intakes of animal food products in improving the nutritional quality of rural diets.

ity of the diet can be increased substantially by relatively small amounts of animal protein, and if the supplement is chosen correctly, the availability of other nutrients also increases. Legume and cereal grain mixtures can also achieve this. For example, supplementing maize with 15% soybean will increase protein quantity and quality and also energy because of the oil provided by soybeans. This approach can be carried out commercially or at home. Similar examples are the addition of iodine to salt, vitamin A to sugar, and the like; however, it would appear that some of these nutrients could be more effective in overall programs if they were included with other nutrients deficient in the diet, as demonstrated in the experiment with weanling pigs. The incorporation of single nutrients may be considered short-term solutions, while the more complete system is a long-term approach.

If formulated foods are to be useful, they should be based on an understanding of the quality of the diet they are supposed to improve, and a formula can be made to supply as many nutrients as possible, even to the extent of being a complete food. Many examples of this have been tried and a few are economic successes, although not in terms of reducing malnutrition as originally believed.

Although formulated foods have been highly criticized during the last few years, the requests from countries for such products are actually increasing. At present, there are no problems with their formulation, industrial manufacture, or acceptability. The problems probably lie in cost, distribution, and knowledge of how to use them as well as in the socioeconomic background that exists in areas where there is malnutrition. Although they have been designed as infant foods—this must be emphasized—they should be foods capable of feeding all family members. Analysis of the success of any intervention, whether of supplementary feeding or formulated foods, is limited in scope and relates only to the food itself, with little consideration given to the multiple factors that contribute in varying degrees toward reducing the beneficial effects of the food that are observed under more controlled conditions. Actually, the need for controls should be indication enough that malnutrition cannot be solved by a single approach. Although multicausality is recognized, food and nutrition policy makers tend to consider the problem from the standpoint of their particular interests.

Weaning foods or formulated foods do not comprise systems peculiar to man; on the contrary, such an approach to feeding young animal species was first devised for swine and calves. The feed products available commercially are of a high quality, prepared by technologies as good as those used for the manufacture of foods for man, and what is even more important, they have been very useful. The reason is that instructions on their use have been provided, and these are closely followed by farmers. Obviously, food and nutrition policy had nothing to do with the development of these products because there is a strong economic interest and a well-established infrastructure for their manufacture as well as benefits for those who make use of them. This implies that food and nutrition policy should stimulate the same kind of interest in the use of *food* products by emphasizing the benefits to be derived. This latter activity is probably the most important factor in stimulating use of a food product, yet it is often disregarded. Thus, the final approach toward reducing malnutrition with such foods is to demonstrate their potential for doing so.

This approach is defined here as the home-economics–nutrition-education solution. It has really not received enough attention, and it is probably the solution that would be the most effective, because it is concerned with providing knowledge directly to those who are in need. It should be remembered that the final decisions about how to improve their diets are the privilege of people themselves, and nutrition and food technology know-how should be catalysts through appropriate channels for influencing these decisions so that people can improve their diets.

The quality of maize–bean diets can be improved by methods described previously and by the consumption of local resources, such as green vegetables. These foods, particularly the leafy vegetables, contain proteins rich in the amino acids limiting the quality of maize diets, especially lysine, and they also provide other nutrients.

Supplementary feeding programs and formulated foods can also provide the nutrients missing in the diet. However, use of formulated foods can be accomplished only if they are properly promoted and their value for the whole family is demonstrated, an activity that can be done best by home economics workers who, at present, are not available in many developing countries. Food and nutrition policy makers should analyze this problem and develop the infrastructure needed to transfer to the rural home level the agricultural, nutritional, and food-processing knowledge that has already been developed.

Many institutions are training nutritionists, but, although they are needed, the home economist is, without doubt, more useful and effective. Just as extension workers in agriculture have proven to be useful for farmers, home economists could be extremely helpful to home makers, particularly for introducing supplementary feeding, demonstrating the use of formulated foods, and imparting know-how in utilizing resources available in the home. The home economists could integrate very well the knowledge available from agriculture, food technology, and nutrition, as indicated above. Just as agronomists are taking their experiments to the farmers' fields, home economists could bring nutrition, food processing, and conservation knowledge to the kitchens and tables of rural inhabitants.

All the activities described above have been developed scientifically for the purpose of contributing to the solution of the malnutrition problem. Under controlled conditions, they have proved to be very effective. The solutions, however, have not in practice been as effective as expected. This lack of success has been attributed to many factors, but not to the one really responsible for the problem, which is the existing gap between the solutions proposed and the resources actually available for poor people. This suggests that food and nutrition policy makers should take into consideration the implementation, at the national level, of solutions that have already been developed, and should establish the infrastructure required to disseminate such knowledge, on a practical level, for the benefit of those in need.

Comment

GRETCHEN BERGGREN

In considering the papers presented in this section, a few issues deserve further comment, based on my experiences in both Zaire and Haiti, where we were able to participate in maternal and child health nutrition programs. First, on the subject of positive deviance, that is, where there is evidence of mothers in an area who are coping, we have shown in Haiti that the mother with one or two young children can manage considerably better than mothers with three or four. While the subject of coping versus noncoping deserves further study, it is important that matched groups be observed, based on socioeconomic status, marital status, and number of small children in the family.

Second, we have found that in the most malnourished populations of Haiti, infants grow relatively well from birth to 6 months, then begin to fall behind. However, there are always mothers who cannot provide the infant with adequate breast milk. These children demand special attention.

Concerning what anthropometric measurements to employ in a nutrition program, it seems necessary to distinguish between their use as screening and research instruments versus as an education tool. I see the "Road to Health" weight-for-age card as an educational tool in the hands of the mother. I have not seen the weight-for-height card, although it has been tried, used adequately by mothers. Therefore, even if it is agreed that the weight-for-age card is useful in the early months for screening purposes, thereafter the weight-for-height might be the better screening instrument.

Regarding the utility of these techniques as educational instruments, I do not think it has been demonstrated anywhere in the world that any better educational tool exists than weight-for-age health cards. The mother can see that line progressing up or down and is capable of inter-

GRETCHEN BERGGREN • Department of Population Sciences, Harvard School of Public Health, Boston, Massachusetts.

preting what is happening. Mothers do respond to it, and, I might add, fathers are equally interested and should not be left out of the educational process when children are weighed. In fact, if the father is not supportive of the mother, it can be a difficult situation for her at home.

In reference to the actual distribution of food and proper services, there are a few points to be emphasized. While I would agree that doctors are not the best people to hand out food supplements, it is vital that medical and health professionals be integrally involved in the project. Community committees should be considered as an alternative to involving the doctor in the handling and logistics of food distribution. Similarly, we found that distributing supplements in smaller quantities, and products that are not organoleptically acceptable to adults, proved effective in targeting the supplement.

Finally, in response to the discussion of nutrition centers for malnourished children, it is first necessary to distinguish between two types of demonstrations as educational tools. In one instance, the mother actually has her hands, her eyes, and her ears involved in learning, which is far better than sitting across the room and looking at a flip chart that she does not understand anyway. In Haiti, we have found that demonstration education in nutrition for 2 weeks, moving from village to village, is a modification of the mothercraft rehabilitation approach that may prove very useful. Although these nutrition centers cannot be labeled nutrition rehabilitation centers—no child is completely rehabilitated—it was amazing to see how much change occurred in children within 2 weeks. They did begin to brighten. They did lose their edema. A mother can see some improvement even in 2 weeks, and she is involved very personally in helping prepare her child's food using *locally available* items.

Comment

HOSSEIN GHASSEMI

Recently, I have been looking at evaluation reports available in the literature on the nutritional impact of supplementary feeding programs for the young child. Our findings suggest that they have not been as effective as anticipated in reducing the nutritional problems of young children. We have been able to locate around 100 relevant reports. Many of them reflect data from either research programs or pilot studies, and almost half of them report data from ongoing projects.

While lessons learned from pilot and large-scale operations are different, some consistent themes emerge. First, the take-home food distribution system, which is a more manageable and feasible way of delivering nutrients to young children, has not been quite efficient, with only 40–60% of the intended nutrients reaching the target population. This has been partially due to sharing of the food within the family, substituting for foods that would have otherwise been purchased, a generally low level of participation within the community, and sometimes insufficient ration size.

Why the participation problem? Many of the target population who potentially could have been reached did not respond, partly because of the lack of motivation of the program implementors and partly because of the social stigma of participating in a feeding program. In addition, the physical difficulties of reaching the distribution site constrained participation.

As far as program impact is concerned, most programs had on the whole small benefits for the cost. On the average, daily supplementation of 300–400 cal produced an additional weight gain of about 0.500–1 kg/year. Program duration and regularity in participation seemed to be

HOSSEIN GHASSEMI • UNICEF, United Nations Headquarters, New York, New York.

among the key variables influencing the impact level. In most of the programs, measurable impact was observed only after 6 months of operation.

Program costs varied between programs and between countries. On the average the annual cost of providing 300–400 cal/day would amount to US $20 (1976 equivalent). Possible effects of supplementary feeding programs on breast-feeding and disincentive effects on local food production caused by changing food habits and/or introduction of exotic foods were considered and no evidence was found to indicate that either of these effects was extant.

While the evaluation reports of supplemental feeding programs allowed us to glean a range of information and insights into the effectiveness and costs of programs, there were also some overt gaps in knowledge that require clarification. For example, what is the health significance of that additional 0.5–1 kg weight gain among program participants? How are the extra calories portioned among different channels, e.g., growth, physical activities, and readaptation of metabolic function? Physical activity may be the main variable affected by increased intake, although to date it has not been frequently addressed in evaluations. But even more important, little is known about the consequences and functional significance of marginal malnutrition, and even less is understood about what indicators should be used to measure benefits accrued to such a population.

Our study showed that the more successful the project is in screening potential beneficiaries, the better the response to the supplement. While this is to be expected, it raises the issue that, as screening criteria become more stringent, programs become stronger in a curative sense while the desirable approach to feeding programs would be strong emphasis on preventive aspects. Obviously criteria for selection of target beneficiaries would then be different.

It is also important to distinguish between small-scale research or pilot projects, which were generally found to be more effective, and the larger-scale, ongoing projects. In the latter case, insufficient motivation among the staff, poor supervision, and inadequate project design limited their effectiveness. All of these problems can be construed as a function of insufficient financial input compared with that available for intensive, research-oriented activities.

To conclude, it is only appropriate to comment on future directions for supplementary feeding programs, given all the problems and uncertainties indentified. For future policy purposes, there seem to be two options open to the decision maker. First, accept a broader objective for feeding programs and consider it as a means to redistribute income and reduce deprivation among the low-income segment of the society. Second, accept the current narrow nutrition and health-specific goals and redesign the program accordingly. There is a general argument that programs would be more cost effective if the family were taken as a target unit rather than individual children. If we want to maintain the objective of improved nutrition status, it is necessary to consider the congruence between the target group and the nature of their individual deficiency, and the ration provided; that is, the type of food provided, the timing of enrollment, and the length of participation must be given more attention.

Finally, if feeding programs can be integrated into the overall nutritional and development activities of the country, including primary health care and attempts to improve the socioeconomic setting supported by community participation, then chances of greater impact would be much higher.

Discussion

Determining the age at which to introduce supplementary foods to the diets of infants, in what quantity, and which types of food should be provided was the major focus of discussion. Emphasis was also placed on the issue of targeting—what criteria to use in the selection of beneficiaries and, thereafter, how to target the food to the designated women, infants, and children.

It was suggested by one participant that malnutrition is characteristically associated with the weaning period, when the malnutrition–infection cycle takes hold. Therefore, it was argued that supplementation should not introduce artificial feedings before 6 months; to do so will only discourage breast-feeding and subject the child to diarrhea, respiratory disease, and other infectious diseases. As a viable alternative, mothers could be provided with supplementary foods for their own diets both while pregnant and during lactation to promote good child growth and development.

While the concept of maternal supplementation was endorsed, a number of objections were raised to a policy that designates a definitive age for supplementation. For example, a study done in Nigeria found that 10–25% of the infants were malnourished by 6 months. By delaying the introduction of food supplements until 6 months or later, one allows a significant percentage of infants to "fall between the cracks," because their nutritional status has already deteriorated.

A further statement on the issue of the proper age for supplementation provided some resolution to the question of when to introduce supplementary feeding. Specifically, there is little doubt that in many societies at present breast milk must be complemented before 4–6 months in order to avoid growth faltering and its related consequences, this, despite the fact that studies of many other populations indicate that it is not necessary to complement before 4–5 months, and in some cases, before 6 months. The desirable solution would be to improve the nutrition of the mother so that no infant would need supplementary foods before 4 months of age. Indeed, that should be the long-term objective of any program, but that does not help the child who is already faltering at a given time.

The optimal response to growth faltering is for the mother to provide a suitable complementary food to the child, using her own resources and know-how, although programs of supplementary feeding represent an alternative.

Besides the issue of when to begin supplementation, debate ensued as to how carefully the food ration should be targeted. It was pointed out that, by increasing selectivity of participants, programs become more rehabilitative or curative. Although no consensus was reached on the appropriate degree of targeting, a series of interesting points was raised.

First, emphasizing supplementary feeding as a preventive tool, covering the entire population, will prove expensive on the basis of cost per child at risk. If a planner or country is willing or able to accept that cost, this kind of program could work. But it should be understood that resources are scarce and that the ability of feeding programs to prevent malnutrition remains debatable.

Second, although the state-of-the-art in targeting to individuals remains imperfect, strides are being made in identifying at-risk indicators that increase selectivity of recipients. In addition, successful examples of targeting to communities with high levels of malnutrition are well documented. By selecting geographical areas for intervention, increased cost-effectiveness may result. Similarly, it was suggested that programs should be targeted seasonally. It is more effective to provide supplementary feeding at particular times of the year, when food is scarce, rather than at harvest time, when it is abundant.

Third, if targeting to individuals is deemed appropriate, experience in many countries indicates that the health delivery system fails to reach a sizable portion of the needy population. Hence, alternative and innovative outreach mechanisms will have to be identified and utilized in many instances.

Fourth, highly targeted feeding programs, such as nutrition rehabilitation centers, can also teach prevention of malnutrition. However, the success of prevention attempts is contingent on the effectiveness of nutrition education designed to prevent the recurrence of malnutrition in the patient, while at the same time preventing it in siblings and other members of the community through the dissemination of knowledge and information. Unfortunately, the documentation of success in this area is limited.

Fifth, although school-age children as a group are often less at risk than preschoolers, consideration should be given to using more than nutritional targeting criteria in enrolling them in a feeding program. Evidence indicates that a school supplementation program may reduce the number of children who drop out of school. If education is given priority, school feeding may represent a worthwhile endeavor, regardless of nutritional considerations.

Active discussion also took place concerning the appropriateness of the theoretical basis for supplementary feeding programs and the various alternative to feeding that may be considered. It was generally agreed that nutrition programs should be designed to eliminate the need for supplementary feeding programs. However, opinions varied; some argued that supplementary feeding programs are the most effective strategy for alleviating malnutrition, while others felt that, whenever supplementary feeding is a part of a community nutrition program, it almost guarantees failure of the program. This is because once supplementation is terminated, little if anything remains in the rest of the program.

Much discussion was directed toward qualifying these two extreme positions. For example, periodic weighing of infants and young children was considered a vital component of any nutrition program. The value of such an effort as a vehicle for nutrition education of the mother was stressed.

The possibility of providing money, rather than food, was also debated. While it was considered an interesting option, especially given reports of the cumbersome and inefficient design of feeding programs, it was asserted that dispensing money is politically and socially difficult for governments. In fact, it is likely that governments and donor agencies do not trust poor householders to dispose of available income wisely. Moreover, the opportunity costs associated with donated food rations are much lower than those imposed by giving money. This is attributable to agricultural surpluses in a country like the United States.

Finally, it was emphasized that more attention must be focused on the return on the investment associated with feeding programs, coupled with an awareness of possible disincentives to agricultural production. All too often countries or regions accept food aid without considering that they could provide food for themselves. This point is especially germane when supplementary feeding efforts involve spending money on costly processing of foods with technology inherited from more industrialized nations. This can prove economically and socially disadvantageous. This is particularly true when local commodities and technology could be employed to produce adequate amounts of indigenous foodstuffs.

IV

Integrated, Multisectoral Village-Level Interventions

In the 1960s, disillusionment with the effectiveness of conventional nutrition education and supplementary feeding programs led to a strong effort in support of so-called integrated, multisectoral nutrition interventions at the village level. The logic of bringing to bear, at the grass-roots level, the resources of agencies concerned with environmental sanitation, health, education, and agriculture, among others, is that a unified approach ought to be more effective than uncoordinated, sector initiatives. But the implementation of such efforts has proved difficult, and this has, in turn, resulted in major questions about their effectiveness. Both arguments for the integrated approach are advanced in the section that follows. The papers and discussion of this section examine the integrated, multisectoral approach, and the problems encountered in its implementation.

The issue paper by Johnston emphasizes that nutrition planning and policy analysis have not proved as effective as expected. Moreover, the dramatic increase in international attention to nutrition has not been matched by significant progress in reducing malnutrition in the villages of the less-developed countries. He suggests that the reasons include the lack of good research and policy analysis, faulty diagnoses, lack of consensus, equation of the desirable with the feasible, and attempts at shortcut solutions as well as severe resource constraints and administrative problems that limit the scope for direct action to alleviate poverty. It is argued that an integrated or systems mix is necessary to understand the multiple causation of malnutrition, but should result neither in the forced administrative integration of diverse activities nor in the neglect of potentially effective single-sector interventions.

The case studies in Indonesia by Hendrata and Rohde, in Colombia by Fajardo, and in the Philippines by Florentino provide examples of somewhat more successful interventions than Johnston's paper predicts.

The description of development from below in Indonesia is particularly interesting, since it is an example of successful implementation in a country where the integrated approach had previously had only limited success. It suggests that perhaps the principle is right, and that it is in the implementation of such programs where difficulties are encountered.

Integrated Multisectoral Nutrition Interventions at the Village Level

Bruce F. Johnston

Introduction

In considering integrated and multisectoral nutrition interventions at the village level, two general propositions should be emphasized at the outset. First, we need to recognize that in the low-income developing countries where nutritional and related health problems are most serious and intractable, the great majority of the population still lives in rural villages. Hence, as we consider the issues related to the design and implementation of policies and programs capable of having an impact at the village level, we must not lose sight of the fact that this target population represents some 70–80% of the total population and is located in thousands of villages—indeed, in something over 500 thousand villages in the case of India alone. Second, I believe that we must face up to the fact that the actual progress to date in reducing malnutrition in most of the developing countries has not measured up to the high expectations expressed at the 1971 MIT Conference on Nutrition, National Development, and Planning (1) and at other international forums.

Moreover, the shortcomings, in terms of practical results, have been paralleled by limited progress in reaching an agreed upon view concerning the type of food and nutrition strategies that will be most effective in achieving more substantial progress in the future. An alumnus of MIT's International Nutrition Program, John Field (2, p. 230n) has stated

Bruce F. Johnston • Food Research Institute, Stanford, California.

that, unfortunately, in the " ... typical case ... nutrition programs are little more than palliatives, in effect if not in intent." Even in those instances in which nutrition interventions have been implemented effectively, they have usually been little more than token programs because they reach such a small section of a country's rural population. In brief, the dramatic upswing in international attention being accorded to nutrition and the related enthusiasm for nutrition planning have *not* led to any significant progress in the reduction of malnutrition in the villages of developing countries, especially in the low-income countries, such as India, Bangladesh, Indonesia, Kenya, and Tanzania.

I will concentrate on the problems to be confronted in eliminating, or at least substantially reducing, village-level nutrition problems in low-income countries, using the World Bank definition of that subset of developing countries as those with a 1976 per capita GNP of $250 or less.* These countries, which account for approximately one-third of the world's population, face especially severe constraints because of an acute lack of financial resources and of trained manpower relative to the magnitude of the interrelated problems they encounter in accelerating economic growth and in reducing malnutrition and other serious manifestations of poverty.

Certain structural and demographic features impose additional constraints on the feasibility of alternative development strategies. In virtually all of the 34 low-income countries, between 70 and 80% of their populations and labor force still depend on agriculture for employment and income (3, p. 102; 5, Chapter 2). This means that the success or failure of efforts at the village level will be the major factor determining the extent to which nutritional and other severe deprivations are reduced. Furthermore, the present dominance of agriculture in their populations and labor force, in combination with high growth rates in their total populations and populations of working age, means that the great majority of their people will continue to reside in villages for at least several decades. The effects of this arithmetic of population growth and structural transformation are illustrated by a comparison with the experience of the industrialized European countries at the turn of the century. Because of a much slower decline in mortality, the upsurge in their rates of population growth and numbers in their labor force was moderate. Their labor force was growing at less than 1% per year, and growth of industrial employment at that time was sufficient to absorb nearly half of the

---

*See World Bank (3, pp. 77ff). The *World Development Report, 1979* (4) uses a 1977 per capita GDP of $300 as the cutoff between low- and middle-income countries and includes 37 countries in the category as compared to 34 in the 1978 report.

annual increments to the total labor force. In contrast, today's "Low-income countries, because of their much higher labor force growth rate, have absorbed less than 20% of their additional workers into industry each year . . ." (4, p. 46).*

A major thesis of this paper is that faulty diagnosis and, closely related to this, the lack of consensus concerning the basic requirements for a feasible and effective food and nutrition strategy, are significant factors underlying the failure to make any significant progress in the reduction of malnutrition and related deprivations. Field's description (2) of "the ideology of nutrition planning" is a useful point of departure for identifying the reasons for the present impasse and also for identifying more feasible policies. He argues that nutrition planners face an agonizing choice between a probably futile effort to promote "multisectoral reform" and "a significant re-structuring of socio-economic relations and an often major re-distribution of wealth" versus settling for promoting "creeping incrementalism" within the framework of an established political order (2, p. 237). Field asserts that, within the noncommunist developing countries, malnutrition " . . . is being addressed, if addressed at all, by nutrition planning" (2, p. 239). Although he argues that nutrition planning is becoming the "dominant mode" of approaching nutrition problems in today's developing countries, Field emphasizes that there is considerable ambiguity concerning the meaning of the term because the "intellectual establishment view" and the "bureaucratic view" of nutrition planning are fundamentally different. His description of the former is worth quoting at length because, as he rightly suggests, it is a widely shared view:

> Nutrition planning covers anything and everything that is thought to impinge upon nutritional status. There may be certain discrete interventions which, by common consensus, are nutrition interventions (fortification, child-feeding, mother education, etc.), but nutrition planning—potentially at least, and ideally—covers much more: from micro-level activities to macro-level planning designed to influence the production, distribution,

---

*Actually, the outcome is influenced powerfully both by the initial weight of agriculture in the labor force and by the rate of growth of the total labor force. Thus, in a country that has 70% of its labor force in agriculture in the initial year, associated with growth rates for its total and non-agricultural labor force of 2.5 and 4.0%, respectively, it would take 52 years to reach the turning point when its farm work force begins to decline. But if agriculture's share in the total labor force in the initial period had already declined to 50%, only 16 years would be required to reach that turning point. However, with 70% of the labor force initially dependent on agriculture, and with non-agricultural employment increasing at the same 4.0% rate, it would require 96 instead of 52 years to reach the turning point, if the total labor force were increasing at 3.0% rather than 2.5% per year (6, p. 127).

consumption, and absorption of nutrients. One's purview is sweeping, embracing food policies in their entirety, also much in the realm of public health, environmental sanitation and the like, and extending all the way to export-import policies and a country's overall development strategy. Good nutrition planning analyzes the entire "nutrition system" and seeks to intervene, as appropriate, at any point where improvement can be postulated as important to the nutritional well-being of clearly specified vulnerable groups. This mental set assumes that malnutrition is a reasonably high-priority concern of public policy and that the nutrition planner's duty is to determine the most cost-effective means of addressing it. The basic question asked is, How can we best remedy an observed nutritional deficiency in a particular setting? In search of an answer, one's professional gaze spans virtually the entire range of public policies, resources, and constraints that might apply.

In contrast, the "bureaucratic view" is " . . . quite restricted: supplementary feeding, child-care education of mothers, and food fortification especially, and perhaps exclusively" (2, p. 230).

It is my contention that the intellectual establishment view is a striking illustration of the tendency for " . . . many otherwise competent and reasonable people . . . to equate the desirable with the feasible" (7, p. 50). By proposing to subsume a vast range of socioeconomic policies and programs under "nutrition planning," one is advocating an approach that is neither politically feasible nor administratively workable. The more limited "bureaucratic view" is feasible in the sense that food fortification, supplementary feeding, and similar schemes can be, and are, undertaken in a number of developing countries. However, they cannot be expected to add up to a food and nutrition strategy that will be effective in reducing the malnutrition that is such a serious and widespread problem in low-income developing countries.*

What the two views have in common is " . . . the working premise . . . that a few resources plus good planning and programming inputs can make a meaningful impact on nutrition regardless of the nature of society, the distribution of political power, control over wealth, even the broad pattern of development" (2, p. 238). That view had a certain plausibility so long as the "protein gap" view of the world's nutrition problem held sway. Even now it is important to recognize that there is scope for reduction of specific nutrient deficiencies. In particular, in regions where goitre is a serious problem, allocating a few resources and providing the good programming required to insure that the inhabitants of those regions use iodized salt is a very cost-effective means of eliminat-

---

*It is suggested in the following section that redistributive measures, such as free or subsidized distribution of food, probably have a more important role to play in middle-income countries such as Brazil or Mexico.

ing goitre. Similar possibilities appear to exist with respect to vitamin A and iron deficiencies. A strong case can be made, however, that a more self-reliant approach, emphasizing expanded local production and consumption of leafy green vegetables and other good sources of those nutrients, is a more promising alternative for coping with vitamin A and iron deficiencies in rural areas.

To the extent that, in most situations, protein–energy malnutrition (PEM) is associated with inadequate intake of *food*, it becomes apparent that both the "intellectual establishment" and "bureaucratic" views of nutrition planning are based on faulty premises. It is time, I believe, to say bluntly that at least for low-income countries, these views are based on defective analysis and that they divert attention from policy designs that might be feasible and effective. The major thesis of this paper is that the mix of policies and programs that constitute a country's food and nutrition stragegy *must* be concerned with the *rate* and *pattern* of agricultural development in order to expand the availability of food *and* the ability of low-income households to raise their levels of food intake. Depending upon the sociopolitical situation in a particular country, this may or may not require radical changes in the distribution of political power and in control over wealth; but changes in the broad pattern of development are a *sine qua non* whether achieved by radical or reformist means. It also seems likely that broad-based agricultural strategies must be supplemented by an integrated nutrition, health, and population program capable of achieving broad coverage of the rural population.

POLICY ANALYSIS AND THE DESIGN OF EFFECTIVE FOOD AND NUTRITION STRATEGIES

Reducing nutritional problems at the village level clearly involves a number of sectors, but it is important to simplify the problem by focusing on two of these sectors—agriculture and health. I interpret "nutrition interventions," whether or not they carry the label "nutrition," as activities that have a significant impact on the nutritional status of village populations. I will argue later that it is important to take an integrated or "systems" view of the determinants of the well-being of a country's rural population; but in general, efforts to integrate a range of activities *administratively* should be avoided. I am persuaded, however, by the evidence and arguments suggesting that nutrition, health, and family planning activities are so closely interrelated at the village level—and potentially so mutually reinforcing—that the benefits of linking them within a single program seem to outweigh the costs and complexity of creating and managing a program that attempts to span a range of activities.

Good Policy Analysis and "Learning to Plan — and Planning to Learn"*

I have asserted that "nutrition planning" has failed and will continue to fail, but I want to state as emphatically as possible that I am in complete agreement with the viewpoint espoused by "nutrition advocates" that nutritional objectives can and should receive a high priority in the design of development strategies in low-income countries. The failure of past development efforts to have a greater impact in reducing malnutrition has no doubt been influenced to some extent by a tendency to ignore or deemphasize the extent and seriousness of nutritional problems in developing countries.

It seems likely, for example, that awareness of and support for nutrition and nutrition-related activities in the Philippines have been increased by Operation Timbang, a nationwide program organized by the Nutrition Center of the Philippines to assess the nutritional status of all preschool children on the basis of weight-for-age measurements. However, I see little evidence to support the implicit assumption underlying the recent emphasis on nutritional surveillance that failure to adopt and implement effective policies for the reduction of malnutrition is mainly a result of ignorance concerning the extent and seriousness of nutritional problems. But I do argue later that integrated nutrition, health, and population programs that include nutritional screening procedures to identify malnourished infants and small children within a village can increase the likelihood that effective action will be taken by the local community to reduce the incidence of malnutrition.

Past shortcomings have also been influenced by the resistance of various social groups that have been opposed to economic and social changes that might affect their interests adversely, and who have been able to wield substantial political and economic power. Migdal (9, p. 193) expresses this aspect tersely and well when he states that

> Policymaking takes place within a highly politicized environment. It demands choosing a particular direction for action when various groups in the society might prefer action in different directions while other groups want no action at all.

*This phrase is the title of a provocative book by D. N. Michael (8).

Also, his assertion that

> Policy scientists have often tended to analyze and formulate population pol-
> icies for Third World societies in a political vacuum, focusing on techniques
> and ignoring the political context within which policies are first formulated
> and later implemented (9, p. 188)

is equally applicable to nutrition planners and others concerned with the
design of nutrition policies. I believe, however, that it would be oversimplified and misleading to conclude that failure to adopt policies and programs that would serve a broader national interest, such as the reduction
of nutritional and other severe deprivations of the poor, is simply a consequence of the resistance of groups opposed to change that might
threaten their vested interests.

A major theme running through the literature on organizational
choice is to emphasize the extreme and often misleading simplification
that characterizes the usual models of decision-making, such as the Rational Actor Model, which assumes that policy decisions, organizational
actions, and their impact on society are adequately explained as being
" ... the more or less purposive acts of unified national governments"
(10, pp. 4,5). Even when it is recognized that decisions and outcomes may
be determined either by a bureaucratic–administrative procedure or by
bargaining–political procedures, it is usually assumed that decision-making is related to (1) objectives that can be stated with considerable precision; (2) a set of technologies that enable us to know the outcomes that
will be associated with alternative choices; and (3) well-defined preferences of the various participants in the decision-making process. The
reality is much more complex and ambiguous. All three assumptions are
perhaps especially dubious in the context in which decisions are made
with respect to food and nutrition strategies. But the fact that such a
naive model of decision-making " ... under-estimates the ambiguity of
self-interest" and that " ... beliefs and preferences appear to be the
results of behaviour as much as they are determinants of it" are certainly
among the important deficiencies.*

It is my contention that a major reason for the failure of past efforts
to identify and mobilize support for effective policies and programs to
reduce malnutrition is because development decision-makers have not
benefitted from useful research and good policy analysis to the extent

---

*The quotations are from a recent book (11, pp. 15,24) by March *et al.* that is an important
recent addition to the rich literature on organizational choice and behavior. Their
emphasis on "participant attention" is also highly relevant to the issues discussed in this
paper; see especially Chapters 1 and 3.

that it is possible and desirable. Morgan (12, p. 971) states that the object of good policy analysis " . . . is to evaluate, order, and structure incomplete knowledge so as to allow decisions to be made with as complete an understanding as possible of the current state of knowledge, its limitations, and its implications." Because the design of development strategies must take account of a host of variables and complex, changing interrelations among those variables, complete knowledge and understanding are impossible. Moreover, decisions will unavoidably be influenced by opinions, preferences, values, and vested interests. Nevertheless, good policy analysis can, as Morgan argues (12), order and structure incomplete knowledge " . . . in ways that are open and explicit" and it can avoid drawing " . . . hard conclusions unless thay are warranted by unambiguous data or well-founded theoretical insight."

I will argue shortly that some of the implications that can be derived from our knowledge of the economic, structural, and demographic characteristics of the low-income countries point to certain "hard conclusions" and that our efforts to achieve the multiple and interrelated objectives of development are bound to fail if those implications and conclusions are ignored. I will, however, be putting forth some additional conclusions for which the underlying evidence is incomplete and frequently ambiguous.

There is clearly a need for both better research and better analysis to assist decision-makers in formulating policies and programs that are well designed, feasible, and capable of commanding sufficient support to be implemented effectively. But no amount of research and analysis will eliminate uncertainty and avoid the mistakes that are inevitable in such a complex undertaking. Hence, it is essential to stress the importance of "planning to learn" and the need for a continuing process of policy design and redesign and for a monitoring of policy implementation to provide feedback and guidance for revising policies and programs in order to increase their effectiveness.

Implementation cannot even begin, however, until there is sufficient consensus for the adoption of recommended policies and for the political leaders and government decision-makers and administrators to provide the resources required to translate those policies into operational programs or projects. It would be naive to underestimate the difficulty of reaching the degree of consensus concerning development policies and programs that is a necessary condition for effective action. Those difficulties are so great in the field of nutrition planning that it is hardly surprising that, with very few exceptions, the nutrition programs that have been adopted are, as Field put it, " . . . little more than palliatives, in effect if not in intent" (2).

In designing development strategies, attention should be given to the *composition* and the *distribution* of the goods and services that are produced as well as to the *rate of growth* of average per capita income. It is precisely for that reason that the debate about development strategies is bound to be influenced so strongly by conflicting interest groups and by the political and economic power of those groups. However, substantive disagreement will also arise because of divergent views about the weight to be given to various objectives, and because of different perceptions concerning the policies and programs that will be most effective in attaining given goals. Even when there is general agreement that a very high priority should be given to the objective of reducing nutritional and other serious deprivations, judgments will differ with respect to what is possible and desirable in both general and specific country situations.

In brief, it is not easy to agree on what is, in fact, good policy analysis of the complex issues that arise in designing food and nutrition strategies. Even the economic analysis of the issues relevant to the choice of food price policies is extremely complex (13).

An important source of difficulty in reaching agreed upon conclusions derives from trade-offs between short-run and long-term effects. Thus, Timmer's review of the symposium volume edited by T. W. Schultz (14), *Distortions in Agricultural Incentives*, concludes that

> Schuh in particular, and the other authors in general, are saying that higher food prices in the short-run are needed to provide lower food prices in the long-run and that sharply improved incentives for agricultural production will ultimately raise productivity and incomes sufficiently for poverty to be eliminated.

But Timmer goes on to suggest that even though a "cheap food" policy has adverse effects on incentives and on the rate of increase in food production, politicians may well be right in the weight they give to the short-run objective of holding down consumer prices, because higher food prices have such severe adverse effects on the food intake and nutritional status of the poor. He clinches that argument to his satisfaction by recalling a statement made by Harry Hopkins during the New Deal: "People don't eat in the long-run; they eat every day or they starve."

Clearly, an important part of the appeal of nutrition planning is the hope that it can make possible short-cuts in eliminating malnutrition in low-income countries. Thus Berg (15, p. 12) argues that

> 150 million Indians must at least double their current incomes if they are to be able to buy even the minimum acceptable diets. Unless a new strategy is evolved to shortcut the traditional means of providing nutrition, it will be near the turn of the century before the poorest third of India's population can afford a minimum adequate diet.

The common tendency among nutrition advocates to disparage the role of development—"the traditional means of providing nutrition"— is reinforced by the widespread tendency to condemn "trickle down" policies. The persistence of poverty, and indeed the continuing increase in the magnitude of malnutrition and other manifestations of poverty in many developing countries, constitute a severe indictment of the development strategies that have been pursued in those countries.*

CHARACTERISTICS OF THE LOW-INCOME COUNTRIES AND THEIR POLICY OPTIONS

There has been a lively debate as to whether there has been an increase in the percentage of India's population falling below a poverty line that has been defined in various ways. There seems little doubt, however, that the absolute numbers subject to poverty have increased substantially during the past two decades in spite of considerable, and in some ways impressive, efforts to develop the Indian economy. This is obviously not the place to explore the strengths and weaknesses of India's development strategies.† It is useful, however, to emphasize two features of India's experience that are of great relevance to the problems confronting most of the low-income developing countries.

First, in spite of the very considerable industrial growth that has occurred in India, there has been only a slight decline in the percentage of the population and labor force dependent on agriculture.‡ Especially for the postwar period, when there was accelerated growth of the country's population and labor force, this is largely a consequence of the arithmetic of population growth and structural transformation that was emphasized earlier. One implication of the continuing dominance of agriculture in India's population and labor force, which is supported by direct evidence, is that poverty is, to a considerable extent, concentrated in rural areas.

---

*Recent World Bank publications (3, p. 33; 4, p. 19) estimate the "number of absolute poor" at 750 million and the projections for the year 2000 range from 470 to 710 million. The large differences in estimates of the extent of malnutrition in the developing world emphasize the conceptual as well as the statistical difficulties of quantifying even such a relatively clear-cut manifestation of poverty as malnutrition (16,17).

†The relevant literature is huge, but I find Bhagwati and Desai (18) and Mellor (19) especially useful.

‡Available statistics suggest that the agricultural labor force was 67% of the total in 1931 in prepartition India; the postindependence figures for the Indian Union are: 72% in 1951, 73% in 1961, and 69% in 1970 (20, Appendix Table 5; 3, p. 102).

Second, there has been a substantial reduction in the average size of farm holdings in India—from 6.3 acres in 1953–1954, to 3.8 acres in 1971–1972. More directly relevant to the increase in absolute poverty is that over the same period, the number of marginal holdings of less than an acre increased from 15.4 million to 35.6 million households; and the average area in those marginal holdings has declined from 0.27 to 0.14 acre. Many factors have been involved in that doubling of the number of marginal households, including increases in the size of many large ownership units and probably a somewhat more pervasive increase in the size of operational units where the profitability of high-yielding varieties and the availability of tractors at relatively cheap prices has encouraged large landowners to evict tenants and go in for direct cultivation. However, these changes pointing to an increasing concentration of agricultural land in large units have been more than offset by other forces. A 66% increase in the number of farm households that was associated with a negligible increase in the cultivated area from 305 to 311 million acres appears to have resulted in a considerable subdivision of large holdings as well as a large increase in marginal holdings.

To be sure, the increase in the number of marginal holdings and the degree of landlessness of those households could have been mitigated to some extent by more vigorous implementation of India's land reform legislation. The evidence, however, seems to support Vyas's conclusion that "... a combination of legislative, market-induced, and extraconstitutional moves ..." has challenged the traditional " ... hegemony of large landholders" (21, p. 18). Between 1953 and 1954, and 1971 and 1972 the number of "big" landowners (15–50 acres) declined moderately in number from 4.3 to less than 4.1 million units, and the number of "large" holdings (50 acres and above) was reduced sharply from 604 to 350 thousand. Moreover, the share of the area owned by "big" farmers was also reduced moderately from 35 to 31% of the total, and the share of land in "large" holdings declined dramatically from 18 to 8% of the total (see Table 1).

There is, of course, considerable variation even among the low-income developing countries in the operation of these structural and demographic factors that impose significant constraints on the development options that are feasible. The pressure of rural population growth on the land and the resulting subdivision of holdings have created considerably more acute problems in Bangladesh and in Java than in India, whereas limits on expanding the area under cultivation have been much less severe in the countries of tropical Africa. Nevertheless, the problems that lie ahead in absorbing a growing labor force into productive employment are perhaps more acute in Africa than in India because of

TABLE 1. Estimated Number of Households and Area Owned by Different Size Groups of Holdings (All India)[a]

| | Number of households and area owned (×10³) | | | | | | | | |
| | 1953–1954 | | | 1961–1962 | | | 1971–1972 | | |
Size group of ownership holdings	No. of households	Area owned (acres)	Average area (acres)	No. of households	Area owned (acres)	Average area (acres)	No. of households	Area owned (acres)	Average area (acres)
Marginal (below 1 acre)	15,360 (31.43)[b]	4,166 (1.36)	0.27	23,579 (36.84)	5,062 (1.59)	0.21	35,640 (43.99)	4,910 (1.58)	0.14
Small (1–4.99)	17,448 (35.71)	45,670 (14.95)	2.62	22,468 (35.11)	58,645 (18.39)	2.60	27,415 (33.84)	71,158 (22.86)	2.60
Medium (5–14.99)	11,145 (22.81)	95,230 (31.18)	8.54	13,002 (20.32)	109,703 (34.52)	8.44	13,564 (16.74)	112,464 (36.13)	8.29
Big (15–49.99)	4,306 (8.81)	106,795 (34.97)	24.80	4,514 (7.05)	109,252 (34.37)	24.20	4,058 (5.01)	98,856 (31.12)	23.87
Large (50 and above)	604 (1.24)	53,580 (17.54)	88.71	437 (0.68)	35,379 (11.31)	80.96	350 (0.43)	28,856 (8.31)	73.87
Total	48,863 (100.00)	305,441 (100.00)	6.25	64,000 (100.00)	317,861 (100.00)	4.97	81,027 (100.00)	311,244 (100.00)	3.84

[a] Reproduced from Vyas (21, p. 4). Based on data from various rounds of the National Sample Survey: NSS No. 36, 8th Round for 1953–1954; NSS no. 144, 17th round for 1961–1962; and NSS No. 215, 26th Round for 1971–1972, Tables on Land Holdings, Cabinet Secretariat, Government of India.
[b] Figures in parentheses are percentages of the total.

the small size of the fledgling industrial sectors in those countries and the higher rates of natural population increase that prevail.

The longer-term prospects in Kenya, for example, point to even more difficult problems than in India, if only because of the considerably higher rate of population increase—some 3.5% compared to about 2.1% in India—and the great difficulty of bringing about a reduction in fertility in Kenya, where more than 80% of the population is still dependent on agriculture, and the traditional attitudes that reinforce the large family norm appear to be considerably stronger. Although Kenya was one of the first African countries to adopt a population policy, the efforts to promote family planning have not yet had much impact. The development plan for 1979–1983 (22, p. 130) expresses the hope that sufficient progress has been made in building up an infrastructure for the delivery of family planning services that the current plan period will see the beginning of a reduction in the country's rate of population growth. Because many of those who will be added to the labor force by the year 2000 have been, or will be, born before the anticipated increase in family planning will have its effect, the 118% increase in the potential labor force between 1978 and 2000 with a declining birth rate is only a little less than the 125% increase anticipated with a constant birth rate. On the other hand, the projected increase in the number of primary school age would be a relatively manageable 75% with a declining birth rate, compared to a 141% increase between 1978 and the year 2000 with a constant birth rate. A similar marked contrast applies to the resource requirements for achieving more adequate coverage of rural areas in the provision of health services, especially if priority is given to the needs of infants and small children (22, p. 63).

The implications of continued rapid growth of a country's population and labor force obviously become more dramatic as the time horizon is extended because of the compounding that characterizes population growth. A recent set of projections for Kenya traces the effects on population growth until the year 2024 of six scenarios of possible changes in fertility and mortality that might take place between 1969 and 1999 (23). The most likely estimate according to projections by Shah and Willekens (23) is for a nearly sixfold increase in Kenya's population, from 10.9 million in 1969 to 64.3 million in 2024. Their projections, which are broken down by age group and by rural–urban location, are also interesting in their implications concerning the problems of labor absorption and of transforming the structure of Kenya's overwhelmingly agrarian economy.

On the basis of fairly optimistic estimates concerning the growth of nonfarm employment, they project that the share of the rural work force in the total would decline from 87 to 65% between 1969 and 2024. A six-fold increase in the total population of the economically active age group would be associated with a sixteenfold increase in the active-age population in urban areas; but even so there would be a fourfold increase in the rural work force (23, p. 29; 24, pp. 36–37).

The evidence from India and Kenya provides a useful background for examining the issues raised earlier with respect to food price policy and the trickle down view of development. Although I am equally critical of Schuh's essay (25) on basic needs and equity, I believe that his analysis is defective for reasons that are more fundamental than Timmer's criticism (14) of his neglect of the adverse short-run welfare effects of moving away from a cheap food policy. After all, the more numerous rural poor are more likely to be harmed than helped by policies that depress agricultural prices. They are not likely to have access to rationed or subsidized distribution of food at artificially low prices, and those farm households that have little or no marketable surplus of food are likely to be affected adversely, because artificially depressing agricultural prices and incomes will tend to reduce the employment opportunities available to them in rural areas. In fact, such policies are typically an important manifestation of the urban bias that has often had harmful effects on the well-being of rural populations in developing countries (26).

I agree with Castle (27, p. 328) that "Schuh's major thesis is that policies to promote the generation of additional income streams should be uncoupled from policies to redistribute income or wealth." Schuh is here expressing the orthodox view based on the compensation principle of modern welfare economics, that is, to argue for the "efficient choice" and then to supplement that decision with " . . . the necessary distributional adjustment through a tax-transfer mechanism" (28, p. 804). But where poverty is a pervasive phenomenon and fiscal constraints are severe, distributional adjustments through a tax-transfer mechanism almost certainly will not be carried out on any significant scale. Furthermore, conclusions with respect to the "efficient choice" are likely to be inappropriate in terms of the broader and more dynamic concept of efficiency that should guide the design of agricultural development strategies in low-income countries.

My other principal criticism of Schuh's analysis relates to the common tendency of both economists and technical specialists to ignore constraints that derive from the structural and demographic characteristics of low-income countries. Thus, Schuh asserts that it is misguided to believe that the choice of production technology should be influenced by the relative abundance of labor in agriculture. He argues that " . . . to increase employment in agriculture rather than to attack the fundamental problems causing low labor absorption in the industrial sector . . ." is " . . . to deal with symptoms rather than fundamental causes" (25, p. 321). His general conclusion (p. 322) is that

> Policies for alleviating rural poverty must be directed to giving rural workers the skills they need for alternative employment, to promoting more efficient labor markets, and to removing the anti-employment bias of development policy by reducing the factor-price distortions in the economy at large.

Schuh's assertion that the fundamental problems pertain to low-labor absorption in the industrial sector ignores the structural/demographic characteristics of low-income countries.

However, the elimination of price distortions that have an antiemployment bias, such as an overvalued exchange rate and underpricing of capital, is clearly an important concern in many developing countries. Moreover, distortions of factor and product prices have been among the forces that have so often encouraged premature tractor mechanization and dualistic development of agriculture, in which increases in productivity and output are confined to a large-scale, relatively capital-intensive subsector, and, therefore, yield very slight benefits in expanding employment opportunities and reducing rural poverty. The "trickle" of benefits that reaches down to the poor is bound to be very small indeed under those circumstances.

But it is a hard conclusion in the case of countries where the economically active population is increasing rapidly, and where a large share of the labor force still depends on agriculture, that the bulk of the annual additions to the country's labor force must be absorbed by the agricultural sector. Also, given the severe resource constraints and administrative problems that limit the scope for direct action to alleviate poverty through income redistribution, it also appears to be a hard conclusion that the design and effective implementation of a broad-based strategy for agricultural development is the most fundamental requirement for reducing poverty and malnutrition at the village level. Therefore, it is absolutely essential for the goal of accelerating the increase in agricultural output to be coupled with a pattern of agricultural development that enables a large and increasing fraction of the farm population to participate in gains in productivity and output. Simply to rely on a continuation of traditional labor-intensive technologies is not a viable solution. The challenge is to identify and foster the diffusion of combinations and sequences of technological innovations that will achieve the twofold objectives of expanding food production and reducing rural poverty.

Rapid growth of agricultural output is a necessary condition for meeting the requirements of a growing population and for raising the food intake levels of the low-income households where malnutrition is concentrated. But it is not a sufficient condition. Poor households must either acquire increased purchasing power or increase their capability to expand home production, or the need for increased food intake will not be translated into effective demand and higher levels of food consumption.

It is my contention that the economic, structural, and demographic characteristics of the low-income countries and the constraints they impose lead to the conclusion that the design of development strategies should be guided explicitly by the need to achieve multiple objectives. As a minimum, those objectives should include: (1) accelerated expansion of agricultural and nonagricultural output; (2) expansion of farm and nonfarm employment opportunities (including improved income-earning opportunities for self-employed family labor, which is such an important part of the total labor force in the low-income countries); (3) reduction of malnutrition, excessive morbidity and mortality, and other especially severe manifestations of poverty; and (4) decrease in population growth. Failure is inevitable if we continue to equate the desirable with the feasible and assert that easy, shortcut solutions are available. Constraints cannot be wished away, and external aid can supplement, but not substitute for, national policies and programs that are well designed to achieve these multiple objectives.

This is an argument *not* in the defense of trickle-down policies, nor is it a defeatist view of the prospects for rapid progress in attaining the economic and social goals of development. Taiwan, South Korea, and the People's Republic of China (PRC) are notable examples of countries that have made rapid progress in achieving all four objectives under very different economic and political regimes. Legitimate questions can be raised about the applicability of their experience in today's low-income countries. The progress achieved in the PRC clearly has depended largely on a high degree of social regimentation and control, including a drastic redistribution of land and other productive assets, combined with a great deal of pragmatism, for example, in the willingness to modify policies in order to secure a workable balance between equity objectives and production incentives.

Extraordinarily rapid growth of nonfarm output and employment in Taiwan and South Korea has been related to the rapid expansion of production for export and to the availability of substantial external assis-

*See Hsing (29) for a careful assessment of the influence of foreign aid on Taiwan's rate of growth.

tance, although the importance of the latter should not be exaggerated.* The success in narrowing differentials in income distribution was also influenced favorably by their postwar land reform programs. However, the broad-based pattern of agricultural development in Taiwan and South Korea was mainly a legacy from the period of Japanese colonial rule when the Japanese model of broad-based agricultural development was introduced in order to accelerate the growth of agricultural production in the former colonies to provide expanded food imports to Japan as well as to meet the growth of local demand. Agricultural research institutions that generated a sequence of divisible, yield-increasing innovations, and expansion and improvement of irrigation and drainage that facilitated multiple cropping as well as better water control for individual crops, were critical elements in the progressive modernization of the uniformly small-scale farm units that dominated agricultural production.

Progress in eradicating rural poverty in the PRC has also owed a great deal to the priority that was given to a broad-based strategy of agricultural development. Recent modifications of agricultural policies suggest that the present leadership in China is convinced that production incentives have not been sufficiently strong to elicit the effort and the initiative required for accelerated growth and production. Nevertheless, it seems clear that the decentralization of agricultural decision-making in the early 1960s did much to overcome the acute problems that were encountered in the first phase of launching the rural communes as a key organizational innovation for rural development. Instead of individually operated farm units, the key farm management unit in the PRC has been the production team of some 30–40 households, but the emphasis on labor-using, yield-increasing innovations associated with substantial expansion and improvements in irrigation and drainage has been similar to the strategies pursued in Taiwan and South Korea. It is also noteworthy that the positive interactions between agricultural and industrial development made an important contribution to the decentralized development of small- and medium-scale manufacturing enterprises in all three countries.*

The other notable similarity in the experience of Taiwan, South Korea, and the PRC is that the development of health services appears to have achieved broad coverage of their rural populations by emphasizing low-cost preventive and promotive measures, including immunization, environmental sanitation and hygiene, and the use of health auxiliaries.

*For the Taiwan experience in agricultural development and agriculture–industry interactions, see Reference 20 (Chapters 5 and 8). For the PRC, see Perkins *et al.* (30) for the decentralized development of small- and medium-scale industry, and Timmer (31), Chinn (32), and Tang (33) for summary analyses of the pattern of agricultural development.

China's "barefoot doctor" program has received a great deal of attention in recent years. However, simple but effective public health measures had achieved a substantial reduction in mortality levels in Taiwan even during the period of Japanese rule (34). A significant achievement of this broad coverage of the rural population is that the large reductions in crude death rates (CDRs) in these countries seem to have included a reduction of infant and child mortality to levels only moderately above those prevailing in the high-income, developed countries.

Finally, it is important to note that in all three countries, the decline in mortality has been followed by extraordinarily rapid reductions in fertility. In the case of Taiwan and South Korea, for which the data are relatively good, the decline in the crude birth rates (CBRs) between 1960 and 1977 greatly exceeded the reductions in CDRs. For South Korea, a decline in the CDR from 13 to 8 per thousand was associated with a reduction in the CBR from 41 to 21 per thousand. In Taiwan, the CBR dropped from 40 to 21 per thousand, while the CDR declined from 7 to 5 per thousand. Thus, the rates of natural increase in 1975 were reduced by 1.5 and 1.7 percentage points, respectively, compared to the rates that would have prevailed with constant fertility. The estimates of vital rates for the PRC are much less reliable, but according to the latest estimates published by the World Bank (4, p. 161), the 1960–1977 decline in the CBR from 36 to 22 per thousand was also substantially larger than the estimated reduction in the CDR from 16 to 9 per thousand.

Although the contemporary low-income countries have experienced substantial reductions in overall mortality, infant and child mortality levels are frequently shockingly high—often 100–150 per thousand compared to approximately 15 per thousand in Taiwan and in the high-income developed countries. Although mortality data for the 1–4 age group are sketchy, it seems clear that the differentials are even higher during that period of life in which mortality rates are so strongly related to nutritional status.

The significance of these unacceptably high levels of infant and child mortality in the low-income countries is accentuated by two closely related factors. First, these high mortality levels are associated with appalling levels of morbidity. According to a recent study in a Guatemalan village, just over half of the 1- to 3-year-old children were sick on an average day (35). A British pediatrician who has been studying the health problems of developing countries for many years estimates that child morbidity rates in these countries tend to be some five to ten times higher than in the developed countries (36).

Second, the two-way interactions between poor nutritional status and frequent bouts of infection and other health problems have serious adverse effects on both the physical and mental development of children. Particularly in the case of severe malnutrition in infancy, the impaired mental development may be a result of physiological factors. But the most persuasive evidence is related to the behavioral conse-quences of the syndrome of malnutrition, frequent illness, and apathy (37).

Fortunately, there is encouraging evidence that retarded mental development that is mainly a consequence of these behavioral effects of malnutrition and ill health need not be permanent. Thus, a highly sig-nificant conclusion of a major study carried out in Columbia is that " . . . combined nutritional, health, and educational treatments between 3.5 and 7 years of age can prevent large losses of potential cognitive ability, with significantly greater effect the earlier the treatments begin" (38, p. 277). That study did not include children younger than 3.5 years. How-ever, because a large deficit in cognitive ability was already apparent in the children subjected to nutritional and other poverty-related depriva-tions, it seems probable that this initial cognitive deficit could have been reduced significantly by action to improve the nutritional status and health of the children during the critical period from birth to age 3.5 years.

This brief account of the characteristics of today's low-income coun-tries, and of the experience of three whose economic, structural, and demographic characteristics were similar to the low-income countries until their recent success in reducing rural poverty, clearly directs atten-tion to the central importance of a country's strategy for rural develop-ment. Their progress toward realizing the half-completed demographic transition that typifies the contemporary low-income countries by reduc-ing fertility at a rapid rate is also noteworthy. It is scarcely a hard con-clusion, but the presumption is strong that the progress that they have also achieved in completing a partial health revolution by providing broad coverage of rural areas and dramatically reducing infant and child mortality were major factors contributing to the rapid decline in fertility.

Leaving aside the "city states" of Hong Kong and Singapore, there were ten other developing countries besides Taiwan and South Korea that significantly reduced their rates of population increase between 1960 and 1975, defining a "significant" decline somewhat arbitrarily as a CBR reduction that exceeded the decline in CDR by more than 5 per thousand. By that definition, Sri Lanka was the only low-income country to experience a significant decline in the rate of population increase between 1960 and 1975; reduction in the CBR from 36 to 27 per thousand was associated with a decline in the CDR from 10 to 9 per thousand. The infant mortality rate in Sri Lanka in 1975 was 45 per thousand, compared to an average of about 120 per thousand for the 34 low-income countries. In addition, its literacy rate was much higher, and the percentage of the labor force dependent on agriculture was much lower than was typical of other low-income countries. (See Table 2 for these and other comparisons among the 12 countries with significant declines in fertility, and average figures for 34 low-income countries, 58 middle-income countries, and 11 centrally planned economies).*

Although Costa Rica's per capita GDP is well above the levels prevailing in the low-income developing countries, it is noteworthy that a substantial strengthening of rural health services and a decline in the country's CDR from 10 to 6 per thousand between 1960 and 1975 was associated with a remarkable reduction in fertility—from 47 to 29 per thousand.

Trinidad experienced an equally large net change in its rate of population growth between 1960 and 1975, but its experience is of limited relevance to the low-income countries because agriculture's share in the labor force had already declined to 22% in 1960, and the 1976 per capita GDP was some 15 times the average for the low-income developing countries, and the literacy rate was about 4 times higher.

AGRICULTURAL AND HEALTH STRATEGIES IN THE REDUCTION OF MALNUTRITION AT THE VILLAGE LEVEL

The analysis of some of the most significant characteristics of the low-income developing countries, and of the major implications of those characteristics, has directed attention to the central importance of a country's strategy for agricultural development. The development experience of Taiwan, South Korea, and the PRC provides additional support for that finding. Their experience also suggests that the ability of a country's health strategy to achieve broad coverage of rural areas is a critical factor in reducing unacceptably high levels of infant and child morbidity and mortality. It also seems probable that the effectiveness of efforts to reduce fertility and population growth rates can be enhanced considerably by completing the health revolution that has already reduced overall mor-

---

*As noted above, the latest estimates for the PRC published by the World Bank (4, p. 161) indicate that the decline in China's rate of population increase was also significant. However, this is not included in Table 2, which is based on estimates indicating that the decline in the CBR between 1960 and 1975 was only from 31 to 26 per thousand, i.e., slightly less than the estimated reduction in CDRs from 16 to 9 (3, p. 105). The considerable change in the 1960 figures for China's CBR emphasizes the wide margin of uncertainty concerning vital statistics.

TABLE 2. Crude Birth Rates (CBR) and Crude Death Rates (CDR) (per 1000) and Related Statistics in Various Groups of Countries, and in Individual Countries with Significant Declines in Population Increase Rates[a]

Country/group average	1960[b] CBR	1960[b] CDR	1975[b] CBR	1975[b] CDR	1960-1975 Change in natural increase (% points)	1975 Infant mortality (per 1000)	1974 Adult literacy rate (%)	1976 Per capita GNP (U.S. dollars)	1960 Agriculture's share in labor force (%)	Percent of national income received by lowest 20%	Family planning effort[c]
Average of 34 low-income countries	48	26	47	20	+0.5	122	23	150	88		
Average of 58 middle-income countries	45	17	40	12	0.0	46	63	750	60		
Average of 11 centrally planned economies[d]	24	10	18	9	−0.5	NA	NA	2280	48		
Average of 12 countries with significant declines[e]	41	11	28	8	−1.0	43	82	1129	46	5.1	
Sri Lanka	36	10	27	9	−0.8	45	78	200	56	7.0	M[c]
Colombia	45	12	33	8	−0.8	56	74	630	51	4.0	M
Korea, Republic of	41	13	24	8	−1.2	38	92	670	66	10.0	S
Tunisia	47	19	34	13	−0.7	63	55	840	57	NA	M
Costa Rica	47	10	29	6	−1.2	38	89	1040	51	5.0	S
Chile	37	12	23	8	−1.0	79	90	1050	30	5.0	M
Taiwan	40	7	23	5	−1.5	14	82	1070	56	NA	S
Jamaica	39	10	30	7	−0.6	20	86	1070	39	NA[f]	S
Panama	41	10	31	7	−0.7	36	82	1310	51	3.0	M
Trinidad and Tobago	38	9	23	6	−1.2	38	90	2240	22	NA	M
Venezuela	46	10	37	7	−0.6	46	82	2570	35	2.0	W
Cuba[g]	33	9	21	6	−0.9	—	—	860	39	NA	M

[a] Data from World Bank (3, pp. 76, 102–105, 108–111); except for column 10, which was taken from World Bank (4, pp. 172–173), and column 11, taken from Cassen (61). NA, not available.

[b] A CBR decline that exceeded the CDR decline by more than 5 per 1000 is arbitrarily defined as "significant."

[c] Family planning effort is based on a classification of countries by Lapham and Mauldin (62), where S = Strong, M = Medium, W = Weak.

[d] In the Soviet Union and Poland, the CBRs declined from 24 to 18 and their CDRs remained constant at 8 and 9 per 1000, respectively. However, as industrialized countries that already had low rates of natural increase in 1960, their inclusion did not seem warranted. According to the estimates for China included in this source, the rate of natural increase had already declined to 1.5% in 1960. The estimated reduction in the CDR, from 16 to 9 per 1000 between 1960 and 1975, slightly exceeded the estimated decline in the CBR from 31 to 26.

[e] Hongkong and Singapore, with declines of 1.5 to 1.7%, respectively, in their rates of natural increase, are excluded because of their predominantly urban character.

[f] Estimated at 2% for 1960.

[g] The source gives no estimates for infant mortality in Cuba, but reports that in 1960 the population per physician was only 1200 compared to the 1960 estimates of 3050 and 37,000 for the middle-income and low-income categories.

tality sufficiently to give rise to the unprecedentedly high rates of population increase of from 2.5 to 3.5% that now prevail in most of the low-income countries.

But how does this relate to integrated, multisectoral nutrition interventions? The conclusion I draw is that the most feasible and effective approach to improving nutrition at the village level in the low-income countries requires a two-pronged approach that takes account of the significant difference between the determinants of nutritional status among older children and adults on the one hand, and among infants and small children on the other. For the former, there is strong evidence that malnutrition is related mainly to inadequate levels of food intake as a consequence of poverty. Hence, the most effective strategy for reducing undernutrition among those segments of the population is one that enhances the productivity and incomes of poor households by broad-based, employment-oriented development strategies. Moreover, increasing the availability of food at the household level obviously facilitates efforts to improve the nutritional status of infants and small children.

It seems clear, however, that to rely solely on production-oriented measures is an inefficient strategy for reducing the especially serious malnutrition prevalent among infants and small children, even when those measures are effective in ensuring broad participation in the gains in productivity and income. This conclusion is based on the considerable body of evidence suggesting that inadequate knowledge about child-feeding practices, and the two-way interactions between malnutrition and infection, are particularly significant causal factors responsible for the high morbidity and mortality, and the retarded physical and mental development of so many small children in poor countries.

Those causal factors derive, in part, from past effects of malnutrition on the stature and health of mothers that impair their ability to deliver a healthy child. Unfortunately, the effects on the stature of mothers, which increase the frequency of low birth weights among newborns, appear to be largely a consequence of malnutrition that the mothers experienced during their first two or three years of life. There is also evidence to suggest that reasonably adequate energy intake by mothers during pregnancy can substantially reduce the number of low birth-weight babies.

According to a recent study of rural Guatemalan women carried out by INCAP, 20% of the women with energy supplementation of less than 10 k cal during pregnancy gave birth to low-birth-weight babies, i.e., less than 2.5 kg. In contrast, less than 10% of the women who had an energy supplementation of 20 k cal or more had low-birth-weight infants. The significance of low birth weight is emphasized by a related study indicating that over half of the babies with birth weights of 1.5–3 kg and about a third of those averaging between 2 and 2.5 kg died, compared to only 2.3% of those with birth weights of 3 kg or more (39).

Malnutrition during infancy and early childhood affects mortality and morbidity first of all because it impairs many of the body's defense mechanisms against infectious disease. In addition, frequent bouts of diarrhea and other health problems contribute directly to malnutrition. This is in part a result of decreased food intake because of loss of appetite, or the common cultural practice of withholding solid food and even liquids when a child is sick. In addition, there is commonly reduced absorption of nutrients because of vomiting or malabsorption *per se*. In many cases, altered metabolism or parasitic infestation accentuates the nutritional deficiencies of infants and small children.

The other principal conclusion that emerges from the earlier discussion on policy analysis relates to the need to design development strategies so that they will be as effective as possible in attaining multiple objectives. Specifically, it was argued that there is a need to be concerned with at least four interrelated objectives: (1) accelerating the rate of growth of output; (2) expanding employment opportunities for a rapidly growing, working age population; (3) reducing the malnutrition and high rates of mortality and morbidity, especially among infants and small children, that represent such serious deprivations in low-income countries; and (4) slowing population growth.

Furthermore, it was suggested that this requires giving explicit attention to the *composition* and *distribution* of the goods and services made available in the development process, as well as to the rate of increase in output. Preston (40, p. 14) has offered persuasive evidence demonstrating that "unstructured" economic development is generally inefficient at reducing mortality levels compared to a more "structured" development, in which a larger fraction of a country's output of goods and services is allocated to educational expenditure and preventive health measures. It seems clear that efforts to improve nutritional status and to slow population growth are also influenced strongly by the composition and distribution as well as the rate of growth of output (5).

It needs to be recognized, however, that to design strategies to achieve multiple objectives, and with explicit concern for the composition and distribution as well as output growth, is a formidable undertaking. Complexity is increased because of the need to be concerned with numerous and interacting variables. As previously noted, the problem of reaching a workable consensus becomes more difficult because of the political factors involved. Harold Lasswell's well-known definition of politics as "who gets what, when, and how" is obviously even more relevant to decisions that influence the composition and distribution of national output than to those that influence the rate of growth.

I have argued elsewhere that analysis and decision-making related to the design of rural development strategies can be facilitated by focusing on the problem of determining an appropriate balance between production-oriented activities and consumption-oriented ones (41). Subsequently, I have tried to clarify further the analysis by presenting a "systems view" of the determinants of rural well-being (5, pp. 80–91). Figure 1 facilitates the analysis of the major causal linkages and the feedback effects that jointly and separately determine the well-being of a country's rural population. This is a highly simplified portrayal. The influence of price policies, for example, is largely ignored.

Obviously, the rate and pattern of a country's agricultural development will be influenced greatly by policies affecting the prices of farm products and of fertilizer and other inputs. A "cheap food" policy, based on either an explicit subsidy or on artificially depressing prices to farmers, e.g., through restrictions on interzonal movement and sale of farm products, is in practice one of the most important devices used to redistribute current income. In that case, however, the redistribution is usually in favor of urban consumers, and the costs are typically borne mainly by the farm population. Moreover, the trade-offs in the allocation of scarce financial and manpower resources for programs to expand and strengthen health and other social services, as compared to schemes for income redistribution, may be even more significant that the trade-offs between the general categories of production- and consumption-oriented activities.

This systems view of the determinants of rural well-being underscores the importance of complementary as well as competitive relationships among the various components of a country's strategy for rural development. The need to determine priorities among alternative policies and programs in the low-income countries is especially critical because of the severity of the resource constraints they face. Undertaking low-priority programs, however desirable they may appear to be when considered in isolation, will have a high opportunity cost because the commitment of resources they require will almost inevitably be at the expense of higher priority objectives. Thus, Lele (42, p. 123) has emphasized that " . . . the substantial allocation of central resources to social services frequently occurs at the cost of more immediately productive investments in rural areas and, therefore, may prove self-defeating in the long run."

In my judgment, however, it is also important to recognize that failure to give serious attention to the nutrition, health, and population

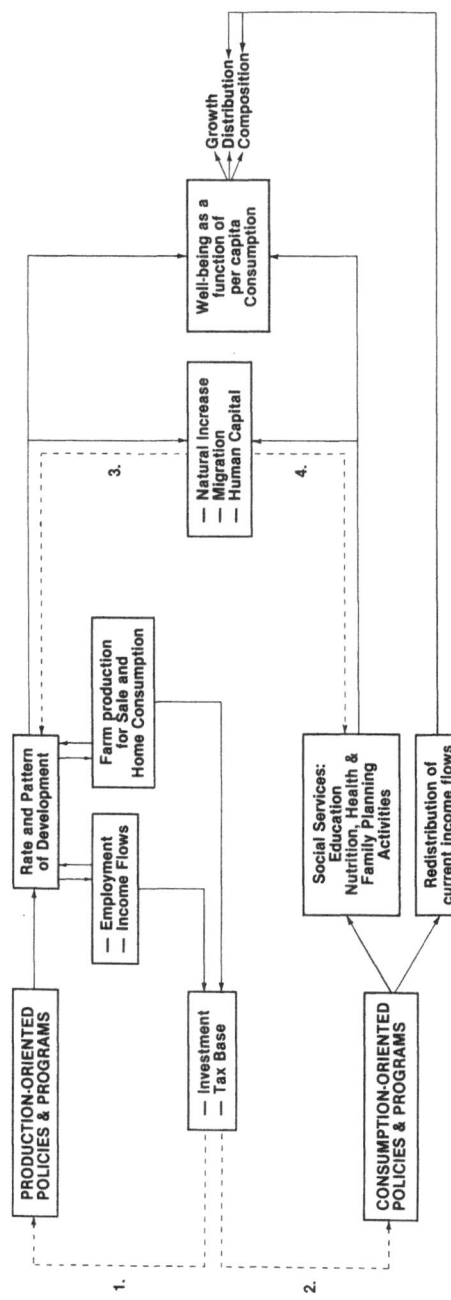

FIGURE 1. A systems view of the determinants of rural well-being. Solid lines denote important causal linkages. Dotted lines indicate major feedback loops.

aspects of the development process is also likely to be self-defeating. To reiterate, the problem is one of striking an "appropriate" balance among the various components of a rural development strategy. Progress in achieving the multiple objectives of development may be unsatisfactory either because policies and programs are focused too narrowly on growth *or* because decision-makers opt for an unrealistically wide range of activities so that plans and pilot projects are not translated into programs that have a significant impact on the mass of the rural population.

STRATEGIES FOR AGRICULTURAL DEVELOPMENT

It is a favorable omen that there is now a considerable consensus concerning the feasibility and desirability of emphasizing broadly based, employment-oriented strategies for agricultural development [see, for example, References 3, 22 (Chapters 2 and 6), 43 (p. 45 and Chapter 9), and 46 (Chapter 5)]. Unfortunately, there are very difficult problems to be overcome in translating intentions, and even a strong commitment into policies and programs that will be effective in achieving a pattern of agricultural development that enables a large and growing fraction of the farm population to benefit from improved income-earning opportunities, and that also stimulates more rapid growth of output and employment in a country's nonfarm sectors.

On the one hand, there is still a common tendency to assume that the technical superiority of "modern inputs," such as tractors and even combine harvesters, means that large-scale, mechanized technologies are also superior in terms of economic efficiency. Large farmers and those who identify with them for personal or political reasons obviously have a vested interest in strategies that continue to concentrate scarce resources in a large-scale, highly commercialized subsector. Coalitions of medium- and large-scale farmers are frequently able to block or evade land reform legislation aimed at a more nearly equal distribution of agricultural land.

These problems are not confined to market economies where profit maximization provides a clear motive for the beneficiaries to encourage emphasis on the large-scale sector. In socialist Tanzania there are strong interests within the government that seek to expand the role of large-scale, capital-intensive state farms. Indeed, there is reason to be concerned that a heavy emphasis on such state farms may jeopardize the prospects for raising the productivity and incomes of the village sector on which the great bulk of the population depends for its livelihood (47, pp. 77–79).

The persistent support for dualistic agricultural strategies is also related to a common failure to recognize that, to a considerable extent, pursuing policies that create a dualistic pattern of agricultural development and successful implementation of a broad-based strategy represent mutually exclusive alternatives. The existence of a trade-off between the two alternatives is relatively obvious in land-scarce countries. If a large percentage of the arable land in such a country is cultivated by a subsector of large farm units, the average size of the great majority of farm households will be even smaller than necessitated by the fact that the number of farm households is very large relative to the land area available for cultivation.

However, as a result of the structural and demographic characteristics of low-income countries, pursuit of a dualistic strategy also tends to foreclose the opportunity for effectively implementing a broad-based strategy, even in countries where land is relatively abundant. This is a consequence of the cash income constraint that severely limits the purchasing power of the average farm unit when some 60–80% of a country's population is dependent upon agriculture, so that the domestic commercial demand for farm products is relatively small. In fact, the common emphasis on promoting production of export crops in developing countries is motivated in part by the fact that the rate of expansion of farm cash income based on production for export is not limited by the restricted size of the internal market.

One of the most important reasons for failure to implement broad-based strategies for agricultural development successfully derives from deficiencies in the level and orientation of agricultural research. The historical experience of Japan, Taiwan, and South Korea demonstrates clearly that a labor-using, capital-saving agricultural strategy can be the efficient, low-cost expansion path in economies characterized by the structural/demographic patterns that formerly prevailed in those countries and that are still prevalent in low-income countries. However, national research programs in many of the developing countries have failed to generate a stream of profitable technological innovations adapted to local environmental conditions and to the needs of small-scale farmers subject to a severe cash income constraint.

I have belatedly come to the conclusion that those shortcomings also derive, in part, from the fact that the physical environments in which farming is carried out in many of today's low-income countries allow relatively limited scope for increasing productivity and output by the heavy reliance on seed–fertilizer combinations and hydrological innovations and investments that were of such overwhelming importance in Japan, Taiwan, and Korea.

Because of greater dependence on rain-fed agriculture, also because of the existence of extensive areas where rainfall is marginal and erratic, many of these countries appear to have an important need for simultaneous introduction of improved seed–fertilizer combinations (with relatively low levels of fertilizer application) and mechanical and tillage innovations that will increase the efficiency of land and water management. Unfortunately, the methodologies for carrying out the research and development required to identify and diffuse mechanical innovations are not nearly as well developed as the plant-breeding techniques and other activities involved in developing productive seed–fertilizer combinations (24).

There is neither the space nor the need in this chapter for detailed examination of the complex issues relevant to the design and implementation of effective agricultural strategies. There are, however, two points that I believe are especially pertinent to the objectives of nutrition advocates.

First, it is important to recognize that the resource requirements and technical problems involved in achieving broad-based agricultural development are formidable, and that past shortcomings are not to be explained as simply reflecting a lack of political will or a failure to recognize the advantages of labor-intensive technologies. Progress in achieving national development objectives depends on a rapid pace of technological progress as well as on the need for innovations biased toward a labor-saving, capital-saving direction. The diagnosis and prescriptions of quasi-experts such as Lappé and Collins (48) are too oversimplified to be of much value.

Second, it seems to me that, because of the close linkage between successful pursuit of broad-based agricultural strategies and improvements in nutritional status, nutrition advocates have an important role to play as part of the coalition of support for the policies and programs required to achieve broadly based agricultural development. This relates not only to an issue such as land reform, but also to the more prosaic but fundamental requirements, i.e., improving the level and orientation of agricultural research, increasing investments in irrigation and other types of agricultural infrastructure, and resisting the effects of "urban bias" that often seriously depress agriculture's terms of trade, which may deprive farmers of the resources and incentives required for accelerated expansion of agricultural production.

INTEGRATED NUTRITION, HEALTH, AND FAMILY PLANNING PROGRAMS

In several papers (5,41,46,49), I have argued that a high priority should also be given to integrated programs designed to enable the rural populations of low-income countries to have access to a composite package of nutrition, health, and family planning services. I continue to be persuaded that such programs offer a great deal of promise as a means of achieving broad coverage and promoting improved nutrition and health, together with better child-spacing and lower fertility. There is evidence of a growing consensus that such programs are feasible and desirable, which enhances the prospects for achieving the support required for effective action (16,50–52). A particularly noteworthy development was the launching of a Rural Health Scheme in India in October 1977, including a program for village-level " . . . reorientation training of uni-purpose workers engaged in control of various communicable disease programs into multi-purpose workers . . ." (45).

It is essential to recognize, however, that the design and effective implementation on a national scale of such integrated programs is an extraordinarily difficult undertaking, and evidence concerning the feasibility and effectiveness of this approach is limited. Moreover, there is still a great deal of controversy about the advantages and disadvantages of an integrated approach to the provision of nutrition, health, and family planning services. Many nutrition and population specialists either are opposed to such programs or give only lip service to that approach.

Some population specialists, for example, have expressed concern that family planning activities may be " . . . neglected, weakened, or rendered inefficient by too much dilution with other programs . . ." (53, p. 113). A more important concern, in my opinion, is that community health workers tend to concentrate on curative activities, such as responding to requests for drugs, while the more cost-effective preventive and promotive activities related to nutrition, hygiene, and immunization, as well as family planning, will be neglected because they are more difficult and not in strong demand in most village communities. Problems also arise because of strong resistance among the medical profession to this new model of health care that is such a sharp departure from the Western model emphasized in their medical training (54,55).

More generally, it is important to face the fact that there are significant disadvantages as well as advantages in administratively integrating a set of activities, even when they are complementary and mutually reinforcing. The insightful analysis by Pressman and Wildavsky (56) of the failure of an employment-oriented poverty program in the United States—an account of " . . . how great expectations in Washington are dashed in Oakland" because of problems of implementation—emphasizes the importance of simplicity in the design of programs in order to improve the prospects for effective implementation. They also argue that "co-ordination," which is so often invoked as the answer to weak implementation, " . . . is a term not for solving problems but for re-naming them . . ." (56, p. 128). I attach particular importance to their observation that failure to recognize the seriousness of the obstacles of implementation inhibits the learning process that is essential if policy design and implementation are to achieve their goals (56, p. xii).

Inasmuch as there does not appear to be any promising alternative to an integrated approach for achieving broad coverage of the rural population in low-income countries in order to provide improved access to nutrition, health, and family planning services, it seems to me that there is an urgent need to maximize the process of learning from the mistakes and successes of both pilot projects and national programs. Although my knowledge of Costa Rica's rural health program is very limited, it appears to offer some useful lessons. Certainly there is a great deal to be learned from the efforts to implement the Rural Health Scheme and Community Health Worker Programme in India. Fortunately, the Indian government has already commissioned a series of evaluation studies (57).

Study of the design and implementation of integrated health delivery systems represents a major undertaking, but the stakes are also very high. It is one that calls for a genuinely collaborative effort among scientists, policymakers, and administrators. The greatest need is probably for in-depth research in individual countries, but comparative studies could facilitate learning as much as possible about key problems, such as fostering effective community participation in planning as well as implementation, ensuring and sustaining the motivation of village-level workers, and devising methods of financing that include contributions from the local community (and perhaps private payments to cover the cost of drugs, except in the case of the poorest families).

A critical problem that could benefit from several types of research concerns the choice of activities to be given priority in the initial and subsequent phases of an integrated program. Giving priority to the nutritional health problems of infants, small children, and mothers seems to be in order because their problems are especially severe, and interventions can be so effective and yield such large, long-term benefits. The complex but undoubtedly significant relationship between infant and child mortality and receptivity to family planning also lends support to an initial concentration on those groups. In my opinion, this should include giving a high priority to the use of simple nutrition screening procedures—weight-for-age or mid-arm circumference measurements if scales are too costly—to identify *all* infants and small children in a village with moderate or severe malnutrition, because such knowledge can increase the prospect that external, and especially local, resources will be used to correct the deficiencies that are identified. As Chambers (58, p.

2) has aptly observed, the poor rural households that contain a disproportionate share of the malnourished are "relatively invisible." National-
level studies and comparative analyses could facilitate the learning process and provide feedback for improving the implementation of ongoing
programs, and could also assist in the diffusion of the hard-earned
knowledge and understanding that is being acquired.

CONCLUDING REMARKS

I will not attempt to summarize the numerous and controversial
issues examined in this chapter. I have argued, in effect, that the attempt
to define a new and powerful role for nutrition planners may have given
the illusion that we had created an emperor who would find appropriate
shortcuts via direct nutrition interventions to the new land in which
malnutrition had been eliminated. Alas, the emperor wore no clothes.
The magic path that would fulfill the universal declaration of the 1974
World Food Conference by leading to the eradication of hunger and malnutrition by 1985 has not been found.

I anticipate that many will condemn this chapter as being pessimis-
tic, reactionary, or defeatist. Those who have worked hard at becoming
nutrition planners will almost certainly be critical, and some of those in
the wider community of nutrition advocates may feel that I have underestimated the importance of nutritional objectives. I think not.

In his retrospective on the 1977 International Symposium on Nutrition at Berkeley, Joy (59, p. 142) states that "for many people, including
myself, the immediate experience of the Symposium was depressing."
He then concludes on an optimistic but ambiguous note: "Perhaps our
depression has become a necessary precursor and a true augury of
enlightenment." I share that hope, but I contend that the fundamental
need is for realistic, careful, and constructive analysis of the complex
determinants of malnutrition.

I have suggested first of all that this requires some attention in
developing a useful typology of the variety of country situations to be
found in the heterogeneous world of developing nations. Specifically, I
have argued that the low-income countries (and some of the lower-middle-income countries, such as Nigeria, Thailand, and Honduras) share
some common characteristics that have significant implications for the
design of strategies for the reduction of malnutrition and other manifestations of poverty. These include the severity of the constraints they face
because of a shortage of skilled manpower, as well as the lack of financial
resources, the overwhelming importance of agriculture as a source of

employment and income, and the pervasiveness of poverty and its concentration in rural areas. Hence, the task of eliminating malnutrition is beyond the reach of specific nutrition interventions.

The evidence seems irrefutable that broad-based agricultural development is a necessary condition for substantial and sustained progress in eliminating malnutrition and poverty for low-income countries. The problem is not merely one of distribution. There must be progress toward the interrelated objectives of accelerating the growth of output of food and other services, expanding employment opportunities, reducing malnutrition and related deprivations of poverty, and slowing population growth. In addition, I have suggested that considerable, although less conclusive, evidence suggests that a high priority should also be given to the design and implementation of rural health programs that are focused on improving the nutritional status and health of infants, small children, and their mothers and are linked to efforts to spread both the knowledge and the motivation to limit family size.

I have spoken critically of a number of specific nutritional interventions, such as schemes for free or subsidized distribution of food, not because I lack sympathy for their objectives, but because they have a high opportunity cost in diverting attention and resources away from higher priority objectives.* I readily concede that many of the judgments and conclusions that I have put forth rest on insufficient or ambiguous evidence. However, I assert emphatically that our analysis and policy prescriptions for eliminating malnutrition will continue to be defective unless we face up to the magnitude of the task and the complexity of the underlying causal factors, and recognize that trade-offs are severe when the requirements for scarce resources greatly exceed their availability.

REFERENCES

1. Berg, A., N. S. Scrimshaw, and D. Call (Eds.). *Nutrition, National Development, and Planning.* MIT Press, Cambridge, Massachusetts and London, England, 1973.
2. Field, J. O. The soft underbelly of applied knowledge. *Food Policy* 2:228–239, 1977.
3. World Bank. *World Development Report, 1978.* Washington, D.C., 1978.
4. World Bank. *World Development Report, 1979.* Washington, D.C., August 1979.
5. Johnston, B. F., and W. C. Clark. Food, health, and population: Policy analysis and development priorities in low-income countries. *Working Paper WP-79-52.* International Institute of Applied Systems Analysis (IIASA), Laxenburg, Austria, June 1979.

*For a brief statement of a contrary view see Gavan (60). Gavan recognizes, however, that because the cost of food subsidy schemes exceeds the resources of low-income countries, " . . . foreign assistance must meet a major part of the burden," and he further suggests that " . . . funds to help maintain farm prices must be forthcoming as well."

6. Food and Agriculture Organization of the United Nations. *Demography for Agricultural Planners.* Food and Agricultural Organization, Rome, 1975.

7. Majone, G. The feasibility of social policies. *Policy Sci.* **6**:49–69, 1975.

8. Michael, D. N. *On Learning to Plan—and Planning to Learn.* Jossey-Bass, San Francisco, California, 1973.

9. Migdal, J. S. Policy in context: The intended and unintended in migration policy in the Third World. In: *Patterns of Policy,* J. D. Montgomery, H. D. Lasswell, and J. S. Migdal (Eds.). Transaction, New Brunswick, New Jersey, 1979. (pp. 187–209).

10. Allison, G. T. *Essence of Decision: Explaining the Cuban Missile Crisis.* Little, Brown & Co., Boston, Massachusetts, 1971.

11. March, J. G., and J. P. Olsen, *Ambiguity and Choice in Organizations,* Universitetsforlaget, Bergen-Oslo-Tromsø, 1976.

12. Morgan, M. G. Bad science and good policy analysis. *Science* **201**:971–972, 1978.

13. Mellor, J. W. Food price policy and income distribution in low-income countries. *Econ. Dev. Cult. Change.* **27**:1–26, 1978.

14. Timmer, C. P. Review of *Distortions of Agricultural Incentives.* [T. W. Schultz (Ed.), Indiana University Press, Bloomington, Illinois and London, England, 1979] in: *Science* **205**:385–386, 1979.

15. Berg, A. (portions with R. J. Muscat.) *The Nutrition Factor.* The Brookings Institution, Washington, D.C., 1973.

16. Food and Agriculture Organization of the United Nations/World Health Organization. *Food and Nutrition Strategies in National Development.* Report of the 9th session of the Joint FAO/WHO Expert Committee on Nutrition, FAO Nutr. Mtgs. Ser. No. 56 and WHO Tech. Rep. Ser. No. 584, FAO, Rome and WHO, Geneva, 1976.

17. Reutlinger, S., and M. Selowsky. *Malnutrition and Poverty: Magnitude and Policy Options,* World Bank Staff Occasional Papers, No. 23. World Bank Publications Unit, Washington, D.C., 1976.

18. Bhagwati, J. N., and P. Desai. *India Planning for Industrialization: Industrialization and Trade Policies Since 1951.* Oxford University Press, London, England, 1970.

19. Mellor, J. W. *The New Economics of Growth: A Strategy for India and the Developing World.* Cornell University Press, New York, 1976.

20. Johnston, B. F., and P. Kilby. *Agriculture and Structural Transformation: Economic Strategies in Late-Developing Countries.* Oxford University Press, London, England, 1975.

21. Vyas, V. S. Some aspects of structural change in Indian agriculture. *Indian J. Agric. Econ.* **34**:1–18, 1979.

22. Republic of Kenya. Development Plan: For the Period 1979 to 1983, Part I, Government Printing Office Nairobi, 1979.

23. Shah, M. M., and F. Willekens. *Rural-Urban Population Projections for Kenya and Implications for Development.* International Institute for Applied Systems Analysis, Laxenburg, Austria, 1978.

24. Johnston, B. F. The Socio-Economic Aspects of Improved Animal-Drawn Implements and Mechanization in Semi-Arid East Africa. Paper prepared for the Workshop on Socio-Economic Constraints to Development of Semi-Arid Tropical Agriculture, International Crops Research Institute for the Semi-Arid Tropics (ICRISAT). Hyderabad, India, February 1979.

25. Schuh, G. E. Approaches to "basic needs" and to "equity" that distort incentives in agriculture. In: *Distortions of Agricultural Incentives,* T. W. Schultz (Ed.). Indiana University Press, Bloomington, Illinois and London, England, 1978 (pp. 307–327).

26. Lipton, M. *Why Poor People Stay Poor: A Study of Urban Bias in World Development.* Temple Smith, London, England, 1977.

27. Castle, E. N. Comment on G. E. Schuh, Approaches to "basic needs" and to "equity" that distort incentives in agriculture. In: *Distortions of Agricultural Incentives*, T. W. Schultz (Ed.). Indiana University Press, Bloomington, Illinois and London, England, 1978 (pp. 328–334).

28. Musgrave, R. A. Cost-benefit analysis and the theory of public finance. *J. Econ. Lit.* 7:797–806, 1969.

29. Hsing, Mo-Huan, J. H. Power, and G. P. Sicat. *Industrialization and Trade Policies.* Oxford University Press, London, England, 1971.

30. Perkins, D. H. (Ed.). *Rural Small-Scale Industry in the People's Republic of China.* University of California Press, Berkeley, California, 1977.

31. Timmer, C. P. Food policies in China. *Food Research Institute Studies* XV(1):1976.

32. Chinn, D. L. Income Distribution in a Chinese Commune. *J. Compar. Econ.* 2:246–269, 1978.

33. Tang, A. M. Food and Agriculture in China: Trends and Projections. A study prepared for the International Food Policy Research Institute, Vanderbilt University, Nashville, Tennessee, May 1979.

34. Barclay, G. W. *Colonial Development and Population in Taiwan.* Princeton University Press, Princeton, New Jersey, 1954.

35. Martorell, R. Nutrition-Infection Interactions and Human Growth. Paper presented at the Annual Meeting of the Human Biology Council, San Francisco, California, 5 April 1979.

36. Morley, D. Personal communication, July 1979.

37. Levitsky, D. A. Ill-nourished brains. *Nat. Hist.* 85:6–11, 1976.

38. McKay, H., L. Sinisterra, A. McKay, H. Gomez, and P. Lloreda. Improving cognitive ability in chronically deprived children. *Science* 200:270–278, 1978.

39. Martorell, R. Responses to Chronic Protein-Energy Malnutrition: Adaptation or Malady? Paper presented at the 48th Annual Meeting of the American Association of Physical Anthropologists, San Francisco, California, April 1979.

40. Preston, S. H. Mortality, Morbidity, and Development. Paper prepared for the Seminar on Population and Development in the ECWA Region, Population Division of the United Nations, New York, September 1978.

41. Johnston, B. F. Food, health, and population in development. *J. Econ. Lit.* 15:879–907, 1977.

42. Lele, U. *The Design of Rural Development: Lessons from Africa.* Johns Hopkins University Press, Baltimore, Maryland and London, England, 1975.

43. World Bank. *The Assault on World Poverty: Problems of Rural Development, Education and Health.* Johns Hopkins University Press, Baltimore, Maryland and London, England, 1975.

44. Asian Development Bank. *Rural Asia: Challenge and Opportunity.* Praeger Publishers, New York, 1978.

45. Government of India, Planning Commission. *Draft Five-Year Plan 1978–1983*, New Delhi, India, 1978.

46. Republic of Philippines. *Five-Year Philippine Development Plan, 1978–1982*, Manila, Philippines, September, 1977.

47. International Labour Office (ILO). *Towards Self-Reliance: Development, Employment and Equity Issues in Tanzania.* ILO Jobs and Skills Programme for Africa, Addis Ababa, 1978.

48. Lappé, F. M., and J. Collins. *Food First.* Houghton Mifflin Company, Boston, Massachusetts, 1977.

49. Johnston, B. F., and A. J. Meyer. Nutrition, health, and population in strategies for rural development. *Econ. Develop. Cultural Change* 26:1–23, 1977.

50. World Health Organization. *New Trends and Approaches in the Delivery of Maternal and Child Care in Health Services*, Sixth Report of the WHO Expert Committee on Maternal and Child Health, WHO Tech. Rep. Ser. 600. WHO, Geneva, 1976.
51. World Health Organization. *Primary Health Care. Report of the International Conference on Primary Health Care*, Alma-Ata, USSR, September 1978.
52. International Institute for Applied Systems Analysis (IIASA), *Health Delivery Systems in Developing Countries.* Committee Report to IIASA by participants in an informal meeting, Collaborative Paper CP-79-10, IIASA, Laxenburg, Austria, July 1979.
53. Bogue, D. J., and A. O. Tsui. Zero world population growth? *The Public Interest* **55**:99–113, 1979.
54. Maru, R. M. Paper presented at an IIASA meeting on Health Delivery Systems in Developing Countries, Laxenburg, Austria, July 1979.
55. Bose, A. Paper presented at an IIASA meeting on Health Delivery Systems in Developing Countries, Laxenburg, Austria, July 1979.
56. Pressman, J. L., and A. Wildavsky. *Implementation: How Great Expectations in Washington are Dashed in Oakland.* University of California Press, Berkeley, California, 1973.
57. Bose, A. *An Assessment of the New Rural Health Scheme and Suggestions for Improvement.* Demographic Research Centre, Institute of Economic Growth, University of Delhi, Delhi, May 1978.
58. Chambers, R. Simple is Practical: Approaches and Realities for Project Selection for Poverty-Focused Rural Development. Paper prepared for a Seminar on the Implications of the Employment and Income Distribution Objectives for Project Appraisal and Identification, Kuwait, April 1977.
59. Joy, L. (Ed.). *Nutrition Planning: The State of the Art.* IPC Science and Technology Press, Guildford, England, 1978.
60. Gavan, J. D. Commentary: Food Subsidies—Imperfect but Expedient. International Food Policy Research Institute (IFPRI) report, September 1979.
61. Cassen, R. H. Current trends in population change and their causes. *Pop. Dev. Rev.* **4**:331–353, 1978.
62. Lapham, R. J., and W. P. Mauldin. National Family Planning Programs: Review and Evaluation. *Stud. Family Planning* **3**:29–52, 1972.

Development from Below

Transformation of Village-Based Nutrition Projects to a National Family Nutrition Program in Indonesia

Jon Eliot Rohde and Lukas Hendrata

Introduction

Although many agencies around the world have devised successful pilot projects in nutrition, relatively few of them have seen these projects transformed into national programs. Costs are too high, technologies are not readily universalized, key personalities provide motivation and management that cannot be expanded on a broad scale, and communities tend to view their role as one of recipients of food (a view shared by many politicians and health professionals). These and other factors affecting replication and expansion of pilot projects to a national scale have provided nutrition and development planners with few experiences on which to base strategies and plans for nutrition.

Activities in Indonesia offer an exception to this pattern. During the five year plan of 1979–1984 (REPELITA III), the National Family Nutrition Programme is scheduled to cover 40,000 of the 65,000 Indonesian villages. The evolution toward this program over the past 10 years provides the opportunity to examine the process of program development. While in retrospect there appears to have been a logical sequence of interacting activities, in fact, the many participants in this evolution, both government and private, followed no preconceived plan or pattern to reach the

Jon Eliot Rohde • Gadjah Mada University, Yogyakarta, Indonesia. *Present address:* c/o Agency for International Development, Department of State, Washington, D.C. Lukas Hendrata • Yayasan Indonesia Sejahtera, Jakarta, Indonesia.

goal of a common program. Frequent meetings and field visits between government, academic, and private-sector workers, coupled with a genuine commitment to flexibility and innovation, led to a coherent formulation of an affordable and implementable nationwide program.

In our review of this process, simultaneous development of three crucial areas has become apparent:

1. The understanding, acceptance, and articulation by planners and decision makers of the importance of nutrition to national development, resulting in formulation of policy, political will, and resource commitment to specific nutrition goals.
2. The development and field perfection of an appropriate technology that not only proved to be effective in terms of nutritional goals, but also proved to be pragmatic and affordable within the means of the country.
3. The formation of a comprehensive, intersectoral organizational structure capable of systematically administering and managing a populationwide program at the village level. The organization had the means to provide training, supervision, information flow, logistical support, and outreach to guarantee coverage of specific targeted groups.

Although in this paper we review these three elements separately, we should reemphasize that the elements evolved simultaneously and synergistically. As in all living structures, the whole exceeds its individual parts.

POLITICAL COMMITMENT

Wide awareness by government decision makers of the extent of malnutrition in Indonesia dates from Sayogyo's evaluation of the Applied Nutrition Program (ANP) 1972–1973 (1). Physicians and nutritionists alike had long recognized, treated, and researched malnutrition, but their approach, which was reflected in scientific writings, viewed it as a clinical or a biochemical problem of individual patients. Sayogyo's sample survey demonstrated undernutrition on a massive scale; he showed that one-half of Indonesian children were malnourished, that poverty and malnutrition are closely linked, and that existing programs aimed at increasing protein consumption were largely irrelevant. The report called for specific actions in home food production, nutrition education, and targeted preventive measures.

Of considerable importance, these findings were expressed not in medical–nutrition terminology, but rather in broadly understandable lay terms focusing on poverty, inadequacy of food, and resulting poor child growth and ill health. The complex web of causation was clearly seen to involve economics, social inequity, traditional behavior patterns, and agricultural stagnation, as well as ignorance and disease. The nutrition issue began to be seen as an integral part of the development process itself, both as a means and an end to the nation's development. Nutrition entered the political arena.

In 1974 President Soeharto called upon 10 ministries to join in a coordinated effort to " . . . improve the nutritional health of the populace . . . as an effort important for national development . . ." (2). A National Committee on Food was founded, and during REPELITA II a large number of approaches were initiated that involved agriculture, education, health, information, religion, industries, and internal affairs. While sectoral efforts were limited in extent and impact, momentum was building as more ministries and departments of the government accepted a role in addressing the nutrition problem.

Several groups worked diligently to educate the public and move the nation toward concerted action. UNICEF–Indonesia sponsored a sound–slide show that highlighted both the problems and various program options. Open dialogue in the press, in seminars, and in other forums kept the issue in the public eye and contributed to the critical reeducation of policy makers and top bureaucrats about the issues involved. The importance of these communication strategies in obtaining the needed political commitment cannot be overemphasized. Armed with clear data on the problem and with the increased public interest in nutrition, decision makers could grasp with confidence the issue of nutrition as a major social need with positive political impact.

Following the formulation by Parliament of the development strategy for REPELITA III, emphasizing "equity," the planning board, BAPPENAS, has given particular attention to multisectoral approaches to nutrition. With the major plan emphasis on social and economic equity, improved nutrition has become a specific goal of Indonesian development policy, which focuses heavily on the poor. No longer considered as an adjunct program facilitating national growth through its effect on the economy, good nutrition is accepted as an end in itself, a legitimate and highly desirable outcome to be achieved through multisectoral development efforts. Equitable development means good nutrition.

THE DEVELOPMENT OF A PRAGMATIC FIELD PROGRAM

In spite of the plethora of small field projects in food raising, nutrition education, and supplementary feeding, a successful and affordable nutrition technology for mass implementation was unknown 10 years ago. The cost of food supplements was too high, the results transient at best, and the dependency engendered was damaging to the family as well as to national self-esteem. World Food Program milk and fortified cereals provided through Maternal and Child Health (MCH) clinics have served largely as a reward for clinic attendance and have not been highly focused on those who are undernourished or poor. Considerable evidence exists to suggest that those most in need of such supplements do not attend MCH clinics and therefore are excluded from the program.

The ANP emphasis on production of protein foods was not relevant, given the overall calorie deficit among the poorest groups (roughly 500 cal below the RDA). Sayogyo's finding that protein–energy malnutrition (PEM) was equally prevalent in "food-adequate" and "food-deficit" households gave strong evidence that nutrition education aimed to effect behavioral change within the family should be a central part of action programs. The ANP failed to select target groups in which a measurable and sustained improvement in nutrition could be expected. The ANP did, however, provide the first experience for many government agencies in an intersectoral, community-based development effort and significantly raised awareness of nutritional problems among civil servants in the selected communities where ANP projects were carried out.

During the 1970s, an "appropriate technology" emerged from the combined field experience and innovative projects of both the private sector and the government. One factor was the development of the hardware for program implementation on a massive scale—the DACIN weighing scale and the special weight chart, which have proven simple, practical, economical, and, to a large extent, self-explanatory. But "technology" is now recognized to include not only scientifically sound equipment and information but also certain organizational elements. Some elements found to be essential to an "appropriate" nationwide program are:

1. The program must cover the total population at an affordable cost, with major recurring costs funded by the community itself.
2. The community must be involved, not only in a passive way but also in the development of leadership trusted with continued implementation of program activities.
3. Nutrition goals must be understandable to the lay public as well as to the civil leadership to enable mass involvement.
4. Activities should be targeted to those most in need, and particularly to those subgroups in which a measurable impact can be expected and obtained.
5. A nutrition program should be framed in terms of multisectoral

involvement to insure maximum utilization of existing sectoral manpower and implementation of field activities. It is not, and cannot, be viewed exclusively as a health problem.

6. The emphasis should be on the prevention of PEM rather than rehabilitation of existing undernutrition. This is not only a more efficient use of limited resources but also a more achievable use and, in the long run, more effective on a mass populationwide basis.

While it is not generally considered technological, the inclusion of such social and logistic issues in program implementation is a vital part of "appropriate technology" for a national-scale program. A review of some of the many field experiences leading to these principles highlights the process of the technological transformation from small projects to large-scale program design.

More than 10 years ago, Dr. Gunawan Nugroho, then the Director of the YAKKUM Community Development Foundation in Solo, Central Java, introduced the concept of weighing in the village rather than in the clinic, plus the use of Morley's chart to record growth. In the suburban village of Kerten (population 3000), mothers organized the weighing sessions in each hamlet, but the actual weighing and filling out of the weight chart was done by clinic staff. While it was apparent that mothers were interested in having their children weighed regularly, their lack of involvement in both the measurement and understanding of its implication resulted in a limited impact. The clinic scale, a standard platform Detecto beam balance scale, was impractical in the village setting and was considered as something alien and peculiar. Lack of specific nutrition messages or activities and passive participation of mothers led to marginal results. However, Kerten showed that higher levels of participation in maternal–child-health-promotive activities could be achieved in the village than in the clinic itself.

In Godean, a subdistrict of Yogyakarta Province (population 40,000 in 17 villages), the community nutrition program conducted by the Pediatric Department of the Gadjah Mada Medical Faculty in Yogyakarta brought further improvement to this approach (3). Weighing activities were built into the existing village women's organization, the PKK, becoming a part of the regular "arisan," a monthly social hamlet meeting. Instead of the clinic scale, the locally made market DACIN scale was used. This robust bar scale, costing under $20, was universally available in rural villages, and proved to be accurate and much better understood by the mothers. Sleeping babies could be hung in a sling, while older children were suspended in cloth weighing pants.

Nutrition advice was largely based on the result of each weighing and aimed at achieving gain in weight each month. While surveys demonstrated that roughly 50% were undernourished, those well-nourished were found to be from the same economic and social strata, thereby indicating that the local ecology could sustain good nutrition. The program focus became positive, emphasizing the "wisdom of village motherhood" rather than the "science of nutrition." Successful village mothers whose children demonstrated persistent normal weight gains were asked to advise their neighbors whose children faltered in growth. This "pairing method" sought to replace scientific and clinical nutritional advice with practical, affordable action already practiced in the same village. While this presents a far more culturally acceptable approach, the lack of specific feeding guidance resulted in a haphazard communication strategy.

Emphasis on weight gain was reinforced by recording, on a large wall chart, the percentage of children weighed who gained weight each month. However, the card on which weights were recorded continued to be seen mainly as a clinical record rather than as a communication tool. The three growth lines, based on the Gomez interpretation of static weight, tended to stratify children as "good," "inadequate," or "bad." This type of understanding is detrimental, both from the point of view of nutrition and as a communication strategy. It stigmatized about 50% of the target population as failing in their efforts as mothers, and therefore tended to alienate those most in need of the program benefit. Thus, while the advice attempted to emphasize *growth*, the weight chart, with its inherent emphasis on weight *category*, did not support this concept. The communication strategy was still not consistent.

In Banjarnegara Regency (population, 650,000 in 281 villages), the Godean approach was further integrated into the structure of village development strategy. The approach in all sectors has placed a major emphasis on community participation in the design and implementation of development activites. Working within the existing government staff and budget, but through a strong commitment by the regency leadership to decentralize control of village-based activities, Banjarnegara has developed the Kader system, involving community members as both technical and social motivators for their own neighbors. Chosen by each neighborhood, kaders are trained by each development specialty to provide services to their immediate neighbors in a monofunctional role. As kaders are fully voluntary, they are expected to devote only several hours a week to their tasks as specialists. Tasks are limited in number, time, and obligation. The kaders know one thing, they know it well and do it well, covering 16–20 families with the particular skill that they have been taught. Their responsibility is entirely "down" to the rest of their neighborhood and in no way do they answer "up" to the bureaucracy.

The critical elements of this mobilization of community manpower lie in: (1) selection of kaders by the community; (2) the highly specific nature of their responsibility to the small neighborhood they serve; (3) the totally voluntary nature of the work; and (4) regular supervision and continuous in-service guidance from department field workers who provide their initial training. The small unit of operation is crucial in maintaining the community sense of belonging to any particular action program, and assures the degree of decentralization and flexibility capable of responding to each community's potential and needs. There are at present more than 1500 nutrition kaders working in over 100 of the 281 villages of the regency (4). Kaders chosen for nutrition training are responsible for the monthly weighing program in their own neighborhood.

While the DACIN scale continued to be used, children often cried or fussed about being suspended, relatively immobile, in the cloth pants. Woven baskets or wooden boxes painted to look like an animal, an airplane, or a car suspended under the scale made weighing an interesting and fun game even for shy children and eliminated the tendency of the mothers to avoid the weighing of their children because of the unpleasantness involved. A new weight chart was designed to reinforce the important message of monthly growth (Fig. 1).

In adopting the techniques of "social marketing," a design team was formed that included a communications specialist, an advertising firm, and a group of physician/nutritionists. The marketing goal was set to motivate mothers to seek a monthly increase in the weight of their young children. The goal was understandable, measurable, and attainable. The weight chart became the prime communication tool with a market appeal and inherent emphasis on action leading to growth, replacing its usual function as a clinical record of nutritional status. A variety of "product presentations" were field-tested among potential "consumers," leading to a "sales" approach that regularly affected mothers' perceptions of, and attitudes toward, monthly weight gain. A catchy slogan, "Anak yang Sehat, Bertambah Umur, Bertambah Berat" (a healthy child grows in weight as he grows in age) advertised the new, full-color weight chart on posters.

The care with which the card messages were designed can be seen in the choice of the woman shown on the front, breast-feeding her child. The woman was chosen from a panel of photographs and drawings portraying a wide array of women, poor and wealthy, traditional and modern, each nursing a child. The model chosen represents the image of what the majority of women interviewed stated they would *like* to be: one cut above their own level economically, modern in appeal, but tra-

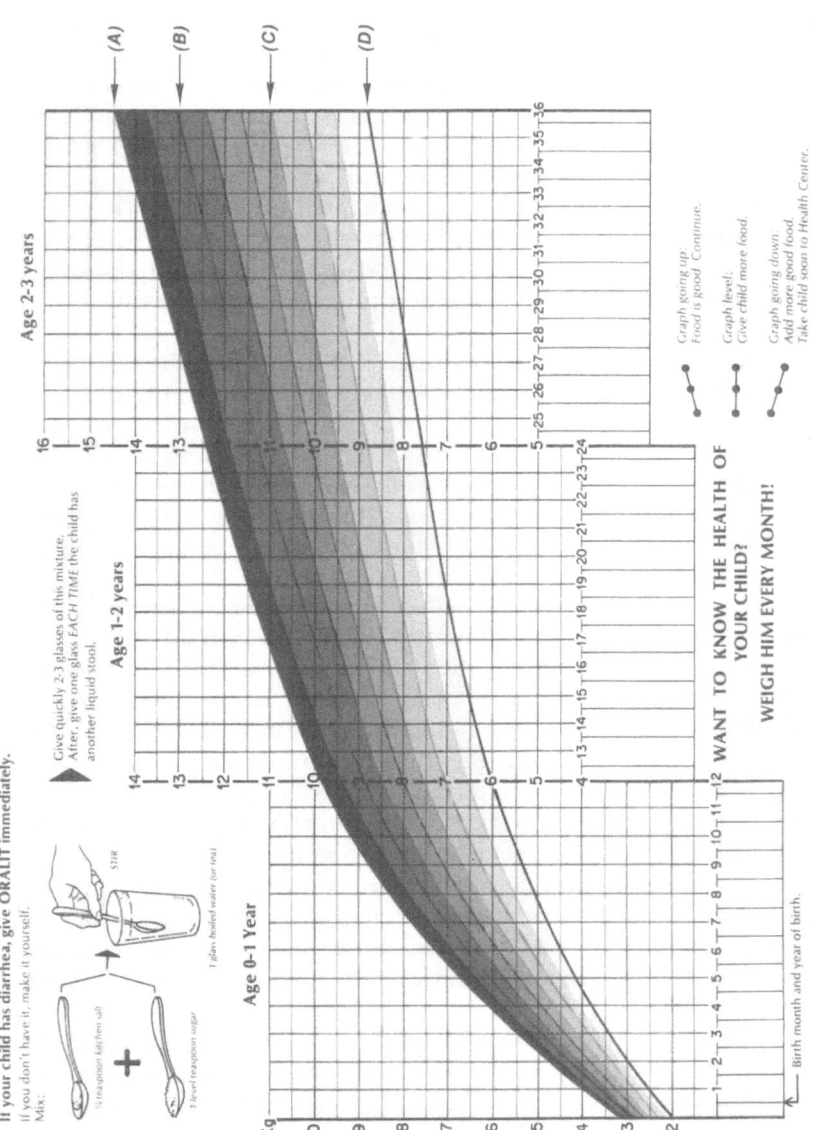

FIGURE 1. Growth chart.

ditional in dress and reserved in composure. The wide appeal predicted by market research has been evident in the demand for posters and fliers of this "national breast-feeding mother."

Of greatest importance is the rainbow distribution of growth curves on the face of the card. Only the first three years are portrayed, as field experience showed that attendance of children above this age fell off considerably, that mothers are most concerned about children in the younger age group, and that children, once they reached 30–36 months, tended to grow consistently at whatever nutritional status they had by then obtained. Thus, the program emphasis falls naturally to the child under three. The rainbow pattern is arrayed as a series of colored channels based on the international (Harvard) standard of weight-for-age, with each channel width 5% of the standard weight. No channel is considered to be normal or abnormal unless the child falls below 60% of the Harvard standard. Each child is said to have his "own colour and he should grow along that channel or above it." Mothers felt that a deeper green color represented greater health (a not surprising finding in this predominantly agricultural society), and so the color arrangement moves from pale yellow to rich green from the lower colors to the upper ones.

However, while growth on higher channels is encouraged, there is no indication that regular growth along a lower channel is not good. Thus, children growing regularly at a weight considerably lower than the international standard continue to receive encouragement and positive feedback. Of even more importance, deviation from the normal trend of growth, even when the child is still above the arbitrary line considered as the "border of malnutrition," is treated as an important sign of faltering growth and indicates the need for nutritional intervention by the mother to assure that the child regains his own growth pattern. Displayed prominently on the face of the card are three trend lines showing growth patterns in children:

1. A rising line accompanied by the statement that the child is healthy and growing well: "Continue what you are doing in the month ahead."
2. A flat trend showing no growth between two months stating: "This is an important sign that the child is not receiving optimal food; give more food daily during the month ahead."
3. A declining growth line stating: "Mother should seek specific health advice and be certain the child is not ill, in addition to providing extra food and nutrition attention during the month ahead."

The new weight chart was not only effective but also inexpensive. The cost of producing the card, when printed in millions of copies, is a mere US $0.05, compared with US $0.03 for the standard WHO card. Many international nutritionists who saw the card without knowing its cost stated that the card must be too costly to justify its publication in full color. This reaction is proof of the appeal of the card, and reflects in a small way the desire mothers have to own such a card and the care with which they keep the card in their homes.

The new weight chart proved to be an effective educational tool, modifying the concept of nutritional health toward one of *weight gain* rather than one of *attained nutritional status* (5). With this card, the attention given to the monthly village "score," expressed as proportion of children weighed who are gaining weight, made obvious sense. The monitoring of the program by this single "score" for each village became both possible and logical to mothers and the village leaders. In Godean, mothers had focused on the location of their children on a weight card (nutritional status), while the village evaluation was based on percentage gaining weight (growth). This new weight card made a consistent and uniform evaluation and monitoring system possible, stressing "growth" of each child and "growth" of the village.

The response to non-weight gain in many Banjarnegara villages was the establishment of a Taman Gizi, or neighborhood nutrition club. This activity was built on the emphasis given in the Godean program of mother-to-mother communication, but placed it in a culturally acceptable context to encourage among mothers both the *specific action* and the *sharing of information* that had been difficult to obtain in Godean. Using food available in their own homes, or produced in their own kitchen gardens, mothers gathered periodically to cook and serve a nutritious meal, discussing food choice among themselves and discovering methods of preparation that would make a well-rounded diet both affordable and acceptable to their children. This *culturally appropriate* forum based on *action* brought mothers together to share relevant experience without having the stigma of "successful" and "unsuccessful" mothers, or advisors and advisees. A Taman Gizi is a group activity based on local resources and local knowledge and it has become a popular social affair. The program extended naturally in Banjarnegara as communities were increasingly seeking action programs that they could carry out themselves. Women in each community became the prime motivators for neighboring groups, and within 5 years weighing programs were established in more than half the villages of the regency.

The Banjarnegara program proved that community nutrition activities are inherently a part of a broader community development program, and thus must adhere to community development principles of self-reliance and genuine, responsible participation. The very absence of material incentives for community nutrition workers and food supplementation, particularly with strange products from outside, proved to be a strength in this program. The Banjarnegara approach showed what the existing government funds could do. The approach to the community and their true involvement in the evolution of this program were not only its hallmark but also its key to success.

During the second five year plan of 1974–1979, the Ministry of Health adapted many of these principles in the revised Applied Nutrition Program covering more than 800 villages in selected sites throughout the country. During a two-week field-training experience, provincial regency and subdistrict nutritionists were exposed to the Godean and Banjarnegara communities, and they initiated the program in one new community during the training course (6). They then implemented, with Government budgetary and logistical support, similar activities in villages of their own provinces. The main components consisted of the following: (1) monthly weighing of children under five; (2) daily food supplements for four months to those 10% of children in the community with the lowest weight-for-age; (3) distribution of vitamin A and iron tablets; (4) nutrition education; and (5) oral rehydration for diarrhea.

A review at a national workshop in 1978 demonstrated a number of common operational weaknesses. The program had no clear objectives, which made evaluation difficult. Locations were extremely scattered and coverage was limited even within project villages; therefore, impact was difficult to see. No training network existed and there was no follow-up to the initial training of the leaders in the program. Thus, implementation frequently deviated markedly from the planned activity. Communication support was weak, with a total absence of manuals for field staff and lack of useful media or even guidelines for clear feeding directions of practical value to mothers.

Attempts to include all children under five in a village led to considerable difficulty with the cooperation from the older children in that age group, whose mobility and general independence made the influence of maternal attention to their diet somewhat marginal. This detracted considerably from the attention that should have been given to the children in the 6-month to 3-year age range, when the choice of food, feeding patterns, hygiene, and the like can have the greatest impact on growth.

Supplementary feeding of selected children overwhelmed both the mothers and program personnel. In many villages it became the focus of the program, the weighing and nutrition messages being of secondary interest. The dependence on outside food sources, even if locally available, made program continuity almost impossible following the 4 months of scheduled free supplementary feeding. Thus, rather than a sustained, village-based nutrition education effort, the program tended to become a 4-month supplementary feeding activity.

From these field experiences, which involved hundreds of health and nutrition workers throughout the country, evolved the specific program for the present national program. The REPELITA III Family Nutrition Programme is aimed at community self-sufficiency, home food production, redistribution of existing food resources within the family setting, and greater emphasis on preventing malnutrition rather than on rehabilitation of malnourished children. By aiming the program at the successive cohorts of nutritionally healthy children under 3 years old, the program hopes to achieve good nutrition in these children throughout, at least, their third year, thereby drastically reducing malnutrition among all children in the areas where the program is operating. On this basis, guidelines for admission to the program are to restrict eligibility to children under 3 years of age, and preferably those who are 6–18 months old. Six critical program elements can be summarized:

1. *Clear, simple, achievable, and objectively measurable program objectives.* These are: (a) all children under three years of age should gain weight every month, and (b) all children who reach the age of 36 months should have reached a weight of 11.5 kg. The development of clear program goals, specific actions, and unequivocal objective monitoring indicators led to a high degree of accountability by local administrators and assured their participation and involvement in reaching program goals. The demystification of nutrition goals, as exemplified in this program, led to commitment on the part of lay persons involved in program implementation. This is a critical element in the success of making a transition to a truly community-based activity.

2. *Emphasis is entirely on behavioral change* leading to the goal, "every child should gain weight every month." Mothers can easily understand, appreciate, and achieve this goal monthly. By contrast, improved nutritional status (or maintenance of "normality") has less psychological attraction, is relatively static, and often leads to complacency or resignation on the part of mothers who see their children classified in a single, broad, nutritional category. Monthly growth is a self-motivating goal with recurring rewards.

A specific series of 12 messages tailored for each age grouping of several months provides a prescription for each mother to follow for any month in which her child does not gain weight. Each message specifies a feeding action, the amount of food, and the frequency with which it is to be given over the period of the next month in order to achieve the desired goal: "weight gain." Each message is printed on one page of a colorful flip chart, in a brief and carefully worded instruction. Thus, desired messages are uniformly transmitted, yet their local adaptation is assured by the directions to the kader to use local practices to illustrate the message.

3. *Kaders are chosen from among, and by, the participating village women.* They are trained in a highly standardized series of five lessons teaching them: (a) how to weigh the children and fill out the weight card; (b) how to interpret the resulting growth line; (c) how to give nutritional advice using the weight chart; (d) what to do for diarrhea; and (e) what advice to give pregnant women. The nutrition kaders are encouraged to "pair" with mothers of children who are faltering in growth and to visit them occasionally in their homes to share their own knowledge and experience in an informal setting.

4. *A high degree of community participation and self-reliance is encouraged.* Program goals embody the principle that *all* children under 3 years of age in the community should be weighed monthly. The monthly report form includes a statement of how many eligible children are in the community, how many have been issued weight cards, and how many came to the weighing that month (Fig. 2). The provision of free food supplements has been avoided, and in its place communities are encouraged to use their own resources for occasional common meals, during which they discuss home food production, preparation, and feeding. Except for the initial investment in equipment: weight chart, manuals, and flip chart, and recurring supplies of high-dose vitamin A, iron tablets, and oral rehydration fluids, the program will be managed and financed by the community.

5. *Highly standardized procedures* have been carefully detailed for the program elements. Use of the weight chart, the DACIN scale, and the flip chart are described in a programmed text for self-learning. Organizational and management aspects of the program in such elements as referral and monthly report forms are standardized in a manual used by the field worker advising the village. This manual is at the same time a trainer's manual for use by these field workers, containing one chapter detailing the specific objectives and methodology to be used in training community nutrition kaders. This 100-page manual forms the basis for training at *all* levels, from the provincial nutritionists and related administrative staff down to the field workers in the village. This "vertical approach" to training was adopted in preference to the more usual

MONTHLY REPORT FOR _____

(month)

Weighing group (hamlet) _____Village _____ District _____
Date of weighing _____ Field worker _____ Number of kaders helping _____
Total hamlet population _____ in _____ families

1. Total children under 36 months old   _____
2. Total children with weight charts   _____
3. Total newly entered this month   _____
4. Total with increased weight this month   _____
5. Total with *no* increase in weight   _____
6. Total weighed with last month weight unknown   _____
   (therefore, do not know if weight increased)
7. Total weighed this month   _____

Participation score   = # 2/1
Activity score   = # 7/2
Growth score   = # 4/[7 − (3 + 6)]
Overall score   = # 4/1

Use of supplies this month:
   Weight charts   _____
   Oralyte packets   _____
   Vitamin A high-dose capsules   _____
   Iron folate tablets   _____

FIGURE 2. Monthly report form for village weighing post. The same form is used for summing results from all hamlets in each village, all villages in each subdistrict, and all subdistricts in each regency. Subdistrict and regency summaries are sent directly for data processing in Jakarta.

approach whereby persons "higher" in the system received a far more complex and detailed training, which was then abbreviated and simplified at each level as it reached down to the village level. Experience through the Ministry of Health showed that such broad-level training at the higher level resulted in considerable variation in program implementation in the more peripheral sites, a problem that has been avoided by uniform training at provincial, regency, and subdistrict as well as village level.

In the community, however, considerable latitude is encouraged in the choice of program activities and implementation. The community is invited to choose its own nutrition kaders and to establish its own program goals for coverage and targets over a given period of time. While the monthly weighing forms the backbone, they may choose to emphasize a variety of activities, such as Taman Gizi, home-garden food production, small-animal raising, treatment of minor illness and nutrition problems, such as vitamin A deficiency and anemia, or improving their own access to the formal health center system through a program of voluntary contribution toward health insurance or Dana Sehat. Family planning clubs are often interested in a variety of welfare activities for their members, among which nutrition may be but one. Nutrition activities complement and enhance interest in village level programs from other sectors and can be flexibly adapted to any village forum or organization.

6. *The monitoring and reporting system is designed primarily as a stimulating and motivating tool* and only secondarily as an information collection device. The colored weight chart retained by the mother remains the basic information tool, and the monthly weight is recorded graphically on this chart. No effort is made to keep a master record of this weight, since such records were generally found not to be useful, and, more importantly, to detract from the nutrition education work of the kaders.

The monthly report form (Fig. 2) is designed to encourage a clear view by the weighing group of their success toward their program goals. The same form is used to summarize all the hamlets in the single village, all the villages in a single subdistrict, all the subdistricts in a single regency, and all the regencies in a province. The total target population, the number holding weight cards, and the number participating in monthly weighing are important participation indicators. Program success is measured by the number of children gaining weight each month, and, for those passing 36 months of age, their attained weight at that one time. The other information on the form facilitates resupply of expendable items. The data from the monthly form are graphically displayed in each hamlet as a single vertical bar for each month, with lines at each level to indicate participation and weight gain. Program goals as set by the community can be easily viewed from such a monthly record.

Thus, through repeated evolution of several field action projects, beginning in a single village and extending through a subdistrict and regency, and refined through experience of several years at the national level, a culturally acceptable and affordable program has been designed. With this "appropriate technology," including field manuals and communication tools, and the basic strategy now known, understood, and accepted by policy makers, the challenge was to find the organization and management approach that could expand the program to reach a substantial proportion of the target population in Indonesia.

ORGANIZATION

While numerous successful pilot projects in primary health care and nutrition have been developed in countries throughout the world, the transition from project to national program is fraught with difficulties and has frequently resulted in failure. The leadership so often found associated with successful pilot project efforts tends to be lost in its transition to a program. This is particularly true where the "grass-roots social qualities" of the program, such as community participation and self-reliance, appear to be key elements. The charismatic leader who provides much of the driving force and inspiration in smaller pilot projects is absent once implementation occurs on a large scale.

In the search for an organizational structure for broad-reaching community nutrition programs, an analysis of the characteristics of the charismatic leader indicates some of the essential qualities of the charismatic organization necessary for mass implementation. Leadership must inspire, motivate, and engender enthusiasm and a sense of purpose for all involved. Leaders offer training, usually of a highly personal and action-oriented nature, that is geared to the level of trainees and that stimulates their responsible participation in an active learning process. Leaders provide ongoing encouragement, technical supervision, and back-up in a flexible way, assuring evolution of the program to meet local contingencies. Leaders give a sense of purpose and accomplishment, both through personal encouragement and recognition of success in all those participating. The leader leads by example, becoming a role model for those around him, who come to realize the importance of dedication to the task and respect for the role of others in program success.

While these are generally personal characteristics, they also describe the elements of a successful organization and management structure. Indonesia's National Family Planning Coordinating Body (BKKBN), today not yet in existence for ten years, has applied many of these characteristics to its leadership in the implementation of the National Family Planning Programme (7). Provided in 1972 with a mandate to coordinate and facilitate all involved sectors of the government in the National Family Planning effort, the BKKBN has evolved a highly successful management structure to meet these aims. BKKBN hired 7000 field workers (FPFWs) to be the major communicators of the family planning message. Recruited from villages in which they would work, these FPFWs were given a short, uniform training course at 16 national training centers and have continued to receive periodic refresher courses as well as continuous education through monthly newsletters and technical bulletins. Their task was highly target-oriented, with recruitment of new acceptors the clear goal. Incentives were paid for new acceptors only until 1974. Since that time, FPFWs have been given targets for the number of visits they would make each month to eligible couples, and they have been constantly reminded of the importance of reaching these targets on a village, subdistrict, regency, and provincial level. The terminology of family planning and its goals were supported by a mass communication effort involving simple slogans through posters, radio, newspapers, and other mass media.

By 1975 the number of current users of modern contraceptives became so high that FPFWs spent a majority of their time in resupply activities. They then established village resupply posts staffed by acceptor volunteers who received and distributed contraceptive supplies for their neighbors. From these posts developed acceptor clubs or Paguyuban KB, which held monthly meetings, and they increasingly became a major factor in the extension of family planning goals and recruitment of new acceptors. These groups became highly articulate in their own communities, branching out into areas other than family planning and involving community members in other issues of common interest, such as health, nutrition, income production, village beautification, handicrafts, village art, and entertainment. Increasingly, FPFWs were called upon to address these groups about subjects beyond the boundaries of clinical family planning. By 1978, more than 40,000 acceptor clubs existed throughout Java and Bali, many of which had changed their name and primary focus to become family welfare clubs.

The Family Planning Programme in Indonesia has achieved remarkable success in the past decade. While 65% of the total population of 140 million crowded onto the island of Java (representing only 7% of the total land area), a crude birth rate of over 40% threatened the future welfare of the population. Over the past decade, 14 million couples in fertile age groups have become new acceptors of family planning. The crude birth rate has declined almost 20% over a 5-year period. In some large areas such as East Java, with a population of 25 million, over 50% of eligible couples are currently practicing family planning.

The organizational factors, contributing to the BKKBN-led success in family planning, are highly relevant for nutrition programming. The BKKBN has achieved:

1. A high level of *political commitment,* starting from the President of the Republic, and extending to all civil leaders and bureaucrats in all sectors.
2. A strong *communication strategy,* exemplified in the recruitment of village workers for face-to-face communication, use of mass media, and the formation of acceptor clubs.
3. A young, *flexible bureaucracy* functioning as a coordinating unit among existing sectors. The BKKBN has endeavored to co-op all sectors to work toward the common goal of fertility reduction. As

a coordinating unit, they must work with and through other departments, providing concise goals and actions for cooperating sectors. They have built on the existing strengths and outreach of the Ministeries of Internal Affairs, Education, Information, Religion, Health, Agriculture, and Cooperatives, and other ministries. The BKKBN has made a national program by actively involving a majority of the population.

4. A high degree of *community* and *local leadership responsibility* in program planning and implementation. It has thus been crucial to formulate program objectives that are simple and objectively measurable and to design an effective program information system to provide feedback to each of these levels, as well as to monitor program effectiveness.

5. An *effective program information system* working in both directions to hold the various levels together. Monthly program reports from field workers and clinics pass rapidly to a central processing office where computer analysis provides rapid, precise feedback that is sent to the administrator of each level in less than a month. Thus, all participating individuals are aware that their performance has been monitored and recognized.

Appropriate as the BKKBN is, it could not implement the nutrition program alone. Several important elements are missing. First, the credibility of any primary health-care effort is closely linked to the availability of secondary backup services for individual cases and situations that cannot be managed at the village level. Technical advice, and particularly management of malnourished or continuously faltering children, is necessary if FPFWs are to command the respect and support of the communities they serve. Second, program focus on additional feeding assumes that such food is available, while in many households it clearly is not. Increased home food production thus becomes an action focus of the program, and specific family-oriented activities are needed. Third, in an Asian agricultural society, the acceptance of a family planning organization is limited, particularly among the more traditional elements of that society. In spite of the widely hailed success of the BKKBN, there still exists in many villages a substantial minority of people who are suspicious of the aims and messages of the Family Planning Programme.

An intersectoral program was therefore designed where Health would provide the technical guidance and clinical backup, Agriculture extension workers would provide inputs for intensified home gardening, and Religion would actively seek social outreach through the mosques and churches of the country; meanwhile the BKKBN assimilated nutrition activities into its large organizational network. For months, the appropriate responsibility of each sector remained a point of contention. Factions within the BKKBN feared that a broadening of the mandate and task of the FPFWs could have a negative effect upon the family planning performance. On the other hand, many Health Department officials believed that nutrition matters should remain in the hands of health professionals, and that a detrimental diminution of program effectiveness would result if FPFWs were given responsibility for village-level implementation. Program proponents replied that a broader view of family welfare would strengthen family planning acceptance and continuation. Also, the current emphasis on primary health care and the present world emphasis on the "demystification of medical technology" strongly supported the concept of turning over nutritional management to the people themselves in the village.

An important turning point in this stalemate came with a national seminar on the community nutrition program that was conducted in a very remote rural setting in Central Java in January, 1979. Top decision makers from BAPPENAS, the Ministries of Health and People's Welfare, and the BKKBN met for several days in the field and visited numerous villages where FPFWs were effectively initiating and nurturing the village nutrition program. Agricultural extention workers and religious leaders and other socially respected figures were actively involved. The health center doctors provided the major motivation and guidance. Integration was *de facto.* This field exposure for top decision makers has been one of the crucial steps in the acceptance of an interministerial national program in nutrition.

By early 1979, the Department of Health, assisted by university and private groups with extensive field and training experience, had defined the details of the program, described in a manual to be used by all workers. They designed a curriculum for a two-week field course for the purpose of retraining all BKKBN staff. Teachers from the 16 BKKBN training centers were the first to follow this course, which was run in Yogyakarta and the surrounding areas of Godean and Banjarnegara.

The Department of Agriculture developed new manuals on home food production and began retraining extension workers in the use of improved seed for vegetable, legume, and root crops. These new services would be made available through the FPFWs to the weighing groups. The Department of Religion has joined in to make the village nutrition program one of its major social messages. Islamic scholars are preparing a booklet indicating passages from holy writings that support good nutrition and child care. There are posters showing a breast-feeding mother that quotes from the Quran, calling upon women to breast-feed for two whole years. The Department of Religion's active support of the national nutrition program is leading to a much broader base of opinion-forming and respected support than had previously been thought possible for a nutrition activity.

Standardized retraining of 2000 FPFWs was carried out in the 16 regional training centers of the BKKBN from July to October 1979, using the national village nutrition workers' manual as the course guide and fieldwork manual. Supplies of DACIN scales, weight charts, vitamin A and iron tablets, rehydration fluids, flip charts, and field manuals have flowed through the BKKBN's well-developed logistic system that effectively meets resupply needs for millions of contraceptive users. The monitoring and information system of BKKBN has been modified to receive and analyze information on monthly participation and on weight gain of children under 3 years of age, thus providing a sensitive index of nutritional status and growth from villages throughout Java and Bali. This rapid information collection system will become a key element of a national nutrition surveillance system, with the percentage of children gaining weight being a sensitive indicator of the need for health and nutrition inputs in food-short or epidemic-prone areas.

During this five year plan, all 7000 FPFWs will be trained to initiate and supervise the village nutrition program. In addition, the Department of Health will continue to expand its own efforts to reach into villages not served by the FPFWs. By 1984 this program should reach into 40,000 villages, providing regular nutrition activities to more than half of the children under 3 years of age in the country. Only then will the transformation of village project to national program truly be a reality.

CONCLUSIONS

The National Family Nutrition Programme in Indonesia was built on the development of a broad-based political commitment extending throughout many levels of government. Founded on representative national data, the importance of the nutrition situation was presented to professionals and policy makers in understandable terms and in a political context in keeping with the national objectives of development. This political commitment, reflected in the current five year plan, is critical to the support necessary for mounting a national effort.

The specific intervention program has adapted and refined a village-level nutrition technology that is at once culturally acceptable, understandable, and effective. Based on clear, simple, and measurable objectives, a communication strategy aimed at behavioral change to reach a national goal of every child gaining weight each month has brought a clear focus to the program. Standardized procedures described in a simple lucid manual insures appropriate program actions, while a high degree of flexibility is encouraged at the field implementation level. Community participation and self-reliance are keynotes to the program. The monitoring and information system is simple, sensitive, and oriented to both the need of the community for self-analysis and to the need to provide operational indicators for the success and extent of program outreach.

The organizational responsibility for program outreach has been accepted by the BKKBN, whose management structure is highly attuned to the needs of a national village-based effort. Their successful experience in training, supervision, information flow, and use of communication strategies in family planning has been adapted for use in the nutrition effort. The institutionalization of charismatic leadership in the form of a charismatic organization promises to extend the benefits of the field nutrition program to a populationwide coverage.

These are the critical elements that have comprised the evolution of the national nutrition program in Indonesia. They are an intricate and complex series of events and interactions among multiple sectors of government and private organizations, bound together by commonly accepted goals and technically appropriate activities, transmitted through a highly focused communication strategy aimed at behavioral change throughout the population. This approach should make the nutrition program in Indonesia a truly national, self-reliant, and living example of the call by Alma-Ata for "Health for all by the year 2000."

ACKNOWLEDGMENTS. While it would be impossible for us to mention everyone whose work and ideas have contributed to this chapter, we wish to acknowledge our special gratitude to Dr. R. Soebekti, Director General of Community Health, to Dr. Haryono Suyono, Deputy to BKKBN, and to Soekirman, BAPPENAS, whose efforts have been vital to the formulation of a nationwide nutrition effort in Indonesia. We thank Kevin Macdonald for help in manuscript preparation.

References

1. Sayogyo, Applied Nutrition Programme Evaluation Study, 1973. Institute of Rural Social Research, Bogor, Indonesia, 1975, 195 pp.
2. Presidential Instruction Number 14, 1974, Republic of Indonesia.

3. Rohde, J. E., D. Ismail, and R. Soetrisno. Mothers as weight watchers: The road to child health in the village. *J. Trop. Pediatr. Environ. Chld. Hlth.* **21**:295–297, 1975.
4. Haliman, A. Indonesia: Community development through primary health care—The Banjarnegara experience. In: *Community Action—Family Nutrition Programmes,* D. B. and E. F. P. Jelliffe (Eds.). UNICEF/Scaro, New Delhi, 1977.
5. Hendrata, L., and J. E. Rohde. Measuring weight gains. *J. Trop. Pediatr. Environ. Chld. Hlth.* **24**:3, 1978.
6. Rohde, J. E., D. Ismail, T. Sadjimin, A. Suyadi, and Tugerin. Training Course for Village Nutrition Programs. *J. Trop. Pediatr. Environ. Chld. Hlth.* **25**:83–96, 1979.
7. Hull, T. H., V. J. Hull, and M. Singarimbun. Indonesia's family planning story: Success and challenge. *Pop. Bull.* **32**(6):52, 1977.

Integrated Multisectoral Nutrition Intervention at the Community Level
The Colombian Experience

LUIS FAJARDO

On March 5, 1976, during a session of the Higher Council for Socioeconomic Policy, the Government of Colombia formally approved the National Food and Nutrition Plan (NFNP) and explicitly made it an essential component of its strategy for development. In 1976 Colombia began the implementation of the NFNP with a set of integrated programs specifically designed for combating malnutrition in the population with the lowest income. The design and implementation of an NFNP was without precedent, since it was the first time that food and nutrition had been a part of the national development policy of Colombia. To implement the plan, the government had to mobilize administrative personnel, institutions, and a budget (1). By 1975, the following conditions had been achieved to facilitate implementation of the NFNP (1):

- Trained personnel with experience in the scientific and administrative fields related to nutrition were available.
- A preliminary diagnosis had been made of the nutritional status of the target population (2) and research had been done on its relationship to global availability of foods.
- Research on primary health care and new models for health care delivery had been developed (3,4).

LUIS FAJARDO • Universidad del Valle, Cali, Colombia.

- There was institutional experience in logistics and administration for the distribution of food to communities and in the operation of nutritional recuperation centers (5,6).
- There had been preliminary experiences in multisectoral nutrition programs (PINA) (2).
- Technology was available for the production of high-protein foods at reasonable cost.
- There was international support for food programs in terms of financial resources, equipment, and technicians.

The NFNP is currently framed within the national development policy of the Colombian government, with the explicit objective of improving quality of life for the poor. An attempt is made in this chapter to describe the components of the nutritional system and to clarify its relationship with development policy.

The government of Colombia views the nutrition system as having three interrelated variables: food, health, and income. These variables occur at three levels: (1) the less disaggregated or individual level, (2) the family level, and (3) the community level. The variables are also discussed at the regional, national, and international levels, but to carry the analysis to these levels would impinge on their general development goals (7).

Characteristics of the NFNP are:

- It is not considered an emergency or palliative plan.
- It is multisectoral; that is, the actions at different levels should simultaneously affect the same set of beneficiaries in time and place.
- It must take into consideration development strategy at the national and international levels because these can have overriding effects. It is necessary that all levels work together toward the common goal of improving quality of life.
- Given all of the above, the NFNP should be funded from the national budget.

The National Planning Office (multisectoral by definition) was chosen to direct the NFNP. Previously, the Planning Office had never been involved with the control and evaluation of projects, only with planning and budget (i.e., macroeconomic variables—general and sectoral—such as credit, trade, and the money market).

The following sections will describe the NFNP program's achievements and impact indicators drawn from villages where the plan was carried out. The current programs are as follows:

- Primary health care program
- Basic rural sanitation program
- Education program
- Production and distribution of food programs:
  1. School and home gardens
  2. Food coupon program
  3. Direct distribution of food (e.g., CARE, Catholic Relief Services, PMA (World Food Program), government of Colombia)

Figure 1 includes the original description of the NFNP.

PRIMARY HEALTH CARE PROGRAM

The objectives of this program, as viewed by the government, are to provide health care through a national regionalization system, to delegate adequately more responsibilities to the nonmedical personnel of the health team, and to rely on preventive rather than crisis services. The system starts at the community level, where a promoter serves the needs of 100 to 200 families. Six or seven promoters report to a health post, where a permanent auxiliary nurse and part-time doctor deliver health care. Each health post is backed by a health center with a permanent doctor and other paramedical personnel. At the regional level there is a hospital, and at the highest level there is a university hospital or other facility with equal technological capacity.

This program is the nucleus of the NFNP, from which the other programs extend or are channeled through the infrastructure, and uses 13.5% of the total budget. Figure 2 shows the levels of the system, and its achievements are shown in Table 1. By December 1978, 297 primary health care modules were in operation, serving 1,500,000 people. In 1979, 406 were operating, accounting for 100% of the community-level services planned for the five-year program (1976–1981).

Although implementation of the program seems to be going smoothly, the quality of the services is still inadequate. The reasons frequently given for this are:

- Lack of physical resources and sufficient supplies, mainly caused by bureaucratic red tape (e.g., often supplies remained in storage for long periods).
- Poorly trained promoters and other paramedical personnel; training has been more technical than practical.

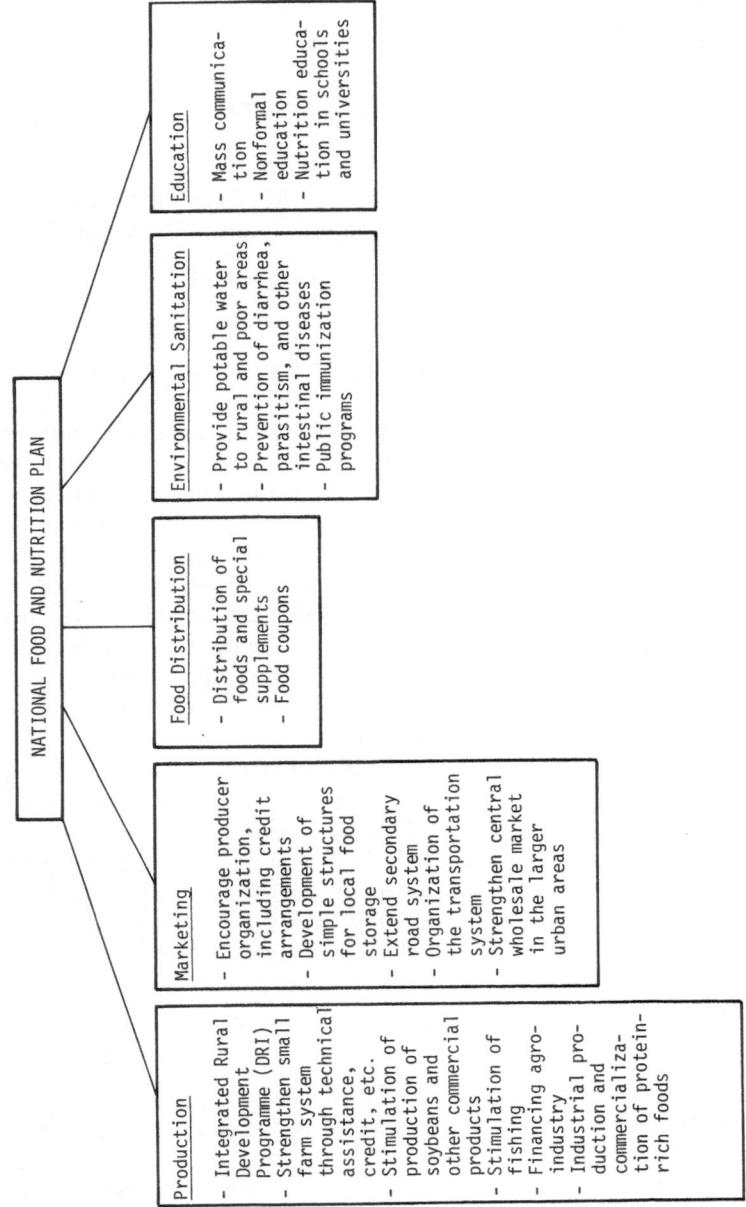

FIGURE 1. Original description of the Colombian National Food and Nutrition Plan.

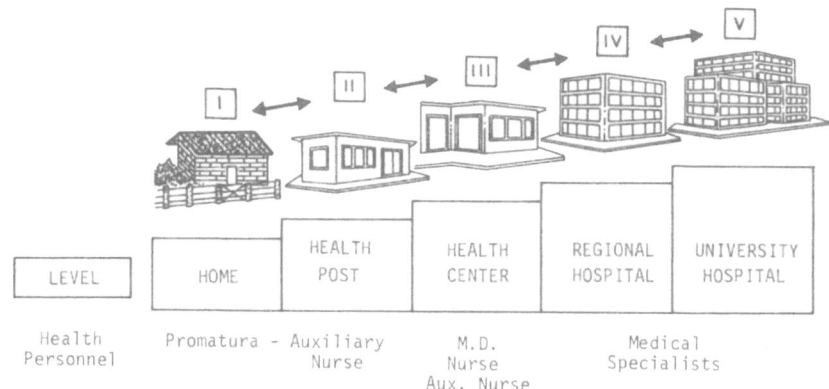

FIGURE 2. Levels of health care available through the government-sponsored National Food and Nutrition Plan.

TABLE 1. Primary Health Care—National Food and Nutrition Plan—Modules of Coverage Started

	Year 1976	Year 1977	Year 1978	Year 1979	Percent achieved of the 5-year goal
Atlantico	6	11	4	2	70
Bolivar	4	9	10	8	60
Bogota	3	9	20	17	136
Caldas	4	8	—	2	87
Magdalena	6	9	11	11	137
Tolima	7	6	5	8	54
Risaralda	3	3	7	2	125
Valle	—	91*	4*	30*	220*
Cauca	6	10	7	6	100
Huila	2	4	11	10	117
Norte de Santander	—	14	13	13	100
Total	41	174	82	109	$x = 98$

*Health post.

- The health establishment has not fully endorsed the promoters or other paramedical personnel, who are therefore given little reinforcement or motivation (8).
- The health department is reluctant to increase the proposed budget of this program, and instead, shifts funds within the health system.

BASIC RURAL SANITATION PROGRAM

The objective of this program is to provide water for 40% of the target population of the NFNP, with construction of rural aqueducts and renovation of existing ones. Of the 478 aqueducts proposed for construction, 118 were finished in 1978, delivering water to 75,100 people. In 1979, 351 were completed, accounting for 90% of the total expected to be in operation at the end of the five-year plan. The cost of this program is 13.5% of the total budget of the NFNP. From a qualitative point of view, it seems there is a low priority for the construction of rural aqueducts by the agencies in charge, again because of reluctance to increase the amount of the proposed budget.

EDUCATION PROGRAM

The objective of the education program is to serve as support for other programs and to find ways to, for example, modify food habits and improve hygiene. Its target population consists of

- People in agencies that carry out the projects, such as health promoters, auxiliary nurses, community-action personnel, business extension workers, and school teachers.
- Professionals who staff the agencies.
- The community in general.

This program has three ways of disseminating information:

- Through interpersonal education directed toward training personnel in agencies in contact with the community.
- Through mass media education directed toward the general population, with emphasis on radio and printed material and with little emphasis on television or film.
- Through professional education directed toward those in charge of agencies, by offering scholarships, training, and research experience.

So far, three projects have been tested by the education program: (1) the prevention and control of diarrhea; (2) the promotion of breast-feeding, and (3) education of the community about nutritional problems.

The cost of the program represents 5–6% of the NFNP's total budget. This program has fallen short of expectations, having completed only 46% of its objectives for 1978. Problems identified during its implementation were: administrative problems with responsible agencies (e.g., delayed flow of funds to the program, lack of expertise in closing contracts), poor conceptualization of what nutrition education is (which literally paralyzed some of the activities), and lack of human resources with multisectoral viewpoints who were capable of integrating knowledge and producing meaningful teaching material.

PRODUCTION AND DISTRIBUTION OF FOOD

The objective of this program is to increase the availability of food with sufficient nutrient content, with the intention of closing an existing or potential nutrient gap. The subprograms include *school gardens*, with an educational rather than a production-oriented purpose, and *house gardens*, whose purpose is to increase food production. The cost of these programs represents 7% of the NFNP budget. They are attempting to coordinate several agro-oriented agencies, nonformal educational facilities, and health and credit agencies for promoting increased food production for the well-being of rural families.

It is still too early to draw any conclusions regarding this program, although the following have been pinpointed as problems:

- Lack of technology for the economical and efficient transfer of agricultural practices to small farmers.
- Lack of appropriate technology for storing perishables in the home.
- Lack of adequate technology for the distribution of potable water to rural families with very low incomes.
- Lack of information regarding credit allowances to these families in order to balance the risk/effectiveness ratio.

Another subprogram, the *food coupon program*, was set up as an innovative response to the problem of food distribution. Its final goal is to increase the income of the beneficiary families, and in turn to increase the availability of food. The idea, which is similar to the food stamp concept, consists of printing a coupon that can be used to buy specific food items and that is worth about two-thirds of the commercial value of the

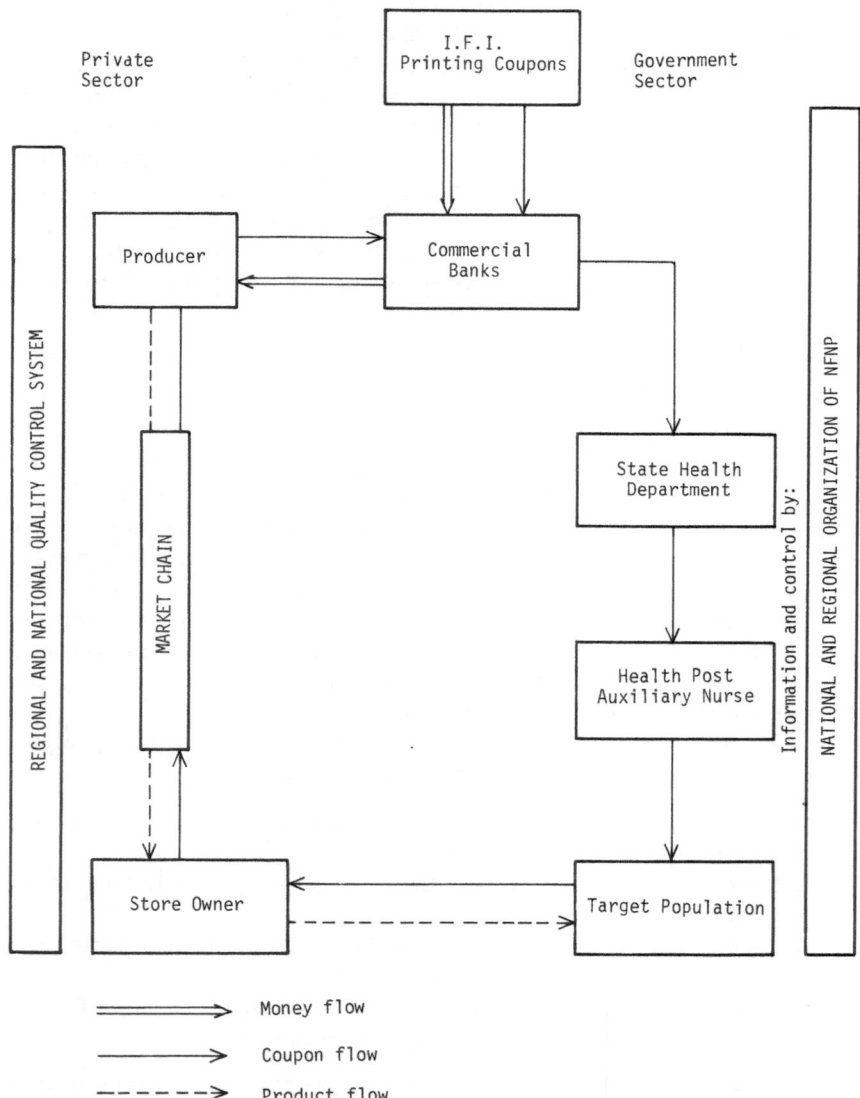

FIGURE 3. Food coupon program, set up to address the problem of food distribution in Colombia.

TABLE 2. Nutrients Available per Coupon

Food group	Grams/coupon	Calories/coupon	Grams protein/coupon
I	250	850	57.7
II	250	845	42.2
III	165	535	82.5

food. The coupons are printed by the government and distributed by commercial banks to the state health system, which then distributes them to health centers, where an auxiliary nurse gives them to beneficiaries. These beneficiaries—mothers of children 6 months to 5 years of age, and all pregnant and lactating mothers—may buy food items in a regular food store by presenting the coupon plus one-third cash of the commercial value. The store management orders the products through regular distribution channels and redeems coupons at an approved commercial bank (Fig. 3). Two types of coupons are issued: those for children 6–24 months of age and those for older children and adults. Food that can be purchased with coupons generally contains 850 cal and between 47 and 56 g of protein (Table 2).

Each month, infants in the target population can receive a total of 10,200 cal and 693 g of protein, older children can obtain 10,620 cal and 853 g of protein, and adults can obtain 19,320 cal and 1791 g of protein. The food subsidy represents 10.8% of calories required and 32% of the protein required for a family of six with two children, three adults, and one pregnant woman. Assuming there is fair intrafamily distribution of food, the mean adequacy of family intake for calories and proteins is 98% and 120%, respectively. However, if intrafamily distribution is not equitable, the mean reached with the present level of subsidy may be only 70% for calories and 87% for protein.

This program was to have a budget amounting to 16% of the NFNP budget, but the program has not been fully developed and has achieved less than 34% of its objectives. A total of 51,380 people are now being covered by it. The problems identified are: inadequate flow of coupons from the state health department to the periphery, inadequate distribution of products to remote townships, insufficient information about the target population, and poor response from the food industry.

The third subprogram is *direct distribution of food*, which is patterned after CARE- and Catholic Relief Service-type programs and shows no innovative characteristics. The cost of it accounts for 40% of the NFNP budget (Fig. 4). The foreign aid that was used to initiate the program has

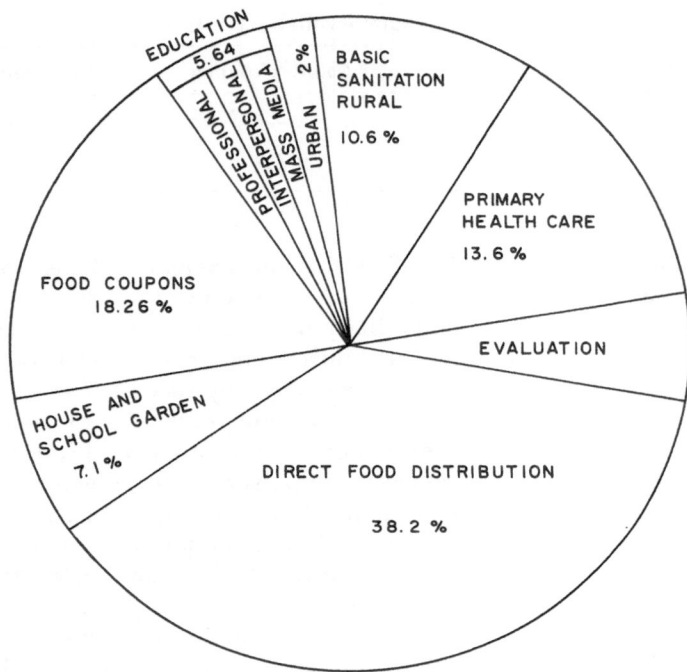

FIGURE 4. Budget of the subprogram for direct distribution of food, modeled after CARE and Catholic Relief Service-type programs. Total budget is 6,138,400,000 pesos, equivalent to US $153 million.

been phased out and the government is making a substantial effort to re-fund it.

GENERAL COMMENT

A review of the activities of NFNP during 1977–1978 (Table 3) suggests several characteristics worth mentioning with regard to the set of programs that constitute it. They are as follows:

- It is a plan concerned primarily with the prevention of malnutrition rather than its cure. Therefore, most of the intervention methods are aimed at healthy, well-nourished children.
- The target population is the family rather than the individual.
- It explicitly considers the interrelated variables of health, food

TABLE 3. Summary of Activities of NFNP during a 2-Year Period, 1977–1978

	Units or constructions in service	People covered
Primary health care		
Modules	297	
Promoters	1,148	1,500,000
Basic rural sanitation	118	71,518
Nutrition education, interpersonal	7,600	1,500,000
Coupons	1,500 tons of food	51,830
School snacks	453	40,678
Direct food distribution	21,668	1,057,000
Gardens at school	445	13,350
Home gardens	80	480

supply, and general development and addresses them simultaneously. The objective is to improve nutrition and the general quality of life.

- Looking at the achievement after 2 years of operation by the percentage of the budget already expended, it can be seen that health-related activities consume 37% (68% if the cost of direct food distribution is not included).
- In its 2 years of operation, the NFNP has spent the equivalent of $19.8 million of its 5-year budget of $153.46 million.

When indicators such as diarrhea, measles, and tuberculosis rates are observed, no positive effects can be seen in specific communities. This implies that, regardless of successful implementation of the NFNP and the impressive budget figures, it remains only an *effort* in the immense challenge of combating malnutrition.

REFERENCES

1. Varela, V. G. El Plan Nacional de Alimentación y Nutricion de Colombia. Un Nuevo Estilo de Desarrollo. *Nutrición,* Departamento Nacional de Planeación, Enero, p. 21, 1979.
2. Fajardo, L. F. Revision Analítica sobre la Investigación en Nutrición Humana 1960–1973. Fondo Colombiano de Investigaciones Científicas Francisco José de Caldas, 1974.
3. Drake, W., and L. F. Fajardo. The Promotora Program. A Colombian Attempt to Reduce Malnutrition and Infection. Presented to AID by the Community Systems Foundation, 1975.

4. Universidad del Valle, Division de Salud, Secretaria Salud Municipal Programa de Investigacion en Modelos de Prestación de Servicios del Salud (PRIMOPS). Componentes Evaluativos de la Atención Primaria, Jaime Rodriguez Ramírez y Jesús Rico (Ed.). Cali, Colombia, 1977.
5. CARE Report, New York, August 1977.
6. *A Practical Guide to Combating Malnutrition in the Preschool Child.* Report of a Working Conference on Nutritional Rehabilitation or Mothercraft Centers, National Institute of Nutrition, Bogotá, Colombia, March, 1969. Appleton-Century-Crofts (Meredith Corporation), New York, 1970.
7. Uribe, T. La Nutrición dentro del Desarrollo. *Nutrición,* Departamento Nacional de Planeacion, Enero, p. 7, 1979.
8. *Informe Anual de Evaluación, 1978.* Documento DNP-PAN, Bogotá, Colombia, July 1979.
9. *Informe Anual de Evaluación, 1977.* Documento DNP-PAN, Bogotá, Colombia, May, 1978.

Comment

RICARDO L. SANCHEZ

Despite the very modest level of implementation suggested by the amount spent, the Plan de Alimentación y Nutrición (PAN) represents a breakthrough in that it has started the process of coordination. This achievement, the very essence of government, is a prerequisite for securing the well-being (nutritional and otherwise) of the nation.

The experience suggests, however, that to a certain degree, slow progress in this multiinstitutional approach is underlined by a less than convincing level of commitment to nutrition and health on the part of the executive branch of government. In this context, it is natural to question the absence of a concise national food policy or national counterpart to the actions directed to the micro level of individuals—families and villages. Without this policy there is a high risk of leaving the *truly* long-range decisions in the hands of those traditionally unaware of, or unconcerned with, the situation of the great majority of the population.

It is also worthwhile to qualify the notion presented by Fajardo as to the confluency of favorable conditions at the time PAN was adopted as part of the Lopez Development Strategy. While it is accurate to say that the PAN staff consisted of "trained personnel with experience in the scientific and administrative fields related to nutrition," it must be noted that this manpower was far from sufficient, and further, that practically no member of this community was directly drafted by PAN. Similarly, while there were certain technological answers in the direction of high-protein, low-cost foods, it must be recognized that generally these solutions have proven to be "culturally uphill." In terms of "institutional experience in logistics and administration for the distribution of food," it is also important to note that this experience was largely negative;

RICARDO L. SANCHEZ ● Department of Nutrition, Harvard School of Public Health, Boston, Massachusetts.

direct delivery is one of the most inefficient and costly programs of the Instituto Colombiano de Bienestar Familiar. Finally, we did not count then, nor could we count now, on a reliable "diagnosis of the nutritional status of the population."

On the political side, a short review of the history of Colombian development plans provides the elements to judge whether inclusion of a certain objective (nutritional, tax, or land reform) can be interpreted as a telling sign of favorable change. Nationally advertised policies are not, historically, reasonably correlated with actual government efforts.

Of the many obstacles that may explain the apparent lack of success suggested by Fajardo, four in particular are worth noting.

FINANCIAL

Although there has been no lack of formal funding, the generous budget figures often do not translate into cash when put through the awkward managerial procedures inherited from institutions or created (for different purposes) by the planning department. This situation is aggravated by the inconvenient "spend now, borrow later" reimbursement policy of some international lending agencies.

CONCEPTUAL

Due in part to the sketchiness of the original documents, and in part to the pressure to get the machinery into motion, a good fraction of the conceptual framework is worked or reworked on demand. Examples of this are community participation and educational programs, and, to a very high degree, evaluation activities. It is with this in mind that one should interpret the proposition to use the incidence of tuberculosis and measles as indicators of the program's nutritional impact.

METHODOLOGICAL

Having bypassed (actually postponed) the pilot stage, PAN was further weakened by its decision to implement the rural development *subprogram* in a separate set of regions. This decision was probably due to regional politics. However, it significantly altered the coherence of the program.

With regard to the food coupons program, it is worth noting that its failure in the rural areas is probably compensated by a clear success in some urban areas to which the program is, by nature, better attuned. With respect to the evaluation program, it is fair to recognize clear methodological limitations due to the imposition of preexisting "information systems" that often have not become functional. Research and pilot project activities have, to date, been severely constrained in an attempt to manage this *support* program in a cooperative fashion involving several committees and alternate routes. The Education Program activities have made significant progress in the design of materials; however, it is clear that the promotion of PAN through the Interpersonal Education Subprogram has had modest impact. The primary health and sanitation programs were really borrowed from preexisting institutions, and it is therefore difficult to separate the influence of PAN.

Superimposed on this picture is a limited ability to coordinate, in a given spot, a significant number of the interventions in accordance with multisectoral theory.

STRATEGIC

Once it became apparent that the President's office would give less than total concrete support, PAN attempted to bypass the formal channels in favor of lower levels of the executive, creating for the planning department a totally new role as promoter/administrator/director. Such a role is not provided for in the formal or informal government structure.

In summary, the role of the scientist as an assistant to the "implementor" has been exemplified (at times by default) in the Colombian experience. Not only does Colombia need appropriate technology development in *all* fields, but it must adopt the systems approach for practically all stages of planning and implementation.

Several participants suggested a distinction between the art and the science of implementing. The Colombian experience suggests that there is only one minor difference: one must be well versed in the "technical" (i.e., skill) aspects of both the science and the art. However, to implement well, one must also put one's heart into it.

Interface Problems between Nutrition Policy and Its Implementation
The Philippine Case Study

R. FLORENTINO, C. ADORNA, AND F. SOLON

INTERFACE ROOTS

Interface problems between nutrition policy and implementation may come about for two major reasons. The first is the limited scope with which nutrition policy is translated into action. The second is the sheer difficulty of effecting a nutrition intervention design because of technical, geographical, financial, and other problems.

Many developing countries have started nutrition programs based on policies that, although not expressed directly as nutrition-oriented, nevertheless conform to nutritional objectives. Most of these programs, however, are only at the pilot stage and thus have not been applied on a national basis to bring benefits to the general population. Moreover, many such programs are highly health-oriented, and their nutritional contribution is easily outweighed by negative forces emanating from other sectors. This chapter will review these two sets of interface problems using the Philippine Nutrition Program as a case study. The chapter is divided into several parts. The first outlines a short rethinking of the etiology of malnutrition, which by definition leads to the formulation of food and nutrition policy. This is followed by a historical review, and

R. FLORENTINO, C. ADORNA, AND F. SOLON • Nutrition Center of the Philippines, Makati, Metro-Manila, Philippines.

then a brief description of the Philippine Nutrition Program. At the end, the chapter offers some positive measures to minimize these interface problems in order to assure better nutrition on a national level.

FOOD AND NUTRITION POLICY REVISITED

Undernutrition has historically been associated with poverty, ignorance, disease, large family size, and other demographic factors. This etiological framework is by no means a distortion of reality. It, however, loses sight of the dynamic nature of undernutrition, the process that brings it about. It fails to answer the very important questions of why families are poor, why mothers are ignorant, why children are affected by disease, and what the conditions are that lead children to undernutrition. This gap is by no means accidental. Classical economics often looks at development from the viewpoint of GNP and ignores the fact that the nutrition and health of children are indeed important aspects of any household's useful function. Adorna and Fernando (1) attempted to put this imbalance into a better perspective, and in the process evolved a comprehensive definition of food and nutrition policy.

A country may have a fine set of nutrition policies, but because nutrition is an intersectoral concern embracing areas such as food demand, food supply, and the biological utilization of food, such policies need to be translated into tangible, supportive action programs and projects in these three areas; otherwise, these policies remain uninterpreted and ineffective (see Fig. 1).

Improved nutritional status can result when these broad policies are translated into specific activities. This often fails because of political and technical problems. A clear example of this is land reform. Even when a country gives nutrition government priority, if it leaves a large number of agricultural households with no land of their own to till, the result is necessarily severe undernutrition.

To be sure, it would be too naive to assert that nutrition should become the central concern of development. Figure 1 simply illustrates that the nutritional status of any country is a product of the conscious or unconscious translation of broad policies into programs and projects. It does not imply that nutrition should be the focal point of the supportive areas or sectors affecting food demand, food supply, and biological utilization of food. Rather, it demonstrates that, because food and nutrition are multisectoral, nutritional well-being is a natural outgrowth of the extent to which nutritional considerations are built into these supportive policies and programs. If these considerations are not included in devel-

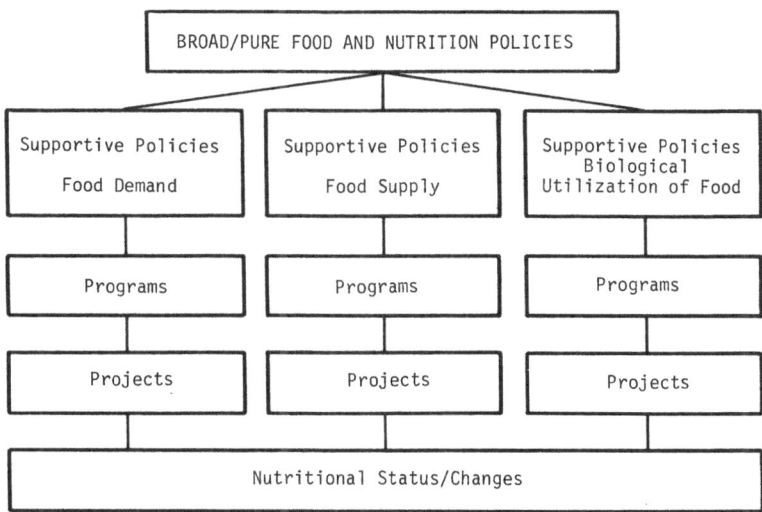

FIGURE 1. Model for translating national nutrition policies into action for improving nutritional status.

opment planning, undernutrition results. This is the framework within which nutrition policy must be defined. This paper rests heavily on this model.

THE PHILIPPINE NUTRITION PROGRAM

Nutrition activities in the Philippines have been going on for many years, even before the last war. These intensified in the 1950s and 1960s in the area of food and nutrition research and applied nutrition programs. Activities at this time, however, lacked a clearly defined nutrition policy originating from the highest levels of national leadership. In 1971, the National Food and Agriculture Council (NFAC) was given the responsibility of supervising all activities in the twin areas of nutrition and food production through Executive Order No. 285. The four-year Philippine Food and Nutrition Program (PFNP) formulated by the Council emphasized the team approach and multiagency participation in program planning and implementation. However, because of limited resources, the PFNP was able to reach only a limited number of provinces and municipalities, and an even more limited number of households.

Initially, the program was confined to 11 out of more than 70 provinces, after which it was extended to other villages and municipalities, according to available resources. The program expanded at the rate of 10–20 provinces per year, so that at the end of June 1974, 42 provinces were covered (2). Although efforts had been made to coordinate all nutrition activities, there was still much to be done to organize a nationwide system that could oversee program implementation from the national to the barrio levels.

On June 25, 1974, Presidential Decree 491 mandated nutrition as a national priority and created the National Nutrition Council (NNC) to coordinate all nutrition-related activities of both the government and private sectors. It took over the task of formulating the integrated Philippine Nutrition Program (PNP) and coordinating its implementation (3). Almost simultaneously, the First Lady, Mrs. Imelda Romualdez-Marcos, established the Nutrition Center of the Philippines (NCP) to represent the integrated nutrition effort of the private sector.

The PNP is the sum total of individual and collective efforts planned and organized to solve the malnutrition problem of the Philippines. As a national integrated scheme to improve overall nutritional status of the Filipino people, the PNP is an integral part of the Government's socioeconomic development program (4).

The ultimate objective of the PNP, improving the nutritional status of the population, especially emphasizes the vulnerable groups identified as follows: (1) infants and preschoolers (0–6 years), (2) school children (7–14 years), (3) pregnant women and lactating mothers, (4) laborers doing heavy manual labor, and (5) those affected with nutrient deficiency diseases such as hypovitaminosis-A, iron deficiency anemia, and goiter (5).

The nationwide PNP, embracing both government and nongovernment efforts, began in 1974 facing a serious malnutrition problem. Its national child weighing survey ("Operation Timbang," or OPT) revealed dramatically that roughly 30% of 4.3 million preschoolers from depressed urban and rural areas were suffering from severe and moderate undernutrition (6). Protein–energy malnutrition, nutritional anemia, vitamin A deficiency, and goiter were the most serious.

Over the past 5 years, the Program has been extremely active. Various evaluations conducted within this period allow PNP implementors an optimistic outlook. An internal exploratory study of changes in nutritional status from 1975 to 1977 for 17 provinces indicated a general improvement. The proportion of children with third-degree malnutrition decreased by 8.6%, while the proportion of normal preschoolers increased by 4.2% from initial weighing to reweighing. The proportion of first-degree malnutrition likewise decreased by 3.6%, with the proportion of second-degree malnutrition increasing by 4.6% (7).

An external evaluation conducted by an independent research group in 1978 supports this earlier finding. On-the-spot weighing of selected OPT participants and comparisons of actual weight results with the latest available OPT records of these participants were undertaken. Anthropometric survey findings indicated favorable results in that 59% of preschoolers with second- and third-degree malnutrition showed improvement in nutritional status. An almost equal number (48%) maintained the same nutritional status, while 3% deteriorated from second- to third-degree status (6).

The above results are further corroborated by the significant decline of severe undernutrition recorded in Albay (a nutrition surveillance project area) in 1979 compared to its 1977 figure (8). Moreover, the periodic Food Consumption Survey conducted by the Food and Nutrition Research Institute exhibits a similar trend. The latest survey of randomly chosen households revealed a 44% decline in severe and moderate malnutrition, from 19.4% in 1976 to 10.9% in 1978, in the entire Luzon area, where seven of the 13 regions of the country are located (9). The same survey showed that the per capita intake of calories and protein had increased over the 2-year period: from 1741 kcal (88% of the RDA) and 47.1 g protein (95.9% of the RDA) to 1861 kcal (89.7% of the RDA) and 54.2 g protein (103.2% of the RDA) (10,11).

While progress seems to have been made, the problem has in no way been reduced to insignificance. Nor are we certain that such results can be sustained. An exploratory study (12) has shown some degree of recurring malnutrition, pointing to inadequacies in the currently existing policies and programs. In retrospect, these inadequacies mainly occur at the interface between nutrition policy and its implementation.

PHILIPPINE NUTRITION PROGRAM STRATEGY

Presidential Decree 491 recognized that nutrition is an intersectoral concern. This is clearly reflected in the *organizational structure* of the nutrition sector. At the national level is the National Nutrition Council (NNC), which is chiefly responsible for formulating an integrated national nutrition plan and for coordinating implementation. The Council is composed of the national heads of participating government and private agencies and is led by the Ministers of Agriculture and Health, who act as Chairman and Vice-Chairman, respectively. A Management Committee composed of representatives from the member agencies of the Council assists the NNC in executing its designated functions. A Secretariat headed by the Executive Director provides technical and administrative support.

To carry out program activities at the different operational levels, nutrition committees headed by governors and city or municipal mayors have been organized at the regional, provincial, city, municipal, and barangay levels. The participating agencies of the PNP work through these committees to plan, implement, and evaluate the nutrition program at the lower levels of the organization (4).

Other strategies employed in the PNP with organizational support are:

1. Provision for nutrition training. Nutrition training orients those involved in the program toward new directions and future developments. Training programs are conducted at the national, regional, provincial, city, municipal, and barangay levels. The "echo training" approach is used, wherein trainees in a particular course become teachers for lower-level trainees. Packaged audiovisual modules are utilized as well. Training is conducted in three areas: (a) local level planning for members of provincial, city, and municipal nutrition committees, (b) program implementation for agency workers, and (c) basic nutrition and health services for Barangay Nutrition Scholars (BNS). The BNS is an indigenous, grass-roots worker selected from within the village, who works on a part-time, semivoluntary basis. He is considered the action officer at the village level.

2. Identification and location of the malnourished in the community. This activity aims to identify malnourished children in a particular locality through OPT, a weight survey of preschool children 0–6 years old.

3. Formulation and implementation of nutrition strategies. A package of nutrition strategies was formulated to implement overall PNP objectives. These are:

    Food Production, to provide families with sufficient quantities of locally available, nutritious foods and at the same time augment family income through production and distribution of selected crops, livestock, and poultry in the homes, school, and community, along with the establishment of seed banks and nurseries.

    Food Assistance, to provide the severely malnourished preschool child with emergency supplementary high-protein, high-calorie foods to save his/her life. Resources of families, local government, and donor agencies are pooled for this program.

Health Protection, to deliver preventive and curative medical services to malnourished children, primarily through the Rural Health Units (RHUs). Immunization, dietary/medical advice to mothers, and health/nutrition/child-care education are provided.

Nutrition Education and Information, to increase the level of nutrition, health, and family planning awareness and knowledge among the people. A person-to-person approach is used, including home visits, individual consultation, and demonstration techniques. Communication through the mass media is also utilized.

PROGRAM ACCOMPLISHMENTS

Over the past 5 years, the above nutrition intervention and program support strategies have been translated into field realities. Local nutrition committees have been established, chaired by the locally elected political leader. Currently, there are nutrition committees in all of the 13 regions, 76 provinces, and 60 cities. Out of a total of 1474 towns and 40,377 barangays, 93 and 74%, respectively, have committees. As of August 1979, nutrition plans were evolved in 81–84% of the provinces, towns, and cities in the country. Such plans were approved by the local development councils, and about half of them had actual local budgetary appropriation (13).

This organizational milestone is matched by the weighing of 5.1 million preschoolers out of an estimated 10.8 million in the Philippines. OPT has thus served as the principal planning tool for local nutrition planners and has greatly contributed to increased nutrition awareness across Philippine society. This was sustained by widespread nutrition education activities aimed at reinforcing correct knowledge, attitudes, and practices among the population. Recently, a novel approach has been introduced in the form of the Nutribus, a vehicle equipped with audiovisual video recording and playback facilities, providing communication support to the BNS. There are now five units based in selected provinces of the Visayas, reaching a total of 300 barangays, or the equivalent of 300,000 mothers within a year. Some 20 more units are being readied for the field.

Extension workers are also conducting nutrition education classes on a steady basis, involving a total of not less than 200,000 homemakers. In recognition of the basic need for nutrition education, more than 20,000 schools have integrated nutrition programs into their curricula.

The potential of the mass media has been proven through the Nutrition Institute for Distance Studies (NIDS). To date, some 883 physicians have graduated from the course. This number, however, is small in comparison to the 150,000 teachers who were also trained under the same programs, but with a module designed especially for them (4).

During this period, the Mental Feeding Program has also gained acceptance among a number of Filipino homes. In its effort to teach parents and child-care workers creative methods for mental stimulation of preschool children, the Mental Feeding Program has reached 7960 preschool children in its pilot phase. About the same number of mothers were also taught by Mental Feeding Parent Educators the rudiments of enriching their children's environment so that they can achieve their full genetic potential as adults.

There have also been significant achievements in the area of health protection. One-hundred and sixty malnutrition wards have been established all around the country. The occupancy figure registered a total of 2952 cases in 1978. Nutrihuts, the malnutrition wards of rural areas, were also constructed to accommodate severe cases of malnutrition. To date, 256 nutrihuts have been built, which housed a total of 891 children for that same year (14).

Recently, the Ministry of Health has started a program of iron supplementation for all pregnant mothers seen in government clinics. Moreover, the Ministry has distributed iodized salt in areas where goiter is highly endemic.

In terms of its food assistance efforts, the PNP, through the Ministry of Social Services and Development (MSSD), has established a total of 4160 day-care centers in all provinces. For the year 1978 alone, some 360,000 moderately and severely malnourished children were served by the Day Care Feeding Centres (15).

The Nutrition Center of the Philippines has developed several food formulations to strengthen the food assistance intervention of the PNP. Of these, a breakthrough has been made by the *Nutri-Pak* (for a detailed description of the Nutri-Pak, see Chapter 9), which also serves the additional purpose of being a subtle educational tool through its packaging concept. Nutri-Paks have been produced in plants set up in strategic locations all over the country. At last count, a total of 133 plants have been providing the food requirements of the target population. Total production is 784,000 packs (1977), meeting 13% of the nutrient requirements of children diagnosed as having third-degree malnutrition in these areas, and 7% (255,436) of all third-degree cases in the country (16).

To make available such food assistance commodities to the most needy in the vulnerable groups, the Ministry of Health instituted its Targeted Food Assistance Program. A total of 336,579 moderately and severely malnourished preschoolers benefited from this program in 1978. To further strengthen this scheme, Mothercraft Nutrition Centres have been established. Some 54,380 second- and third-degree-malnourished preschool children have been listed as recipients in this program for 1978 (17).

Because the availability of a steady food supply is one of the most vital linkages for the solution of undernutrition, this food production campaign was also stepped up during the period under review. The Ministry of Agriculture took the lead, with its Masagana 99 Rice Production Programme at the forefront. Three years after this program began, Masagana 99 made the Philippines self-sufficient in rice. During the first year (Phase I and II), 3.44 million tons of paddy were harvested, a 27% increase over production in previous years, which averaged 2.7 million tons. For the crop years 1974–1975 (Phase III and IV) and 1975–1976 (Phase V and VI), rice production rose to 3.5 million tons and 3.8 million tons, respectively. As of early 1978, rice production expanded by 0.8% over the 1977 output, and even exceeded its target by 4.2% (18). Because of this, the country was able to reap a bumper harvest, and even export the surplus to neighboring countries. The success of Masagana 99 is a reflection of the tremendous effort that we have made to achieve self-sufficiency in food production.

The concern for increased food production did not center on rice alone, but included vegetable production as well. The *Gulayan sa Kalusugan* Project under the aegis of the Green Revolution encouraged the cultivation of nutritious vegetables, particularly legumes. This project produced a variety of crops totalling 193,387 metric tons in 1978. The Bureau of Plant Industry also contributed to the PNP by distributing 67 and 51% of the total seed and plant materials produced, respectively, to families with malnourished children (15).

To ensure integrated delivery of the various services provided by the different intervention schemes, barangay-based and indigenous workers have been trained. The BNS have been charged with the responsibility for basic nutrition and health activities (e.g., OPT, referral of sick and malnourished children). To date, a total of 3972 BNS have been trained and fielded in 41 cities and 57 provinces of the country. They were able to reach no less than 600,000 families, either through home visits or through regular nutrition education meetings.

To serve as an early warning device on local nutrition conditions, a Nutrition Surveillance System was instituted. This consists of: (1) continuous data collection on the nutritional status of high-risk groups, (2) data analysis, and (3) dissemination of analyzed information to policy makers and those who can institute remedial measures. At present, the system is covering all municipalities in five provinces. In addition, a monitoring system has been established in so-called index municipalities where a number of simple indicators on the progress of the program are being gathered quarterly. The system is now operating in a rotating sample of 20 provinces and six cities.

Because nutrition is a national concern, both government and private agencies have allocated funds jointly to support the PNP (17). In 1978, the Philippine government allocated ₱8,481,000* from national funds to support the coordinating function of the Council Secretariat. In turn, funding assistance amounting to ₱1,175,199 in the form of grants-in-aid was provided by NNC to implementors in support of their nutrition projects. In addition, some 19 government and private cooperating agencies spent more than ₱154 million from their own respective budgets to implement projects under the PNP.

Provincial, city, and municipal governments also generously contributed counterpart funding in support of their nutrition programs. Thus, the local governments spent ₱1,338,900 for their BNS in 1978.

INTERFACE PROBLEMS

The PNP accomplishments presented in the preceding section by no means represent the maximum potential of the program, nor have they been achieved with an equal degree of success. This section focuses on the various problems that faced PNP implementation and those inadequacies of the program that affect its level of achievement and chances for continuity. As outlined in the earlier sections, two sets of interface problems are presented: those relating to the actual implementation of the Philippine Nutrition Program and those associated with translating nutrition goals into development programs.

FIRST INTERFACE

The PNP has three basic sources of strength. One is the massive awareness of nutrition it has created. Second is the community level of organization it has established and the interagency participation it has generated. These three sources of strength are equally the PNP's major interface problem breeders. The following discussion mainly addresses these three areas. However, some attention must be drawn to problems related to specific interventions—namely, their outreach.

*₱1.00 - US $0.14.

OPT, the first major success of the PNP in the areas of generating awareness of the importance of nutrition, has also brought its first major problem. Before the weighing began, OPT implementors were not properly instructed that weighing is in itself a service, a diagnostic process. This failure, coupled with inadequate, untimely, or even nonexistent nutrition interventions, has discouraged participation in subsequent weighings. The following excerpt from the SGV evaluation (6) report summarizes major problems in OPT:

> Of an estimated total of 10.8 million pre-schoolers in the Philippines, OPT has covered only 4.4 million, or approximately 41 per cent of the targeted population as of December 1977. No comparisons with historical data can be made since OPT was only instituted in 1976.
>
> The limited accomplishment in both initial weighing and re-weighing is due to the insufficiency of weighing scales (only one-third of the budgeted number of scales was distributed due to lack of funds), slow pace of organization of Barangay Nutrition Committees (BNC), the primary group responsible for the conduct of weighings; and delays in reporting and some inaccuracies found in OPT data.
>
> Operation Timbang is coordinated throughout the country by the Department of Health (DOH), which draws from the various participating agencies and nutrition committees, especially the BNCs. Feedback from OPT participant supports the major role of DOH in OPT-related activities. Rural Health Units (RHU) of DOH, followed by Department of Education and Culture (DEC) and Department of Social Services Development (DSSD) were cited by respondents as the organizations that conducted the weight surveys.
>
> In addition to the actual conduct of weighing, implementors claimed to undertake post-OPT activities (e.g., referrals of third degree cases to rehabilitation centers and extension of Food Assistance). This claim, however, was not corroborated by governors and mayors who reported low admission rates in rehabilitation centers, and OPT respondents' claim that only few referrals were made. Most respondents were not informed of the nutritional status of their chidren after weighing. The omission of this communication process reduces the overall effectiveness of OPT, specifically in instilling among respondents the practice of weighing as a follow-up measure to determine the nutritional status of children.
>
> A greater number of implementors also failed to appreciate OPT as a planning tool, an important component in determining the proper mix of nutrition strategies to be applied to priority groups.
>
> Most respondents were knowledgeable on the OPT objectives and the nutritional status of their children who were weighed. This is also a function of OPT's visibility at the barangay level. In terms of practice and attitude towards OPT, however, a high proportion of the children surveyed were weighed only once against the desired frequency of twice a year. Reasons cited for submitting children to weighing were usually to take advantage of handouts, i.e., food, medicine and vitamins, which usually follow a weight survey.

The awareness generated by the program among local leaders, particularly the governors and mayors, has also served as a double-edged sword in implementation. True, the local leaders became more conscious of building nutrition considerations into their platforms and civic programs, but such action has sometimes been taken by many of the local leaders in order to get themselves on the political bandwagon. What occurred thereafter was automatic institution of only the most visible and impact-creating projects, which failed to consider the actual needs of the locality. Such a display of short-lived nutrition activities and the forced entry of inappropriate technology, mainly for political considerations, have not made the program available to many. It has even caused local level agency implementors to put up defensive mental blocks at the introduction of any new nutrition undertaking.

The imperative delivery of the nutrition package to its final recipients necessitated the formation of Barangay Nutrition Committees (BNCs). The problem, however, lies not so much in making these BNCs come into being as in honing the structure so that they become functional. The rather slow pace of the BNCs is reflected in the amount of material and financial support that has been generated from local sources, especially at the municipal and barangay levels. Although these areas have been high in manpower support, as illustrated by OPT, the same enthusiasm has not been sustained because material and financial support was lacking. The PNP has yet to reach a stage wherein the majority of the barangays are self-reliant, self-sustaining units of nutrition endeavors—a condition that can only be brought about through the presence of active community participation.

This brings us to the problem of the contradiction between the approach to project development and the basic implementational principle that the PNP aims to inculcate—self-reliance of the local units. Over the years, the approach has been notably the "parachuting" type, wherein programs and projects were planned at the national level and then packaged to be implemented at the local levels. This type of approach has not encouraged local participation, and consequently self-reliance has not been achieved by many of these units.

An example of the above is the strategy employed to actualize the BNS Project. By virtue of Presidential Decree 1569, each barangay has been mandated to employ a BNS to act as a catalyst for nutrition activities, and to generate community participation. This is a bit short-sighted because the BNS is not esteemed by the community. He can only be effective if and when the community recognizes that it needs the BNS, thus raising his stature so that he can encourage local participation—a social experience that cannot be brought about through legislation. [To

strengthen this point, one can cite the evaluation done on the BNS project (19). The evaluation revealed a relatively high—30%—annual attri-
tion rate compared to losses of other primary barangay workers.] This is
not to deny the need for the latter, but rather to place in its proper perspective the need to be supportive of the BNS in order to stabilize the
projects.

All of the problems pertaining to community level organization
could be substantially diminished by putting more emphasis on community participation. Program strategies should be designed to encourage such participation as part of the total development framework.

The third problem area that breeds real implementation interface
problems is the interagency mechanism used in service delivery.
Whereas the system has enabled the program to extend its outreach, a
certain amount of laxity in coordination has resulted in an overlap in
activities. For example, the Mothercraft Nutrition Centres of the Ministry
of Health parallel the Day Care Feeding Centres of the Ministry of Social
Services and Development. Both projects have the same main goal of
feeding target preschool children. Examples of overlapping agency activities are many. Although this situation has forged closer links among
some agencies, the overlapping of functions has created petty jealousies
among some of the personnel. This has resulted in a breakdown in coordination, making mutual assistance very difficult.

Recognizing the complementary potential of interactions between
the private sector and government efforts, implementors of the PNP
have involved the private sector in several of its undertakings. The experience has been heartening, to say the least, but various shortcomings
developed. For one thing, the private sector has been given a wide margin of initiative, but, since it is not under any effective organizational
control, its contributions to the program have been rather sporadic and
uncoordinated. So far, the majority of the private sector's fund-raising
activities for nutrition have been unpredictable and seasonal. This has
resulted time and again in short life-spans for projects relying on the
strength of private sector sustenance.

All of these weaknesses in project implementation have resulted in
a major problem that cuts across awareness of needs, organization, and
interagency cooperation: limited outreach. Again, OPT is a very fitting
example of the dialectical relationships of success and shortcomings in
one program. The most massive and far-reaching nutrition undertaking,
OPT has nevertheless reached only a little better than 50% of the target
group. Meanwhile, the rest of the target populations who might be
severely malnourished have not been found, practically obliterating
their chances for rehabilitation. Thus, if the present OPT outreach is the

maximum that can be attained, the extent to which other service projects of the PNP can find and treat the undernourished leaves much to be desired.

Second Interface

The following excerpt from the Five-Year Philippine Development Plan explicitly states the broad food and nutrition policy of the Philippines (20):

> At the head of the Plans is the concern for social justice. The preparation of these plans has been guided by one objective: No Filipino will be without sustenance.
>
> We have therefore set our Development Plans toward a direct and purposeful attack against poverty by: focusing on the poorest of our society, planning to meet their basic nutritional needs, reducing if not entirely eliminating illiteracy, expanding employment opportunities, improving access to basic social services, equalizing opportunities, sharing the fruits of development equitably, and introducing the requisite institutional changes. . . .

This excerpt reaffirms the primacy of nutrition in national development, earlier stated in Presidential Decree 491. The above is particularly encouraging. Its concern for the poorest of the poor (the functional group most seriously affected by undernutrition) happily joins the target group with a goal of nutritional improvement.

Generally, therefore, all is well at *that* policy level. The etiological framework underlying malnutrition, described earlier, shows, however, that there are several other levels for translating nutrition policy into action. The following discussion focuses on the efficiency of this translation process.

Are there policies in the areas of demand for food, supply of food, and its biological utilization that support the above nutrition policy? A scan through the Development Plan reveals that, in fact, supportive policies are there (Table 1), and, provided they are followed vigorously, nutritionists need not worry.

By simply looking at an array of programs and projects, one might easily be convinced that the country's nutritional status is good, or that nutritional improvement is immediately forthcoming. Our nutritional problems are, however, not insignificant, as has been pointed out. Therefore, either some disturbance in translating policy into action, or the translation process itself, suffers from some major pitfalls. Because the reasons for this "translation noise" are not readily apparent, a deeper look into some of these major projects and programs is in order.

One case in point, related to the biological utilization of food, is the development of the health care system and related services. While it can generally be argued that any additional health inputs are desirable, the concentration of such inputs in a particular system may not be advantageous to the nutritional welfare of other groups. The past, and even current (although much less now), concentration of health resources in highly trained doctors and nurses and in high-technology hospitals does not necessarily benefit the rural population and the lower-income groups. The greater Manila area, whose population accounts for only 12.6% of the total Philippine population, benefits from 45.9% of all hospital beds. The concentration of hospital facilities in urban areas may be because the normal tendency of social investments is to seek areas of greater monetary return rather than to form any conscious social policy.

Attempts to redress this inequality are being made through such programs as compulsory rural practice by health personnel, development of paramedical manpower, and the installation of barangay health stations. In any event, Adorna (21) found that the 20% of families with the highest income benefited from 37% of all health expenditures, leaving only 63% of such benefits for 80% of the population. Evidently, there is need to pursue a more vigorous dispersal program for health facilities to areas that need them most.

The situation is not improved by the limited coverage of RHUs, supposedly the pivotal health structure in the rural areas. A probable explanation of this is that RHUs are usually situated in the town proper, generally the residence of the better-off in the rural areas. Partly because of the RHUs' limited catchment areas (the UPSE/PREPF Survey found that 83% of RHU users were within a 0- to 3-km distance) and inadequate numbers of personnel, a substantial fraction of the hard-to-reach, often the poorest, rural population has no access to the rural health delivery system.

It is, nonetheless, consistently observed that RHU expenditures are more available to the poor than are hospitals. While the P0–4000 income group has access to only 36% of public hospital expenditures, its share in RHU expenditure (63%) appears considerable. Tan's study (22) further confirms this. The share of the P0–3999 income group is 49.2 and 54.4% of general hospital and RHU expenditures, respectively. Moreover, in 1974, expenditure data from the Budget Commission and General Auditing Office show that about 63% of public health expenditures (of institutions included in the UPSE/PREPF survey) went to hospital care, while only 31.3% went to RHUs.

The provision of a clean water supply is another major concern affecting biological utilization of food. Only 40% of Filipino households have a potable water supply. On the other hand, there are currently significant numbers of water supply systems lying idle for a variety of reasons. Apparently, one major cause is that the design of the water system

TABLE 1. Policies Supportive of a Broad Nutrition Policy

Demand for food	Supply of food	Biological utilization
1. *Income Policy.* An effective income policy will be followed, taking into account the need to maintain a balance in the growth of incomes, wages, productivity, and prices. Workers will be accorded just compensation that will ensure the maintenance of a minimum standard of living, without prejudice to the efforts to promote a high-employment level in the economy. A high rate of labor absorption will minimize underemployment and assure a steady and upward movement of real wages. Social security will increasingly become an instrument for the protection of workers' welfare.	1. *Resource Use Policy.* The state will promote and regulate the efficient utilization, acquisition, and disposition of land and other natural resources to maximize net public benefit. Land will not be considered as chattel, but as a resource for the benefit of all. As such, the State will institutionalize appropriate organizational structures that will regulate and license the design, usage, location, and intensity of structures and facilities on land and other resources in accordance with desired patterns of national growth.	1. *Human Settlements Policy.* Human settlements will be improved, particularly in the provision of basic amenities and sources of livelihood. A healthy and productive balance between man and his environment will be promoted. Population, services, and facilities will be redistributed to preselected urban areas to diffuse the benefits of development to the countryside.
2. *Employment Policy.* Economic activities that directly or indirectly promote the higher utilization of manpower under just terms and conditions will be encouraged to minimize unemployment and underdevelopment. To enhance labor absorption, particularly in nonfarm activities, the development of manpower skills will be aligned with the requirements of growth. The export of manpower, allowed only as a temporary measure to ease underemployment, will increasingly be restrained as productive domestic employment opportunities are created. This will ensure the availability of talents and skills needed to raise production efficiency in all sectors of the economy. The guarantee of safe, healthful, and humane working conditions will be required from all	2. *Savings Policy.* The encouragement and mobilization of domestic savings are of primary importance for the success of the development plan. This includes the mobilization of rural savings through the organized financial sector and the development of longterm debt instruments. Along this line, the interest rate structure will be aligned with market forces to provide incentives to holders of idle funds, and to promote the application of these funds for appropriate investments. The tax system will be used as a supplementary tool to assist in savings mobilization. Alongside the acceleration of domestic savings mobilization, foreign savings will be effectively utilized.	2. *Social Welfare Policy.* The State will pursue an integrated social program to promote total human social development. Consequently, the national social welfare policy will cover the areas of land reform; health; nutrition; housing; education and culture; manpower development; youth and sports development; children's, women's, and workers' welfare; cultural minorities; social security; and other social concerns. The overall social welfare policy will supplement the economic growth thrusts and ensure a national development consistent with social justice and human dignity. Thus, the living conditions of the general population, particularly the most disadvantaged groups, will be

employers to secure labor welfare. Overseas employment will be better organized to ensure that exported manpower will be accorded equitable and just compensation and treatment in foreign lands.

3. *Price Policy.* Price stability will be promoted to ensure social stability and to provide goods and services that are within the reach of every sector. Likewise, the maintenance of price stability will serve as an incentive for long-term investments. The coverage of socialized pricing will be limited to the most essential goods and services and will be subject to continuing review. Gradual adjustment in the prices of regulated items will be made, taking into account cost of production and accessibility of these goods and services to the low-income group.

4. *Tax and Tariff Policy.* Increasing reliance will be placed on direct taxation and on a more progressive indirect taxation. Stress will be laid on the progressivity of the tax system, with ability to pay as the principal criterion. Apart from the recent improvements in the tariff structure of the country, tariff rates will be further modified to induce local processing and to enhance the efficiency and competitiveness of domestic industries.

5. *Population Policy.* The State will maintain population growth levels most conducive to national welfare. This policy will be pursued without prejudice to the health status and religious beliefs of individuals. A geographical distribution of population consistent with national development will be pursued.

enhanced. Also, the State will implement mechanisms by which the adverse social impact of economic development can be assessed and planned for.

3. *Science and Technology Policy.* The development and widescale application of science and technology will be promoted, especially in the fields of research, local inventions, and adaptation. Technology transferred from developed countries will be adapted to the needs of domestic development. Priority will be given to the dissemination and commercialization of scientific research results.

4. *Agrarian Reform Policy.* Agrarian reform will be a motivating force for social transformation. This program will be vigorously pursued as a concrete measure toward wealth redistribution. The program will emphasize increases in productivity and cooperation to foster the security, welfare, and dignity of the Filipino farmer.

often fails to consider the level of community technology, the beneficiaries' income, and the community preparatory work that needs to accompany installation of a water system. For example, in the design of a metropolitan water system, a third-level system is common practice. One immediate question that can be posed is: Can slum dwellers pay for the service? Such failures often result in (1) an idle water system, (2) water systems turning into sources of water-borne diseases, and (3) very little sense of responsibility among users. While these tendencies have been minimized in recent years, a major strategy reformulation needs to be done.

In the areas of demand and supply of food, some interesting problems are also present. One of these, for example, is the question of exports, particularly of copra. Cooking oil, one major source of calories in the Filipino diet, has become a luxury item in the country. Cooking oil prices have soared beyond the poor man's reach. Part of the explanation is that 80% of the coconuts are exported. While this brings in foreign exchange, these earnings are not necessarily passed down to the actual industry workers and producers.

Another major area of concern is agrarian reform. While the government has pursued this over the years, the impact of such a program needs to be expanded. Lappé and Collins (23), reporting on the land reform program in the Philippines, pointed out not only that the agrarian reform law did not provide adequate coverage and benefits for tenants, but also that its concentration on rice and corn tended to encourage production of nonstaples and export crops. While land reform should not be implemented so drastically as to destroy the middle class and the free enterprise system, the present program would benefit from further study to spread more land to a greater proportion of agricultural producers.

The Integrated Area Development (IAD) Project in the Philippines, currently a major investment area, may also be restudied. A recent experience of the NNC in the area of including nutritional considerations in the plans reveals that, if left untouched, major packages like water supply, irrigation, roads, and agriculture will achieve their primary economic aims, but fall short of nutritional objectives (24).

Another equally important problem stems from the minimum wage. The current minimum wage allowed for industrial and agricultural workers is P13 and P10 per day, respectively. On the other hand, the Food and Nutrition Research Institute's recommended daily food requirements to ensure adequate nutrition for a family of six cost P18.

Masagana 99, the country's success story in rice and corn production, has not been undertaken without pain. According to the Ministry of Agriculture reports in 1979, some 18% of farmers defaulted in their payments in that year. If one were to analyze the Masagana 99 scheme more carefully, it would be noted that it provides credit to farmers *provided* they present some form of collateral. Another aspect is that only production loans are given; consumption loans are disallowed. Such a system screens out those very small farmers who do not have collateral to present. It also makes these farmers, especially those whose consumption is very much dependent on their farm income, fall prey to the middlemen who invest in preharvest trading when hunger periods have set in.

The preceding discussion has attempted to provide some examples of "translation noises" in the three areas affecting nutrition. This was not meant to be comprehensive, but rather illustrative, and should therefore be treated in that light.

These interface problems are basically products of two forces. One major one is the orientation of current agricultural, economic, and health and nutrition planners. Most often these planners and implementors are Western-oriented, either espousing a high-technology approach (as in health), or embracing classical theories of economic dualism and the growth-first-followed-by-welfare theory. Nutritional considerations are not integrated into the planning process. As a corollary to this, food and nutrition policy studies are very scanty, providing little opportunity for on-site planners to learn how to develop a sound nutrition policy.

The absence of any one body that reviews and restructures food and nutrition policies and supportive policies and programs also contributes to this "translation noise." While the NNC is responsible for this task, it does not have a direct link with the National Economic Development Authority (NEDA) and other major development agencies. Neither does the NEDA have a specific body to undertake such functions.

The second major factor is political, referring to the relationship between government and the private sector. Many of the policies and programs in the areas of food demand and supply fall within this relationship. The government's indicative planning power is not strong enough to modify the private sector's motives in favor of government human welfare goals. In some cases, government officials are even in collusion with the private sector's desire to protect its own status quo. Many of these political problems require political solutions, but this does not fall within the scope of this chapter.

SUMMARY AND RECOMMENDATIONS

This chapter has attempted to examine the major problems in the interfaces between nutrition policy and implementation, using the Philippine situation as an example. The case of the Philippines is not unique among developing countries trying to start or pursue their own nutrition programs. A few may be more advanced, but perhaps most are in the earlier stages of development, where the Philippines was not too long ago. Lessons from the Philippine experience will, it is hoped, help the latter countries to avoid the pitfalls and problems that the Philippines faced.

In the light of this retrospective study, some recommendations for the development of a program for food and nutrition policy are the following:

1. *Manpower development.* The development of policy makers, program planners, and implementors who can build nutrition considerations into policy and program formulation and implementation is a prerequisite in food and nutrition policy work. Regional centers for training or graduate work in food and nutrition policy and planning (such as the UPLB-NUFFIC Nutrition Planning Course in Los Baños, Philippines, and the United Nations University Advanced Training Programme on Nutrition Planning being conducted in the Philippines, in Guatemala, and at the Massachusetts Institute of Technology) should be pursued in other areas.

2. *Food and nutrition policy studies.* Thorough country studies should be conducted on existing food and nutrition policies, together with supporting policies and programs, at both design and implementation phases, so that gaps can be identified where nutrition considerations might be included. Guidelines should then be developed on how to incorporate nutrition objectives into agricultural, economic, and health planning.

3. *Nutrition in Integrated Area Development.* IAD projects are being undertaken in many areas. Unless nutrition considerations are consciously built into the design of such projects, they may produce the desired economic effects, but may be counterproductive to nutritional goals. IAD projects, therefore, could very well serve as the entry point for introducing nutrition objectives into development plans.

4. *Organization.* Finally, there should be an organization that would continuously review food and nutrition policies, and recommend, or influence the formation of, relevant policies and the design or redesign of programs to accommodate nutrition objectives. Such an organization should have linkages and influence in the economic, agricultural, health, and social fields.

REFERENCES

1. Adorna, C. L., and A. M. Fernando. Philippine Country Paper on the Food and Nutrition Policy—An Exploratory Study. Manila, November 1978.
2. Solon, F. S. Nutrition and Governmental Policies in the Philippines. Paper presented at the Conference on Nutrition and Governmental Policy in Developing Nations, Bellagio, Italy, September 19–25, 1975.
3. Nutrition Center of the Philippines (NCP). The Philippine Nutrition Program: Building the Community Through Nutrition. Makati, Metro Manila, 1974.
4. National Nutrition Council (NNC). The Philippine Nutrition Program, Five-Year Accomplishment Report, 1974–1979. Makati, Metro Manila, 1979.
5. National Nutrition Council (NNC). The Philippine Nutrition Program, 1978–1982. Makati, Metro Manila, September 1977.
6. Sycip, Gorres, and Velayo (SGV) and Co. Overall and Strategic Effectiveness of the Philippine Nutrition Program, Vol. I, SGV and Co., Makati, Metro Manila, January 1978.
7. Sapinoso, S. Operation Timbang Evaluation of 17 Provinces. Data Bank Section, Nutrition Center of the Philippines, Makati, Metro Manila, August 1978.
8. Adorna, C. L., M. Gonzales, E. de Leon, and G. Montemayor. Nutrition Surveillance: A Brief Review of the UNICEF-Assisted Project in the Philippines. Nutrition Center of the Philippines, Makati, Metro, September 1979.
9. Food and Nutrition Research Institute (FNRI). National Anthropometric Survey, 1978. Manila, Philippines, October 1979.
10. *Five-Year Philippine Development Plan, 1978–1982*. NEDA, Manila, Philippines, September 1977.
11. Food and Nutrition Research Institute (FNRI). 1978 Nutrition Surveys of the Philippines, Preliminary and Partial Results of a Nationwide Survey. Manila, Philippines, July 1979.
12. Daniel, C. Recurrence of Malnutrition. Data Bank Section, Nutrition Center of the Philippines, Makati, Metro Manila, April 1978.
13. Management Planning Division, National Nutrition Council. Submission of Nutrition Action Plans. Makati, Metro Manila, unpublished.
14. Nutrition Center of the Philippines (NCP). NCP Annual Report for 1978. Makati, Metro Manila, 1978.
15. Management Information System, National Nutrition Council. Agency Accomplishments. Makati, Metro Manila, unpublished report, September 1978.
16. Alfonso, M. E., L. Bañez, L. Pineda, R. Florentino, C. Adorna, and R. Guirriec. Organization, Production, Distribution and Utilization of Nutri-Pak—An Evaluation. Nutrition Center of the Philippines, Makati, Metro Manila, July 1979.
17. National Nutrition Council. Philippine Nutrition Program Annual Report—1978. Makati, Metro Manila, July 1979.
18. National Grains Authority. Self-Sufficiency in Rice. *Philippine Farmer's Journal* **19**:5, 1977.
19. Information, Education and Communications Division, National Nutrition Council. Barangay Nutrition Scholar Project Evaluation. Makati, Metro Manila, unpublished report, 1978.
20. National Economic and Development Authority (NEDA). Five-Year Philippine Development Plan, 1978–1982. NEDA Production Unit, Manila, September 1977.
21. Adorna, C. L. The Distribution of Health Resources in the Philippines. Master's Thesis, University of the Philippines School of Economics, Quezon City, 1976.

22. Tan, E. A. Taxation, Government Spending, and Income Distribution in the Philippines. School of Economics, University of the Philippines, 1975.
23. Lappé, F. M., and J. Collins. *Food First: Beyond the Myth of Scarcity*, pp. 354–355, Houghton, Mifflin, Boston, Massachusetts, 1977.
24. Garcia, M. Nutrition Considerations in the Formulation of Project Plans and Designs: A Case Study for Samar Island. Paper presented to the International Workshop on Multi-Sectoral Nutrition Planning and Implementation, Nutrition Center of the Philippines, Makati, Metro Manila, February 12, 1979.

Comment

WARREN BERGGREN

All of the papers on the subject of interventions have emphasized the range of services that must reach the individual, such as primary health care, sanitary water, and family planning, as well as nutrition services. But it is also recognized that, in general, these services are kept administratively or bureaucratically separate at the national, regional, and municipal levels. It is thus the weighty responsibility of the community-level worker, whether it be the Promatura in Colombia, the family planning worker in Indonesia, or the nutrition worker in the Philippines, to integrate the range of services. We should recognize the Herculean nature of this task for the local worker who must integrate an array of services and translate these into useful activities that are responsive to the needs of families and individuals.

WARREN BERGGREN • Department of Tropical Public Health, Harvard School of Public Health, Boston, Massachusetts.

Comment

JOHN O. FIELD

In considering the array of integrated, multisectoral, village-level interventions, we should perhaps be less concerned with what *should* be done, or what *is* done, than with *how* it is done and who does it. My feeling is that doctors and government extension officers are among the weakest pillars on which to build nutrition interventions that are effective in reaching target groups. Therefore, I would emphasize the operational component of nutrition planning in program development. We are very good at diagnosis and planning, and we are getting there on evaluation. However, we are relatively poor in thinking operationally, in viewing nutrition interventions as a process by which change is supposed to happen, in moving from science and technology, where we feel comfortable, to that more murky world of implementation where the idiom is one with which we are much less familiar. It is a world in which you try to apply what you know, but many things go wrong.

A second point the difficulties in implementation suggest is the importance of effective local organizations, as exemplified by the barangay network in the Philippines, in putting nutrition interventions into operation. Effective local organization is necessary to bring about grass roots changes through interventions. Therefore, in order to convert plans into projects, people into a work force, money into credit, and nutrition programs into an instrument of community mobilization and self-help, effective local organization is paramount. The dilemma we face is that effective local organization is such a rare commodity. It is not even the norm; it is not at our disposal.

As planners and implementors, it is incumbent upon us to engineer community organization if we want to make nutrition programs success-

JOHN O. FIELD • Department of Political Science, The Nutrition Institute, Tufts University, Medford, Massachusetts.

ful. Specifically, one of the benefits of an effective local organization is proximity between the programmers on the one hand and the intended beneficiaries on the other. Thereafter, this proximity invites contact and a two-way flow of communication. As a result, participation is redefined from simply attendance or utilization into participation in terms of problem identification, problem definition, and decision-making. Ideally, people in a community will engage in a process of consensus-generation among themselves, so that any endeavor launched has a viable prospect of being sustainable, especially by the people affected by the intervention.

Another ingredient of success in nutrition programs, also an outflow of effective local organization, is flexibility and adaptability in project design so that one does not plan and then ritualistically implement, treating the beneficiaries as targets. On the contrary, it is necessary to build a coalition of interest behind what might be called nutrition goals—which you might define differently to the intended beneficiaries to make the project more meaningful, given their perspectives. By enlisting their support and energy behind goals you will also be able to harness those resources in order to attain those goals and sustain an effort over time.

Based on these notions of community participation and involvement, two propositions emerge. One is that top-down planning and implementation strategies, in which the intended beneficiaries are only targets, are probably doomed to failure. The second is that the key to success is not necessarily the appropriateness or even the adequacy of the nutrition component of a nutrition intervention. Rather, the nature of the system–society interaction that that intervention triggers will be the major determinant of success. Even when a delivery system has worked out all of its intraadministrative, organizational, and logistical quirks, there are countless breakdowns at the level of system–society contact and interaction. I would suggest that this is the Achilles heel of many nutrition interventions all over the world.

Finally, while it may be said that nutrition policy is vital to development policy, it is also true that the development context is vital to nutrition policy, and to the prospects of success of nutrition interventions. I am struck by the fact that the linkage between nutrition and development tends to be raised in the context of advocacy and then forgotten. All too often nutrition interventions are isolated shots in the dark, divorced from anything else that is going on. This should give us pause. Many people accept the premise that, if you have some resources, and if you go through a modestly rigorous planning exercise, identifying need and formulating an appropriate response, you can make an impact on malnutrition. Thus—regardless of the social system, the political system, and how power and influence are exercised and manifested in concerns like land ownership patterns, tenancy, access to credit, and the factors of production—good nutrition planning, it is argued, gets at malnutrition explicitly and directly, *regardless* of that broader environment. I suspect that that premise is wrong because even the best nutrition interventions tend to be overwhelmed by the immensity and the complexity of the problem and provide resources to the malnourished that are minuscule in comparison to their need. Even when nutrition planning and programming are well done, they may not have much impact on a veritable syndrome of deprivation, for which nutrition interventions, almost by definition, are an inadequate response.

It can be concluded therefore that more attention must be focused on structural constraints to adequate nutrition. Unfortunately, we often view those issues as beyond our professional mandate and competence. Therefore, it may be time to reassess who we are, what we are doing, and what contributions we are likely to make.

Discussion

The discussion centered around two points of contention: the interface between research and policy and the interface between policy and politics. Concerning the former, it was noted that there is still a gap between how good science and good research are translated into implementable programs. Greater efforts must be made to determine what "action-oriented people" (implementors, policy makers) can learn from science and, conversely, how science can be made more responsive to the needs of those out in the field.

An example of this science–action linkage concerns the progress that has been made in the field of agriculture. Explicit attention is being given not only to the need for increased production, but also to the questions of who will produce, how will it be produced, and even what will be produced. This is a result of improved technology, coupled with the systematic study of food consumption needs of low-income people and the disaggregation of consumption surveys by income group. The results have suggested that investing in increased production is not necessarily the correct approach to improving a country's nutritional status.

As for the latter issue of policy and politics, it was argued forcefully that underendowment of land and water sources for the poor remains the single most significant cause of malnutrition. Seen in this light, supplementation, fortification, health education, primary health care, and the range of other services that can be provided will not address the fundamental problem. In fact, in the absence of egalitarian and redistributive pressure, the situation will tend to become worse. The poor are inevitably confronted with a decreased variety of foodstuffs, and the migration to the towns only aggravates waste of food due to the logistical problems of transporting it. Therefore, political will and requisite economic policy must underlie any attempt to reduce malnutrition. According to this view, policy will only be effective or have meaning in the context of a country's commitment to structural change.

One participant noted the example of Costa Rica, which has no explicit multisectoral nutrition policy. Nevertheless, it is the only nation in Central America to show marked decreases in mortality and diarrheal disease, and second- and third-degree malnutrition have all but disappeared. The question is: Why? The answer, it was suggested, can be found in the political decision made 15 years ago that health and nutrition are basic rights. Money was raised through taxes to facilitate policies and programs designed to reach those in need. The lesson of this success story, however, is that the evolution of a policy to eliminate malnutrition must be synchronous with the development of political will and commitment, as contrasted with a food and nutrition policy incongruous with other political priorities, or one that is designed to be palliative in nature.

Small Farm Agricultural Systems

V

Without question, one of the most controversial aspects of food and nutrition policy during the past 5 years has been the debate over the efficacy of developing country agricultural producers growing cash crops for export versus staple crops for indigenous populations. A principal element of this discussion has been the role of, and impact upon, small, technically primitive farmers, particularly in areas characterized by increasing concentration of land ownership and growing rural un- and underemployment. Thus, the concern here is both for the positive contribution that small producers can make to the nutritional well-being of less-developed country populations and for the potentially negative nutritional impact on farm families that has resulted, or could result in the future, from changes in national agricultural production policies.

The section begins with a challenging and somewhat controversial presentation by Barraclough on some of the issues inherent in expanding small-farm agricultural production. This is followed by country case studies from Latin America, presented by Fiester, and from Africa, presented by Okigbo, that examine programs designed to reach and benefit the small farmer. The controversial nature of this policy debate is then elaborated upon in the discussant's comments and in the general workshop discussion.

The editors wish to acknowledge the contribution of Nina Schlossman and Patricia Haggerty, who served as rapporteurs for this workshop.

Some Issues in Expanding Small-Farm Agricultural Production

Solon L. Barraclough

Introduction

I have been requested to prepare an "issue paper" on expanding small-farm agricultural production for this volume. This request seems to have some implicit assumption behind it that should be examined critically. In the first place, it assumes that there are issues of expanding small-farm production that can be generalized from experience and usefully discussed in the context of this volume. I am not at all sure that this is the case. In fact, one of the main contentions I wish to make is that conditions are so diverse that the issues can only be treated in relation to specific situations in their own particular historical contexts. I am glad that the volume was planned around case studies; this is the only way to treat the subject in a helpful manner.

The request also assumes that agricultural production, at least in part, takes place on operating units that can be analytically referred to as "small farms," and that these units can be compared usefully from one place to another. In reality "small farm" has a very relative meaning that varies widely from place to place and from time to time. Small farms have to be redefined operationally in each particular context, although I suppose that the editors were referring to some kind of family farm.

Within the context of this volume, the title assigned to me seemed

Solon L. Barraclough • United Nations Research Institute for Social Development, Palais des Nations, Geneva, Switzerland.

to assume that expanding small-farm agricultural production would obviously lead to improved nutrition. This assumption also requires critical examination in each particular situation. I can think of many cases where improving agricultural production on small farms has been accompanied by deteriorating nutrition, both of small-farm families and of many other groups in the particular society where this expansion was occurring.

My own perception of the central issues in "expanding small-farm production" may not be particularly relevant for most decision makers at any level. As I will explain later, I see the central issue as being the terms of incorporation of rural people into societies organized around the imperatives of high-technology, capital-intensive, commodity production and the associated dissolution of self-provisioning agriculture. Another issue that will undoubtedly become more and more central in the future is the search for "alternative developments" that do not encourage the adoption of the high-energy agricultural systems now dominant in the industrialized countries, and, for that matter, imply modification of these systems in the United States and Western Europe, where they originated.

According to Webster, an issue is a debate or a controversy. The two issues that I have just mentioned are not being debated widely by farmers, techno-bureaucrats, politicians, or even most academics. We should commence by asking "issues for whom?"

WHOSE ISSUES?

A problem or an issue arises only when some persons or some groups perceive that their values are being threatened, or that there is something that could be done to attain their objectives that is not being done. This volume of papers by techno-bureaucrats and academics is probably not the best place to discover what small farmers or political leaders perceive to be the issues. But if our work is not to be entirely irrelevant, we must find some way of relating our perceptions to theirs. We do not make decisions affecting small-farm production, although we may sometimes indirectly influence them. I suggest that we should commence by asking ourselves how the different groups involved may perceive the problem of expanding small-farm production.

As small farmers should clearly be the most deeply involved, let us begin with them. But what is a small farmer? Presumably he is an agriculturalist—perhaps an owner or tenant, but possibly with some other form of access to land—who, with his family, produces a surplus for the market and also much of his own food for self-provisioning. He might occasionally hire laborers, or he might work occasionally for other producers, but his basic labor force consists of himself and family members. In other words, it is the "family farm" so dear to the United States and European traditions.

In much of the world, however, these concepts are not particularly applicable. In most of Latin America it is probably more useful to think in terms of "land groups." The land group might be an Indian community or some other settlement of small holders, or it might be a traditional "hacienda," a commercial plantation, a commune or cooperative unit of some sort, or any other rural group defined by its joint occupancy of a given area and its close social interrelationships. In one sense all of these land groups include many small farmers, as even on commercial plantations many laborers have small plots for their own use to produce for family consumption and for the market. None of these land groups, however, closely resemble the groups of small farmers with which most of the agricultural economics literature deals in the United States and Europe. To talk about small farmers without analyzing how their societies developed, who they are, and in what context they are found can lead us to conclusions and speculations that can be highly misleading. In Mexico, for example, "small farmers" are even defined legally, but many who are legally small farmers are, in fact, large commercial entrepreneurs. In Israel, the "moshav" is legally a cooperative farm settlement in which the individual farmer does not own his land, but in reality it is a group of small "family farms" organized cooperatively for carrying out certain functions.

Setting aside these definitional problems, let us assume that we agree on what we mean by small farmers in a particular situation. How do they see the issues of increasing their production? In some cases, the small farmers might not see increasing production as being an issue at all. Their concerns might be more with other matters affecting their livelihood, such as retaining enough of their production for family consumption and marketing the rest on favorable terms without having all their surplus extracted by taxes, high interests, tributes, or any number of other mechanisms. Usually, however, farmers are interested in increasing production, other things being equal. The issues for them can be summarized as: (1) obtaining adequate resources, especially land and water, to provide security of livelihood and productive employment for their labor; (2) marketing of their surplus on favorable terms; and (3) where they have already been partially incorporated into commercial systems, obtaining necessary inputs, credits, technologies, and services as well as consumer goods.

The factors limiting the capacity of small farmers to increase supplies are extremely varied. They may, for example, be technical, socioinstitutional, economic, or cultural. The point to remember is that when one limiting factor is overcome another immediately takes its place. More irrigation and fertilizer may make evident shortages of land, markets, storage and transport facilities, and the like. The small farmer tends to see the issues in terms of immediate limiting factors.

This level of generality, however, tells us almost nothing we did not already know. Again it is necessary to analyze particular cases. What we can predict *a priori*, however, is that resolving favorably for him any of the issues that the small farmer sees as central for increasing his production implies serious conflicts with other groups. Even when we have identified the issues for the small farmer in a particular case, we have done little toward finding solutions.

The issues, of course, are perceived very differently by other social groups. Larger landholders, even when very small by Western standards, often see the issue of obtaining cheap and subservient labor as being central. Landless laborers often see the issues as being their opportunities for secure and remunerative employment, or the access to land for themselves and their families, although again, this varies widely in different historical contexts. To be sure, in large regions of the so-called Third World, the majority of rural people are so close to the margin of subsistence that the major issue for them is how to scrounge a living, especially during periods of scarcity associated with annual and cyclical climatic rhythms.

As small-farm production expands and a land group becomes incorporated into commercial agriculture, what may at the beginning have been a community of more or less equal small farmers usually becomes increasingly polarized between landless laborers and commercial producers. Naturally, the perception of the issues for those affected differently changes radically during this process of market incorporation.

When one asks how other groups in the society perceive "small-farm production" issues, the futility of making international generalizations becomes even more obvious. Each local and national society is unique. One has to study the social structures and processes of each local society and its interactions with the larger national and international systems of which they are a part. Again, all we can do is make some rather trite general observations about how other groups perceive the issues.

The urban poor have a primary interest in obtaining cheaper food. This often creates a contradiction between their interests and those of small farmers, who see the issue as one of higher prices for the agricultural products they sell, although not for those that they have to buy. Higher-income urban groups also often see the issue as one of cheaper food, although their consumption patterns are usually radically different from those of the urban poor. Urban employer groups in particular have an interest in keeping basic food staples cheap in order to minimize social discontent and pressures for higher wages. This kind of approach, however, can only be given analytical content in specific situations. The social groups that are relevant for influencing policies cannot be expected to be the same from one situation to another.

This volume deals with issues of public policy. It grew out of a workshop intended to inform governments about agricultural and nutritional policies that they should change or adopt. Government policies, however, are almost always to some extent contradictory. They depend upon the interactions of numerous social forces—special interest groups and broader supporting class interests—within particular social systems. The state is not a consistently rational, unified and benevolent entity, capable of choosing and entitled to choose a style of development. If we as social scientists hope to contribute to improving policies affecting farm production and nutrition, we have to take the realities of contending social forces fully into account. We might then be able to provide information that would influence the perceptions of the leaders of some of those social forces that, in the final analysis, determine the real strategies of national societies as well as governments.

The demands placed upon government for programs leading to accelerated "development" are growing so rapidly, and the capacities of governments to respond to these demands are so limited, that there appears to be increasing disillusionment about the possibilities of solving complex social problems by established political processes. The politicians must continuously adapt their positions to changing power alignments and other political realities. In this context, the role of technicians and administrators often seems to be crucial in determining policy and implementing it. The "techno-bureaucrats" are frequently seen to be in a position to decide what should be done and how to do it within very wide limits.

One must question, however, how much independence the techno-bureaucrats really have in this respect. The orientation of a particular government is determined by the temporary resolution of contradictory social forces at a given place and time. The techno-bureaucrats who apparently make the key policies affecting agriculture, nutrition, and other matters are selected in a way that tends to make their personal outlooks and objectives coincide with those of the dominant social forces in each society. Even so, techno-bureaucrats do undoubtedly exert a great deal of influence on policy. It is important to ask what their perceptions are of the issues in expanding small-farm production.

Again, it is impossible to make very useful generalizations. The techno-bureaucrat's outlook is, of course, strongly influenced by his class origin and personal experience. This experience often includes studies at a University in the United States or Europe. He may be very aware of issues concerning achievement of more rapid industrial growth and regard the family farm as an anachronism to be eliminated and forgotten as soon as possible. On the other hand, he may emphasize the need to apply the agricultural organizations and technologies that have succeeded with small farmers in certain other countries such as Japan, Taiwan, the United States, Denmark, the USSR, or China. He often sees the issue of whether to have some form of collective farm or a large capitalist agribusiness organization as being a central one. He may view the transnational corporations as a major issue, either as an obstacle to more rapid production increases or as a means for promoting them. He may also have some concern for environmental issues. Most techno-bureaucrats seem to have a penchant for mechanized, high-technology farming systems. Unfortunately, in agrarian countries few techno-bureaucrats have much empathy with peasants or any real knowledge of peasant agriculture and the problems that small farmers actually face. This is one of the reasons that even the best-intentioned policies may have highly negative results for the poorer strata of the rural population, as these poor rural groups usually have little participation in policy making or implementation.

At the level of international organizations and agencies, the perceptions of small-farm production issues tend to reflect those in the governments, and especially the techno-bureaucracies of their constituent nation states. There is an apparent international consensus on development objectives. These include the sustained improvement in individual well-being, the meeting of basic needs for all the populations, a more equitable distribution of wealth for promoting social justice and efficiency of production, the achievement of greater income and employment security, the expansion of health, education, nutrition, housing, social welfare, and measures to safeguard the environment. There is even a formal international consensus on the need for structural changes in society to go hand in hand with rapid economic growth so that existing international, regional, sectoral, and social disparities can be reduced. But the actual programs supported internationally through technical assistance, aid grants, international economic policies, and the like frequently bear little relation to the achievement of these international development objectives. Again, the interaction of social forces and social structures is a much more important determinant than is the perception of the issues by techno-bureaucrats and political leaders. Perceptions of the issues at all levels are an integral part of the social systems and subsystems in which they occur and are not *deus ex machinas*.

When one asks "Issues for whom?" one concludes that it is impossible to write an "issues" paper on expanding small-farm agricultural production that goes beyond banal generalities. When one deals with the implementation of policies this becomes even more the case because the possibilities for different solutions are multiplied. One can cite dozens of examples where certain combinations of policies and implementation mechanisms resulted in highly successful small-farm production experiences. But one can also cite dozens of other cases where about the same combinations were accompanied by resounding failures. It is always possible to analyze in each case why it apparently failed or succeeded. What is not possible is to generalize from one situation to another without studying it first in its own particular social context.

PRODUCTION FOR WHOM?

As I noted in the Introduction, we cannot assume *a priori* that expanding small-farm production will necessarily lead to nutritional improvement for the groups about whom we may be most concerned. We can think of numerous cases where cash crops have been introduced on small farms, such as groundnuts in some parts of West Africa, sugar in the Caribbean region, or cotton in northeast Brazil, that not only displaced basic food staples but did not lead to any improvement in nutrition for the small producers themselves. Their higher output and cash incomes were often associated with the necessity for buying basic foodstuffs of inferior quality at higher costs, and with indebtedness, higher taxes, and other disadvantages.

On the other hand, increased small-farm production may be associated with improved welfare and incomes for many of the producers themselves but with large social costs for other groups. The production of marijuana by peasant groups in Colombia and Mexico or the production of opium by Turkish peasants are good.examples. But one does not have to go to extremes to illustrate.

Several years ago I reported a case in Venezuela in which a handful of "small" farmers obtained access to costly, newly irrigated lands and to highly subsidized credits for machinery and inputs. They were able to produce on a few thousand hectares about one-fourth of the rice that was currently being marketed by local producers in the entire country. As a result, the market for the rice of thousands of small, marginal producers almost disappeared. Similarly, one can point to countless cases where increased production for a particular market of some agricultural commodity resulted in disastrous price declines so that the much larger crop had a total market value inferior to the previous smaller one. Moreover, this phenomenon of local market saturation and price declines can occur easily in countries where a high percentage of total food consumption, including commodities similar to those with market gluts, is being imported or received as "food aid" from abroad. In fact, in one sense the absence of sufficient "effective demand" is almost always one of the chief constraints on increasing agricultural production. How does one generalize about small-farm production issues, given these complexities in the real world?

A basic issue in increasing small-farm production is one of social structure. The power structure in each social system and subsystem determines the small farmer's position and his possibilities of overcoming some of the obstacles facing him. The problems I have alluded to above can seldom be solved piecemeal. The substitution in the cases just mentioned of maize for marijuana, or the limitation of rice producers' freedom to use highly productive, capital-intensive technologies, is certainly not going to make much difference for the different groups that were negatively affected in these situations.

We can assume, I believe, that in any society there is a tendency toward self-organization that permits the most efficient production and extraction of "surplus" for the disposal of dominant social forces. Production for whom and of what are not just agricultural questions and much less questions of small-farm systems, but are rather questions of the organization of the entire local society and its relationships with broader social systems.

THE TERMS OF PEASANT INCORPORATION

UNRISD's Green Revolution studies showed that two of the leading features in the crises of livelihood in most of the developing world are (1) the emergence of more capital-intensive, higher-technology farming, and (2) the accelerating dissolution of self-provisioning agriculture, both as a major element in peasant farming and as a subsistence base for the poorer rural strata.

The commercialization of production and exchange relations, the growing competition for good-quality lands by entrepreneurial farms, and the increasing numbers of landless laborers and of families trying to extract a living from diminishing areas of poor quality lands all contribute to this process of decay. The food systems that have maintained humankind throughout most of its history are disintegrating before other forms of economic activity are able to offer alternative means of livelihood to the displaced peasantry.

The full significance of this transformation is not entirely compre-hended, but it seems to imply deterioration in the nourishment of the already poor who are obliged to purchase food in unfavorable conditions from the market; massive migration to urban centers; growing unem-ployment and underemployment; and a much higher level of conflict, disorder, and repression.

As I noted earlier, for me this is the central issue. What can be done to modify these historical processes of incorporation so that countless millions are not left destitute or worse during the next few decades? This is not an issue that will be resolved by government decrees and laws or by international resolutions. Neither will it be resolved by new technol-ogies, better education, improved credit and extension services, rapid industrialization, or even "economic miracles."

The only long-term solution seems to lie in what has come to be called "another development." In a recent UNRISD publication ("Social Development and the International Development Strategy," published in Geneva in 1979), we summarized three propositions deriving from studies of development alternatives that we believe have a legitimate place in discussions of development strategies. These were as follows:

a) Achievement of the "ultimate objectives" of development requires enhancement of decision-making capacity at the national level, which cannot be confined to decision-making by the state. Organized and informed popular participation is essential, and such participation will entail tension with centralized technocratically-oriented social as well as economic strategies. The proposition that the people must become sub-jects rather than objects of development is not new but its implications can no longer be evaded.

b) A truly international strategy must confront the ecological and interna-tional equity case for modifying patterns and levels of consumption in the high-income industrialized countries. Unless this happens market forces and the demonstration effect will continue to exert nefarious influ-ences on the development of poor countries. The questioning of consum-erist lifestyles by public opinion in these countries makes such a con-frontation more practicable now than only a few years ago. The main legitimate objective is to meet the needs of all the population now and in the future. . . .

c) The dethroning of imported and imitative "consumer societies" for afflu-ent minorities in the developing countries will also be a key component in any development strategy deserving the allegiance of the masses and capable of securing sufficient domestic capital accumulation. There is no way of achieving development goals within the constraints of present-day technological knowledge, natural resource availabilities and organi-zational capabilities while at the same time meeting sophisticated con-sumerist demands of the rich countries and higher income groups in the poor countries while also encouraging their spread to wider strata. . . . Moreover, while consumption and production structures are co-determined, the former can be changed more quickly than the latter. To attempt to reach development goals on a global scale by merely augmenting production without changing consumption and production structures in both rich and poor countries is foredoomed to be an exercise in futility. Achievement of such changes would require massive educational efforts at all levels in coordination with effective supportive national and international policies.

The general propositions, however, say nothing about how to mobilize the social forces necessary to modify social trends significantly toward desired new directions. In my opinion, there can be no general prescriptions just as there can be no general analyses that adequately take into account all the diverse conditions found in the real world. It is a matter of having one's long-term goals in mind and working patiently in given concrete situations to influence those social forces capable of changing social processes and structures. We can contribute in this volume if we analyze the issues of increasing small-farm agricultural production realistically in each case, taking into account the implications for all different groups in the social system.*

BIBLIOGRAPHY

"Food Systems and Society—Problems of Food Security in the Modern World" (Summary of an UNRISD project), June 1979.
"Critical Appraisal of the Chilean Agrarian Reform (November 1970–June 1972)," Solon Barraclough and Almin Affonso, CEREN, Santiago, April 1973.
"No Plumbing for Negroes," Solon Barraclough, *Atlantic Monthly*, September 1965.
"Social Development and the International Development Strategy," UNRISD, Geneva, 1979.
"Seeds of Plenty, Seeds of Want," Andrew Pearse, UNRISD, Geneva, 1980.

Methodological Issues: What has been said in this chapter raises a number of issues concerning the methodologies commonly used to study agricultural production and nutritional problems. At UNRISD we have concluded that a structural system approach is most promising. This approach would look at agricultural production, transformation, distribution, and consumption as a subsystem within larger social systems, which, in turn, are subsystems of other systems. This bibliography explains our ideas of how one might approach more fruitfully than in the past the interface between agriculture and nutrition.

A Regional Approach to Agricultural Development and Its Potential Insights for Nutrition Planning

Donald R. Fiester

The United States has provided agricultural assistance bilaterally to the five countries of Central America—Costa Rica, Guatemala, Honduras, Nicaragua, and El Salvador—since the end of the Second World War. In 1962, upon the creation of the Central American Common Market, the U.S. developed the Regional Office for Central American Programs (ROCAP) to assist in promoting regionwide support for the Common Market. Recently, ROCAP's role has been reoriented toward activities of a research and development nature, of broad interest to all five countries, centering on the area's small-farm problems.

ROCAP programs, working through a group of specialized regional institutions, thus interface with AID's bilateral programs as well as with those evolving nationally in each country. Bilateral programs concurrently focus on issues of local concern. In agriculture, they concentrate on national and area development by providing technical assistance to credit, rural health, land reform, research, extension, and rural education agencies. U.S. bilateral assistance is responsible for working with those

Donald R. Fiester • Regional Office for Central American Programs, Agency for International Development, Department of State, Guatemala City, Guatemala. *Present address:* Office of Agriculture, Development Support Bureau, Agency for International Development, Department of State, Washington, D.C.

institutions that directly contact large numbers of small farmers and the rural poor.

This chapter will describe ROCAP's agricultural programs, some of our experience to date, and ROCAP's implications for the design of future Central American nutrition and agricultural development programs.

THE SETTING

Central America is relatively small—about the size of California and the southern third of Oregon. However, it is complex ethnically, ecologically, and politically. From a developmental standpoint, it is an ideal laboratory for demonstrating new methods and approaches to nutritional, agricultural, and economic development applicable to most other tropical areas of the developing world, because one can easily conceptualize and compare interventions under different conditions and test them at relatively low cost.

Central America's total population is now estimated to be just over 16 million. Rural, per area, population densities vary from roughly 0.1 to over 5 people per arable hectare.* The region's population is expected to increase to over 35 million by the year 2000. Yearly per capita income levels range from $52 for the lowest 50% of the population in Honduras to $2478 for the highest 50% in Costa Rica (1970). Rural income levels are usually less than one-fourth those of urban dwellers, which contributes to a high and increasing level of urban migration. Spanish is the first language for approximately 70% of the area's population; the remainder speak one of almost thirty dialects. Literacy, in spite of major efforts to increase the number and quality of schools, still varies from slightly over 30% in Guatemala to over 90% in Costa Rica.

In Central America, crops and livestock are produced on land ranging from sea level to over 10,000 feet elevation. Rainfall varies from area to area, with a low of about 20 in. per year in the driest areas to over 21 ft in the wettest. Temperature varies from less than 32°F for a very few hours at night at higher elevations to over 95°F during the day on the coast. In contrast, winter and summer variation in daylight is less than one hour. The Pacific watershed is characterized by a distinct dry season of from 4 to 7 months in duration; along the Atlantic Coast, the dry season may be as brief as 1–2 months.

These ecological and topographic differences result in a varied and

---

*1 hectare = 2.4 acres.

complex agriculture. Plants that have economic importance include bananas, plantain, cotton, corn, beans, rice, sorghum, cacao, rubber, allspice, and vanilla near sea level; citrus, corn, beans, cardamom, avocados, coffee, and vegetables at mid-elevations (2000–6000 ft); and wheat, potatoes, apples, pears, cabbage, cauliflower, and pine trees at the higher elevations (over 6000 ft), with animal exploitation at almost all elevations.

The largest farming systems in Central America are the simplest, whereas the small farmer is manager of the most complex systems. The least complicated agricultural management systems are found on large, sophisticated, export-oriented, single-product farms producing coffee, cotton, rubber, beef cattle, bananas, or cardamom. Though relatively simple in organization, these farms currently use (and in some cases misuse) the highest levels of fossil energy and "modern technology," including mechanical land preparation, major and minor element fertilizers, pesticides, weedkillers, improved or selected varieties, and relatively sophisticated product preparation in on-farm or cooperative processing plants. Farm size depends upon type of production and investment pattern, ranging from approximately ten to several thousand acres. By contrast, AID's target group of small farms employs very complex, though less capital-intensive, systems, with greater risk aversion, low levels of production inputs, and more intensive cropping patterns. These result in high land-equivalent ratios (the combined plant density of the group of crops comprising a system compared to the area required for a full stand of the same commodities planted separately), and more intense use of available physical resources.

Small farms have been the traditional source of food crops—corn, beans, sorghum, potatoes, cassava, and a range of fruit species—to meet the needs of the area's rural and urban population. Most recently, vegetables have also become a significant and expanding small- and medium-sized farm output, both as raw sales products and as base material for food processing. In Central America at this time, it is estimated that there are over 1.5 million farms of less than 20 acres in size.

Every market in Central America, in contrast to some other parts of the world, always has food for sale. Regional imports of basic foodstuffs are usually below 10% of annual consumption. That food is available leads one to assume that for most food items farmers are currently meeting effective demand. The volume of sales, however, is small compared to that in more developed countries, because rural and urban purchasing power is low. Too often, unfortunately, only a short distance from the food market, even in the rural sector, people are undernourished and plagued by parasites.

In the overall context, purchasing power, employment, access to land, and use of well-adapted technology appear to be among the key elements in improving rural welfare. However, it is frequently forgotten that farmers do not produce food because someone is hungry, but because they have a market for their production. Therefore, though food production is, and will continue to be, important, it is not necessarily the main ingredient needed to improve the quality of life for the rural poor.

Recognizing that certain areas of Central America already have a high level of rural unemployment (varying from 8 to 30%), with seasonal variations, and low per capita incomes, and that existing rural production systems are not expected to meet future needs, new approaches to agricultural as well as nutritional development are urgently needed.

The ROCAP Regional Agricultural Program

In 1973 AID, through its ROCAP office, began to revise its rural sector program in order to increase its effectiveness and capacity to stay on the leading edge of small-farm agricultural development in the region. Various studies—both internal and performed by such Central American regional counterpart institutions as the Secretariat of the Central American Common Market (SIECA), the Inter-American Institute for Agricultural Sciences of the OAS (IICA), the Institute of Nutrition of Central America and Panama (INCAP), the region's Tropical Agricultural Research Center (CATIE), the Industrial Technological Institute for the region (ICAITI), the region's Development Bank (CABEI), and the private-sector-oriented management center (INCAE)—were undertaken to help us identify a number of new activities. From these, four main project activities in agriculture and agro-industry have thus far been selected for U.S. support. These have been chosen on the basis of:

1. Commonality of the problem.
2. Potential of the activity to complement national efforts or bilateral programs.
3. Flexibility of the proposed activity to develop methods and operational results applicable to different ecological, economic, or social problems or situations.
4. Potential of the activity to make a significant impact on large numbers of the rural poor, especially the small farmer, in a reasonable time frame.
5. Cost effectiveness in the use of high-level regional expertise, as well as financial and other resources.

6. Potential to provide improved, integrative solutions through continuing Central American regional and national efforts after U.S. assistance has been completed.

The ROCAP agricultural program, as it has evolved, covers a considerable spectrum of project activities currently involving several regional institutions and several hundred national technicians in over 30 national agencies. It also interfaces with the work of bilateral AID Missions and their assistance activities, and through them to small farmers and rural labor. Research has now been carried out on over 500 small farms in 14 areas among the five Central American countries and Panama.

Initiating this new program in 1975, ROCAP developed two key projects in the agricultural area. These were the Agricultural Research and Information and Small Farm Cropping Systems projects.

THE AGRICULTURAL RESEARCH AND INFORMATION PROJECT

The project works through the Programa de Investigación Agrícola del Istmo Centroamericano (PIADIC) of the Inter-American Institute for Agricultural Sciences of the OAS. In Central America, PIADIC is concerned with the improved organization, collection, and use of numerical and written agricultural information at all levels of the public and private sectors.

This project was selected because it offers innovative opportunities for directly and indirectly assisting large numbers of small farmers. From the farmer's standpoint, he farms his small holding in a manner that is completely logical within his and his family's frame of reference. He sees opportunities through personal exposure to the local marketplace; in what he learns from his neighbors and outsiders, filtered by his own past experience; and through extension training courses, the radio, and what his father taught him. In order to improve the farmer's decision making, change agents must have good production information that can be adopted or adapted on small farms. This must be accompanied by better market information in order to give producers the confidence required to cultivate their farms more intensively or with a different production mix.

From the national planning, research, credit extension, and marketing agency standpoint, more appropriate data are required to make more effective decisions that can better integrate the best interests of the country with those of the farmer. This demands an improved understanding of farmers and their decision making, as well as of national needs.

Following an in-depth evaluation of some 130 public sector institutions producing, analyzing, or disseminating information in the region,

ROCAP, in 1975, signed an agreement with IICA, located in San José, Costa Rica, for the implementation of this project in Central America and Panama.

The project includes:

1. *Systems for collecting and preserving research results.* It has been said that a researcher's files in Central America contain more about new production methods than does any other source. Little of the research conducted in the region during the past 30 years has been summarized and brought together in a form that extension agents or their clients can use. Unfortunately, too, past research has not been recorded in such a manner that someone, other than the person who conducted the study (if even he!), can later interpret the data, evaluate the quality of the research, or determine where or under what climatic conditions the work was done.

One element of the IICA project is an attempt to develop more complete research reporting systems, so that future data not only will not be lost, but can become available in a form that can be used and evaluated in and of itself and compared to other research in order to produce farm recommendations. The project is also working with national counterparts to bring together past research, evaluate its utility, and store it in appropriate systems for future national and regional use.

2. *The collection of rural sector socioeconomic statistical data using the sample frame methodology.* Sample framing is a tested, cost-conscientious, USDA-stratified, location-specific sampling technique used to collect a range of rural sector data. Sample frame networks are now essentially complete for El Salvador and Panama, complete for the agricultural area of Nicaragua, well advanced in Guatemala, and being developed in Honduras. Production data, data on small-farm land use, cropping patterns, costs, and yields are being collected in five countries and should be available in all six countries by the end of 1982. Costs for data collection, as well as the timeliness and relevance of the data to national resource allocation decisions, are far superior to that under previous improvised "windshield" assessments that were expensive but usually inaccurate, nonreplicable surveys.

3. *Priority data bases are being developed to support research design and agricultural sector planning.* In order to bring together and systematize the most reliable information available on soils, climate, production, marketing, and rural socioeconomic conditions, IICA, with appropriate national institutions, is organizing systems and procedures for the collection, storage, retrieval, analysis, and dissemination of these data in all six countries. Where appropriate, as existing data are brought together

and verified, they are being published or stored for rapid retrieval and use.

Using more compatible basic data systems will permit the exchange of these data among countries, permitting planners to identify sources of food supplies or alternate markets, improve the basis on which price policies are established, identify new areas for public investment, and reduce research redundancy. From the farmer's standpoint, better access to credit, good production recommendations, and more accurate market data can help him to improve his utilization of land, capital, and labor resources.

Using these data, national technicians are bringing together the essential information required to produce 17 area-specific profiles characterizing each area ecologically, socially, and economically. The profile also combines production recommendations for single crops having high income and employment potential for small farms in specific geographic areas.

4. National information centers are being developed with data exchange among countries. Initially these centers are being developed for each country. The key functions are those of planning, research, marketing, and extension. As these develop, and as each country wishes to integrate additional institutions into its system, it may do so. IICA is assisting each country to analyze the various types of data needed, who will collect it, and how, when, and for what reason, and it is also assisting the governments to determine institutional responsibilities within the national system.

As national systems are integrated, collaboration among institutions collecting, processing, or using similar data in the six countries is beginning to evolve. As a result, the climatological institutions already have held meetings in all six countries on the needs and uses of these data for agricultural planning. Similar exchanges are taking place in marketing agencies and among production researchers. In addition, the regional institutions such as INCAP in nutrition, ICAITI in the agro-industrial area, CATIE in production research, and SIECA are determining the types of data required and the manner in which they are collected in their areas, and thus have a new entrée into developing new working relations with their national counterparts.

SMALL-FARM CROPPING SYSTEMS PROJECT

In 1975, ROCAP signed a four-year agreement with the Centro Agropecuario Tropical de Investigación y Enseñanza [Tropical Agricultural Center for Research and Training (CATIE)] in Turrialba, Costa Rica, for a new project, "Small-Farm Cropping Systems," using a new approach to small-farm production research.

After analysis of past research methods and their results, it was concluded that conventional, individual-technician research, conducted in a single discipline on a single crop (e.g., fertilizer levels for corn), and carried out on experiment stations, was not use-effective on small farms. Consequently, the new cropping systems research project concentrates on interdisciplinary research teams conducting research on small farms in various ecologically similar areas and focusing on the total annual production cycle rather than on a single crop for a single season.

Field research was preceded in each area by a macro-sociological, economic, agronomic, and infrastructure study. This was intended to educate researchers about where farmers were in their production practices and to help them understand better the farmer's economic, labor, soil, market, and other constraints, as well as his present profit level. Simply stated, CATIE wanted to start *where the farmer was* in the use of production resources rather than *where the technician wanted the farmer to be.* Also, since most small farms (up to 75% in some areas) were multiple-(or inter-)cropping (growing two or more crops on the same land at the same time), the CATIE/country research teams focused locally on multiple-cropping for the full production cycle. All field experiments, other than methodology studies conducted at CATIE's research station, have been carried out on small farms with the participation of the farmer and his family.

After 4 years, the first packages of new recommendations have now evolved, and a preliminary methodology for conducting this complex type of applied research has been developed. Results have been better than expected. With the new technologies, increases in per-area income of over 300% are frequently brought about by simple changes in cropping patterns, use of closer or different planting configurations, changing varieties, and, in some cases, inserting one new crop into a system. This is usually done with minimal increase in production costs. In some experiments, vegetable protein yields of over 700 kg/hectare or caloric levels (edible portion) of over 100 million cal/hectare have been reported per growing season among selected trial plots.

By shifting from single-cropping to multiple-cropping and using a team approach, the project has led to various other changes. The researcher cannot evaluate differences by simply measuring weight of product, because different crop combinations are involved. Thus, such measures as costs, profitability, calories, protein, biomass, and labor have become essential to compare treatments. The goal of the ultimate production recommendation (i.e., whether to maximize profit, minimize risk, increase labor productivity, augment protein or caloric production, or strive for a mix of these goals) significantly influences the final package offered to small farmers.

Interaction among crops is just beginning to be understood, as are the interactions between multiple-cropping and inputs. Changes in the planting distance between corn and beans, for instance, can change yields significantly, as can changes in the mix of crops and the planting date of different crops. With multiple-cropping, the weed population tends to decrease, total insect populations appear to remain similar, but the number per species changes considerably, usually reducing both the need for pesticides and the incidence of diseases that cause yield depression. The reason for this happy result, however, is still not yet well understood. Also, fertilizer use efficiency appears to increase in multiple cropping.

This year, building on the very promising experience to date, ROCAP has signed a new agreement for a larger and more complex set of activities with CATIE for the next 4 ½ years. Ecologically similar production areas selected with the host country research agency will continue to serve as a basic element, and the program will involve an interdisciplinary team approach and fieldwork carried out directly on small farms. The project will involve both crops and, for the first time, small animals. The goals of this research are to:

1. *Develop an additional ten multiple-cropping systems, six mixed-crop-and-animal systems, and six animal systems with improved production recommendations.* This will expand beyond the initial ten cropping systems produced in the first project and permit CATIE and national researchers to begin to integrate animals into a whole-farm approach. Greater emphasis on meeting family nutrition needs and on more profitable and more labor-intensive farming systems are the objectives.

2. *Conduct research on improved methods of disseminating systems research results.* Almost all present extension activities in the region center on the transfer of one or two new inputs to a single-crop system (e.g., a fertilizer recommendation, control of a pest or disease, a new variety). We have little experience in Central America on ways to introduce a complete, improved system covering the total production cycle for a year to a small farmer in a manner which he can understand and use effectively. This research will employ several of the ten systems just completed and study alternate, cost-sensitive methods of effectively transferring these to large numbers of small producers. Here we expect to interface agronomic, anthropological, and transfer researchers with extension agents in the development of materials, testing the potential of mass media, group

training, and other tools for affecting the decision making of large numbers of small farmers. Concurrent studies of how farmers accept and
apply new methods of production will be evaluated, and the results will
be fed into the transfer system study.

*3. Develop at least one method to extrapolate research results from one area
to another.* Applied production research, as now conducted, is very site-
specific. Its transfer and use in other geographic areas is empirical, based
on the researcher–extension agent–farmer experience and using trial and
error approaches. This means, thinking in terms of specific sites, that the
development of even one improved production system recommendation
for all of the area's small farmers—despite major investments and efforts
by the ministries of agriculture of the entire region—is many years away.
Ways must be found to transfer production recommendations with confidence based on nonempirical systems.

In this research, CATIE will draw on the IICA Agricultural Research
and Information baseline data and test new approaches for the extrapolation of production results and system elements from one area to
another using ecological analogs. At the outset, we will evaluate two different approaches to extrapolating systems transfer with yield production potential. Later, we hope to integrate market and labor data into the
models and conduct further field tests.

4. Train national technicians in farming systems. Over 100 Central American technicians received training in various phases of the cropping systems research project. Under the new farming systems project, this training will continue and expand to include 18 Masters-level degree
scholarships for Central Americans and short-course training for over
200 technicians.

Although it is not possible to discuss this in detail in this chapter,
ROCAP has also been involved in several other important projects that
directly or indirectly relate to small farmers. We have provided loans
totaling over $20 million to two regional banking institutions for agro-
industry development. This is closely linked to the production of agricultural products on small farms for sale in the Central American Common Market or for export out of the region. We have also recently signed
an agreement with CATIE to conduct research on small farms throughout
the region for the production of fuel wood from fast-growing trees and
shrubs. The availability of fuel wood is decreasing rapidly, and the
amount of time needed to collect it, as well as its cost (often exceeding
15% of family income), is soaring. It does little good to produce food if

people cannot cook it. Thus, we feel this work is essential for helping to improve small farm and rural community self-sufficiency in low-cost energy.

Another important ROCAP project focuses directly on nutrition and nutrition planning. This builds on the outstanding research, extension, and training capability of INCAP and assists it to link more closely with national governments in this extremely important area. INCAP is at present working with the member countries to develop a national nutrition planning infrastructure and to implement selected nutritional interventions in each cooperating country to improve the diet and health of rural and urban people.

ROCAP AGRICULTURAL RESEARCH EXPERIENCE AND NUTRITION PLANNING

It should be emphasized that the present focus of ROCAP agricultural research is relatively new. Both we and our counterpart institutions still have much to learn from the approach in agronomic as well as nutritional and human welfare terms. We believe that some of our experiences may have a corollary in nutrition planning, and that some of the results to date should be more closely examined by those planning programs— agricultural as well as nutritional—in other parts of the world. Our regional institutions have learned much in the process about establishing research organizations, developing procedures for systems research, studying their small-farm clients, working with national institutions having different approaches to the rural problem, designing experiments to attain a goal, and developing farmer recommendations. Not all of our experience has been a success story, but the results to date give us confidence that we are aiming in a sound direction.

Our experience may offer some insights into certain factors and approaches needing emphasis in the design and implementation of new programs in nutrition as well as in agriculture. Some of these points are already being used by nutrition planners. Some may be somewhat new. We would summarize what we consider to be the most important insights as follows:

1. *Change the focus.* Although it is often difficult to change direction in an approach to applied research, our experience in dealing with sets of problems, rather than single-element studies, has been extremely useful. Our approach permits researchers of different technical backgrounds to work together and understand better how their concerns interface

with those of their colleagues in the solution of a common problem. It permits them to reevaluate whom they are trying to help, for what reason, and where. A new focus allows both those helping and those who are being helped to see their problems and relationships in a new light. Often, factors that appeared important from a technical point of view, when seen in light of the farmers' concern, become less important. A new focus also permits the breaking of organizational and operational rigor mortis, allowing many of the most potentially effective researchers and change agents stagnated by "the system" to become innovative again and to contribute new ideas to the process.

2. *Where possible, work in a multicountry context.* Most nutrition and agronomic problems are not unique to political boundaries or to areas in a country. Working in a multicountry context permits technicians from different institutions and different countries to pinpoint those problems that are common and those that are site-specific. Working together is frequently more effective in evaluating the national and farmer consequences of food self-sufficiency vs. food interdependency. Those reviews often result in technicians carrying back to their political leaders new ideas and different sets of options that meet both food needs and broader human welfare objectives more satisfactorily.

The multicountry approach can also be used as a tool to permit peer cross-fertilization of technical expertise and more effective approaches and exchange of data on a range of factors that can assist in reducing costs, saving time, and increasing sensitivity to the needs of the ultimate beneficiaries. Few countries have the expertise available with which to be self-sufficient in planning, research, or implementation; thus multicountry-oriented programs can stimulate better use of all available professional talent, resources, and experience.

Multicountry approaches are excellent for training. All of a country's technicians do not have the same experience and professional background. Courses—mainly short-term sessions—are more cost-effective regionally, especially where a few people per country are needed in a specific discipline. Students in these courses usually form professional and personal bonds going beyond the subject matter, and frequently develop continuing collaborative relationships on key problems of mutual concern.

3. *Where possible, use multidisciplinary teams for problem solving.* In agriculture the multidisciplinary approach is extremely important. By training (and this is more significant at higher degree levels), technicians are more concerned with a particular disease, an individual insect, or a spe-

cial variety of plant than with the total system. They too often concentrate on a problem in their professional field rather than on *farmers'* problems. Also, they are more concerned with yield results than with profitability, efficient use of inputs, and the marketability of the farmers' products. Similar corollaries undoubtedly exist in nutrition.

Multidisciplinary and multicountry efforts are not a panacea, nor are they easy. They often require complex and difficult administrative management and depend upon individual willingness to collaborate, exchange knowledge, and develop true give-and-take among peers. They require flexibility in methodologies, permitting local factors to play a role in both planning and implementation. At the outset, it is often difficult to achieve the understanding and interpersonal exchange of ideas required to make the experience effective, taxing the capacity of the assistance donor as well as the recipient.

However, the grouping together of agronomists, economists, sociologists, nutritionists, and other specialists with experience relevant to a problem can evolve approaches and considerations of alternatives that would not otherwise be formulated. Dietary specialists who know local nutritional problems can guide production researchers to integrate crops, animals, or home self-sufficiency subsystems into improved, farmer-accepted production packages. Conversely, agronomists and social scientists working together with nutrition specialists can develop new cost-conscientious, ecologically adapted diets for urban and rural communities. Unfortunately, the use of multidisciplinary teams has thus far not been widely adopted in Central America.

4. Set quantifiable, time-phased goals for both research and implementation of agronomic and nutritional programs. Agronomic researchers and transfer agents working in applied programs appear to have an aversion to quantifiable goals. Well thought-out, concisely framed, quantifiable, targeted goals can focus applied research and its transfer toward more effective use of financial as well as human resources, but time-phased goals are much less effective in guiding more basic research requiring highly intuitive and more abstract solutions to biological problems.

The careful framing of problems and the establishment of quantifiable goals promote more careful selection of applied research interventions and approaches having a greater economic or social impact. Agronomic researchers left on their own too often become involved in studies that may be interesting, but which do not address themselves to target population priorities. Conducting research and transferring results to low-income target populations is an expensive process in itself. In developing countries, where skilled technicians are limited and the demands on capital many, it is crucial to concentrate on fewer well-chosen objectives. Work must be carried out with a sense of system, urgency, and priority for those things that can make a quantum difference to many people in a reasonable time frame. This is true in agriculture and has its corollary in nutrition planning.

To have well-quantified goals is not enough. Social as well as economic changes within, or exogenous to, the area or problem can make periodic revision of the goals themselves as well as their quantification necessary. Thus, a formal periodic process of evaluation of both results and goals must be built into the process. This will permit shortening of the preestimated goal achievement time, increasing the time frame, or abandoning the goal or line of research altogether, should this be necessary.

Agronomic scientists are extremely cautious about their results. Some would say they want to continue experimenting until the "ultimate" has been discovered. Developmentalists, on the other hand, are usually so desperate for change that they are willing to take risks and base new programs on inconclusive and often flagrantly flimsy data. The one who suffers from either extreme in agriculture is the small farmer. Well-designed research programs with clear goals and quantifiable targets can be a means of ameliorating this dichotomy, permitting the applied researcher certain freedom of action, yet promising results which transfer agents can use effectively in their work with small farmers.

5. *The Production vs. income dilemma.* At present in Central America, small farmers produce almost all of the basic food crops used in the region's diet as well as the area's fruits and vegetables. Larger farmers are almost entirely involved in production of higher-profit export products such as coffee, cotton, sugar, and rubber, although some small producers also cultivate these crops.

A major issue is the question of how much small producers should be encouraged to meet national food requirements and relinquish the higher income potential inherent in producing for export. At present, even with subsidies pushing prices well above world levels in all of the Central American countries, small farmers find it difficult to generate profits higher than $200/hectare from basic food crops or animals. In El Salvador and the highlands of Guatemala (possibly the forerunners of things to come in other areas), where the population density is often over four people per hectare, the low income derived from basic food crops and their poor employment-generating capacity offer little opportunity for improving the quality of life of many small farmers and their families.

Looking at the question from a development standpoint we may ask: Should small-farm production be shifted to: (1) a different, high-profit mix of production, (2) self-sufficiency of basic food crops for the farm family and concentration on higher-income and employment-generating activities on the rest of the land, or (3) new levels of subsidization, with continued small-farm concentration on basic food production? Each of these solutions will have political, social, and economic consequences if extended to a significant number of producers. Answers are urgently needed to guide both research and public investment. More comprehensive study of this issue will be necessary before it can be resolved satisfactorily for the farmer and each nation as a whole.

6. Production, employment, and nutrition planning. If the attainment of production levels capable of meeting internal effective demand and the creation of greater employment (with consequent income distribution effects) by farmers are, in fact, the seat of the nutrition problem, this has major potential consequences for both production and utilization of food. The problem is equally social and economic. Unfortunately, the economists have been more articulate than the social scientists in defending their approach. Social scientists, nutritionists, home-improvement extension agents, and agriculturalists who can work pragmatically and approach the employment and nutrition problems in more macro terms are urgently needed. At present, political policy makers are not addressing this difficult issue squarely enough to give rural development specialists the insights required to make our contributions more meaningful. In this area as well as others, the greater use of interdisciplinary team approaches can be extremely beneficial in filtering through alternatives and evaluating trade-offs.

7. Extrapolation and transferability of potential solutions. In agriculture, we are beginning, through several world-wide efforts, to address the dual problems of extrapolation and transferability. Several models are being developed that will test certain hypotheses for the extrapolation of results developed in one location to similar areas where the research has not been conducted. In human nutrition, the problem appears to be less demanding, and extrapolation should be considerably easier. Nutrition planners, however, could provide valuable insights into local problems by geographically mapping nutritional problem areas. Then, working closely with agricultural planners, production researchers, credit agencies, and extension agents, they could focus in each setting on those products having a potential for contributing to the solution of nutritional problems as well as leading to greater family income and employment.

It is recognized that dietary habits also play a significant role in the potential for extrapolation of nutrition solutions. However, in one case, we found that existing dietary habits were limited more by the mix of food products locally available than by dietary preference. In an area in which *Phaseolus* beans to meet local needs were being grown under adverse agronomic conditions with consequent low yields, the introduction of better adapted, high-yielding cowpeas has led to a rapid change to the new crop and has resulted in ready acceptance of it by rural farm families. This step is not only increasing income, but contributing toward improving the diets of small-farm families as well.

Information transfer in agriculture, as well as in nutrition, may be the greatest, most complex, and recalcitrant problem facing developers. We are seriously hampered by a lack of knowledge about producers and consumers and how and why they make decisions. We also lack the capacity to offer new information quickly in a stimulating manner to large numbers of people (many agricultural publications printed today are better sedatives than Valium).

Improving transfer effectiveness will require more penetrating sociological studies and new operational organizations with better transfer tools to meet this serious need. Radio, if one is to judge by recent research studies in Guatemala, offers a tool that deserves much greater attention than it is being given. Also, extension workers must know how to identify progressive farmers and use them more effectively in stimulating others to adopt new ideas. In nutrition, how much has been done to identify women who are leaders in dietary changes, and how much are they being involved by, or as, nutrition transfer agents? Nutrition interventions probably follow the same two-step process of acceptance and use that we find in agriculture. For both, we must learn much more about how to increase *acceptance* of new ideas and about what conditions are required to promote *use* by millions of rural and urban people.

Transfer itself, even with a good product, is a costly, time-consuming process. It is more difficult in Central America because farming patterns are different from what we have been accustomed to in the U.S. As an example, an Iowa extension agent may work with 200 farmers who have 200 acres each. He introduces a change worth $10 of net profit per acre per year, or a total benefit of $400,000. His counterpart in a less-developed country also works with 200 farms and an equal $10 per acre annual improvement. Unfortunately, however, his clients have only two-acre farms, so the total benefit is only $4000. If the U.S. agent is paid

$50,000 a year and the less developed country agent $5000, in one case, we have a large net profit and in the second a significant loss. In many cases in the developing world, it might be better today to discard existing systems and subsidize farmers.

One recently proposed extension model offered for use in Central America would require over 7500 extension agents, over 25,000 farmer leaders, and over $100 million in annual cost. This, in the Central American context, is prohibitive. The question remains: How can we reach all of the people with appropriate, timely information with which they can progress? Mass media are one element in this equation. However, more research needs to be done before they become a really effective tool. Another question is: How can mass media be supplemental to, or integrated with, conventional methods? How can the essential feedback on the effectiveness or misinterpretation of recommendations become a meaningful tool for changing recommendation presentation as well as other elements of the process?

Obviously, we have not gone far enough in looking at either small farms or nutrition in a more comprehensive manner. ROCAP's agricultural programs have only recently begun to bear fruit. Some of these, including both positive and negative results, may yet have value for nutrition planning. Certainly, some of the work in sample framing, farming systems, extrapolation, and transfer can be used or modified to meet nutrition planners' requirements. We, and our counterpart regional and national institutions, welcome the chance for a closer working relationship and a better understanding of nutrition policy and its implementation in order to assist small farmers, rural laborers, and their families— AID's ultimate agricultural clients—to improve their personal welfare and contribute more effectively to society as a whole.

Nigeria's Experience with Programs Aimed at Expanding Small-Farm Agricultural Production

Bede N. Okigbo

Introduction

In Nigeria, as in other countries of tropical Africa, over 95% of the food is raised by small-holders, about 80% of whom farm not more than about 2 hectares in any given year. It is estimated that about 20 million of an estimated population of 80 million have insufficient food to meet their nutritional needs (1). Currently, the average Nigerian nonfarmer spends over 70% of his income on food, and food import costs now amount to over $1300 million annually. Since the colonial era, Nigeria has passed from a period when farming was left to small land-holders, through periods of interest solely in cash crops, with limited emphasis on food crop production on small farms, and increasing reliance on large-scale farms. Since the 1960s, Nigeria has had three development plans whose objectives in each case included increasing agricultural productivity and improving rural welfare. Yet the growth rate of agricultural production has remained below that of population growth. This chapter is devoted to consideration of Nigeria's experience in attempts to increase agricultural production on small farms, the consequent nutritional status of its

Bede N. Okigbo • Farming Systems Program, International Institute of Tropical Agriculture, Ibadan, Nigeria.

people, and recommendations for providing effective solutions to the problems.

HISTORICAL BACKGROUND TO AGRICULTURAL AND SMALL-HOLDER PRODUCTION IN NIGERIA

The existing agricultural or farming systems that have left their mark on the cultural landscape of Nigeria evolved after several centuries of experimentation. Whether they are the results of diffusion or independent farming, there is no doubt that some interchange of ideas, materials, and techniques gave rise to the present mosaic of crops, traditions, and techniques whose origins are obscure (2). After thousands of years of gathering and hunting (some elements of which are still with us), perhaps at about 4000 years B.C., several crops were domesticated in western Africa. These include yams *(Dioscorea* spp.), fluted pumpkin *(Telfairia occidentalis),* oil palm *(Elaeis guineese),* African yam bean *(Sphenostylis stenocarpa),* and African pear *(Dacryodes edulis)* in the southern area, east of the Bandama River in the Ivory Coast; African rice *(Oryza glaberrima)* in the middle Niger Basin, from where it spread to parts of the Ivory Coast, Liberia, Sierra Leone, and other areas west of the Bandama River; and sorghum *(Sorghum vulgare),* millet *(Pennisetum typhoideum),* cowpea *(Vigna unguiculata),* and melon *(Colocynthes vulgaris)* in the savannah areas.

In about the first millennium A.D., Asian crops such as water yam *(Dioscorea alata),* coconut *(Cocos nucifera),* bananas and plantains (*Musa* spp.), citrus fruits (*Citrus* spp.), and cocoyam *(Colocasia esculenta)* began to appear. Later, following the discovery of the New World in 1492, American crops, including maize *(Zea mays),* cassava *(Manihot esculenta),* groundnut *(Arachis hypogaea),* sweet potato *(Impomoea batatas),* papaya *(Carica papaya),* lima beans *(Phaseolus lanatus),* cocoa *(Theobrama cacao),* and cocoyam (*Xanthosoma* spp.) were introduced. Many of these were not only cultivated in the same manner as indigenous yams, but were grafted onto the existing systems.

Associated with the crops were livestock such as chickens, sheep, goats, pigs, ducks, and cattle. Each wave of introduction of new crops and new techniques enhanced population growth.

Following the European explorations along the West African coast, a lucrative trade developed in spices, ivory, palm oil, forest products, and, later, slaves. With the increasing industrialization of Europe, cash crops such as palm oil, cocoa, rubber, groundnuts, and cotton became of major economic importance. As spheres of influence and colonies were established along the West African coast, these cash crops became important earners of foreign exchange.

In Nigeria, Ghana, and Sierra Leone, which became colonies and protectorates of Great Britain, no foreigners were allowed to own land, as they were in South, Central, and East Africa. The land was held in trust for the local people, and only a few plantations were established by English commercial companies. The growing of cash crops was encouraged, and this practice flourished to the extent that it could be supported by the prevailing market prices and individual initiative of largely subsistence small-holders. In the German territories such as the Cameroons, the Belgian Congo, and the then French West Africa (Ivory Coast, Benin, etc.), plantations owned by foreign and local entrepreneurs were encouraged. It is not surprising, therefore, that early British colonial policy encouraged small-holder production of export crops, sometimes at the expense of food crops. In West Africa there was also national or regional specialization in different commodities that, during periods of unstable world market prices, had adverse consequences on productivity and on the economy of the countries or regions. Efforts to stabilize these prices led to the formation of marketing boards in 1944.

Prior to the establishment of the British colonial administration in Nigeria in 1861, contact with Europe ushered in an era of increasing trade in forest products (peppers, spices, and ivory) and slaves. After the abolition of slavery, cash crops such as cocoa, oil palms, cotton, groundnuts, and rubber became major foreign exchange earners. Cocoa was introduced into Nigeria by Chief Squirs Banigo in 1874. Exploitation of wild rubber led to an early establishment of plantations (Funtumia spp in 1894, replaced by *Hevea* in 1903). Increasing interest in oil palms led to establishments of plantations in the Cameroons in 1912. The Moor Plantation, Nigeria's premier agricultural research station, was started in 1899 on land acquired by the British Empire Cotton Growing Association (BCGA). In the late 1930s and early 1940s, interterritorial research institutes such as the West African Cocoa Research Institute (WACRI) at Tafo, Ghana, the West African Institute for Oil Palm Research (WAIFOR) near Benin, Nigeria, and the West African Rice Research Institute in Sierra Leone were started. Early emphasis was placed on research for cash crops, and while individual cash crop commodity research institutes adopted a systems approach for the increased production of the relevant cash crops and had extension, marketing, credit, and infrastructural support, only fragmentary disciplinary research was done on food crops.

Consequently, although from the early 1920s some studies were done to find more permanent food production systems to replace shifts in cultivation, not a single food crop variety was released to Nigerian farmers until the 1950s, when a maize rust epidemic led to the production of NSI yellow maize, a variety not acceptable to farmers because of its color and chaffiness. Similarly, methods to improve soil fertility with herbaceous green manure leguminous cover and fallow cropping have still not gained acceptance among farmers. The reasons for the latter were mainly that environmental conditions and socioeconomic factors affecting production by small-holders were often overlooked in research. Moreover, extension services for food crops were fragile, poorly staffed, and inefficient.

Since gaining independence, Nigeria has recognized the importance of planning as a prerequisite to the execution of economic and industrial development programs. So far there have been three development plans: The First Development Plan (1962–1968), Second Development Plan (1970–1974), and Third Development Plan (1975–1980). Related to these were a series of studies to enhance agricultural development, since before the advent of oil, agriculture was the backbone of the economy in its contributions to GNP, in its role as a source of foreign exchange, as a means of livelihood, and as a source of food and raw materials.

The first long-range plan for agricultural development, *Agricultural Development in Nigeria 1965–1980* (FAO, 1966) was the first attempt to evolve an integrated agriculture development program that gave emphasis to (1) the importance of food production and nutrition in agricultural development, (2) the need for the federal government to play a leading role in the formulation of policies and the coordination of efforts in agricultural production, and (3) the need to strike a meaningful balance between cash and food crop production. Before the recommendations were implemented, the Nigerian Civil War broke out, and the *Strategies and Recommendations* for Nigerian Rural Development was produced. It highlighted the importance of agriculture in rural development and emphasized the need for (1) provision of favorable prices and incentives for export crops so as to enhance increased agricultural production; (2) greater emphasis on private sources of inputs, finance, and marketing services rather than dependency on the public sector; (3) provision of a range of infrastructural supports to farmers; (4) long-range strategy of increased research on food crops, to be followed by production campaigns; and (5) greater emphasis on production by private small-holders. However, this report could not be implemented immediately after the Civil War, and it was revised and replaced by *Agricultural Development in Nigeria, 1973–1985* in 1974, which formed the basis for the Third Development Plan.

THE FIRST DEVELOPMENT PLAN, 1962–1968

Evaluation of the First Development has been carried out by Wells (3). Altogether, about $180 million (13.6%) was allocated to primary agricultural production out of a total budget allocation of $1300 million. At the end of the 6-year period, total spending on the projects was 20–25% short of the allocations. Recurrent expenditure on agriculture amounted to about $72 million, or 7% of total government expenditure. The proportion of capital allocations varied between regions, from 20% in the West to 40% in the East. Details are shown in Table 1. Various activities involved in the projects consisted of (1) government-directed projects, including farm settlements, plantations, cattle ranches, and irrigation schemes; (2) investments in processing and marketing, including storage depots; (3) extension services for small-holders, such as fertilizer distribution, tree development, demonstrations, soil conservation, and pest and disease control; (4) research and investigations, including soil and water surveys; (5) education and training, including farmer training; and (6) provision of credit. The detailed evaluation of the plan from 1962 to 1967 concluded that a capital expenditure of only $79 million was recorded by the end of 1967, compared to the $155 million capital budget

TABLE 1. Subsectoral Allocations and Expenses as Indices of Performance of Projects on Various Commodities in the Third Development Plan

Sector	Original plan allocation (10^6)	Revised plan allocation (10^6)	Actual expenditure 1975–1976 (10^6)	Actual expenditure 1976–1977 (10^6)	Total expenditure to date Amount (10^6)	Total expenditure to date Percent (10^6)
Crops						
All states	754.7	1547.6	162.4	206.6	369.0	24
Federal government	694.8	1212.8	77.1	149.2	226.3	19
Total	1449.5	2760.4	239.5	355.8	595.3	21
Irrigation						
All states	91.6	166.2	15.8	19.3	35.1	21
Federal government	536.6	856.1	73.3	139.0	211.8	25
Total	628.2	1022.3	89.1	158.3	246.9	24
Livestock						
All states	168.0	326.1	25.7	31.9	57.6	18
Federal government	295.2	454.4	8.4	36.2	44.6	10
Total	463.2	780.5	34.1	68.1	102.2	13
Fisheries						
All states	51.2	75.0	5.8	5.4	11.2	15
Federal government	95.0	88.6	2.5	8.0	10.5	12
Total	146.2	163.6	8.3	13.4	21.7	13

allocation; the structure of the budget allocations indicated a strong difference between the southern regions, where emphasis was on government-directed projects, and the northern region, which emphasized extension activities for farmers. Southern capital allocations concentrated on farm settlements and plantations growing cocoa, rubber, and oil palm. In general, the overall results of the projects—especially those involving direct government production and farm settlements—were disappointing. In the north, most of the fertilizers were concentrated on the groundnut crop. Among the projects of nutritional importance was livestock raising, most notably the successful establishment of a poultry industry in the southern states, which made egg imports unnecessary. However, this did not benefit small-holders because it was run by well-endowed urban dwellers and retired public servants or their wives. Otherwise, the First Development Plan had no noticeable effect on available food supplies.

THE SECOND DEVELOPMENT PLAN, 1970–1974

The Second Development Plan accorded priority to agricultural development, and within the agricultural sector the first priority was given to food production. The first of the five objectives of the agricultural policy was to ensure " . . . food supplies in adequate quantity and quality to keep pace with increased population and urbanization, having regard to changing tastes and need for fair and stable prices." Of the total allocated expenditure of $39 million in the agricultural sector, about $13 million (33%) was allocated to food production.

The Second Development Plan bore the brunt of the rehabilitation effort after the Civil War. But its evaluation, based on percentage of expenditure reported after the first half of the plan period, led to the conclusion that overall performance was disappointing. The percentage budget allocation to agriculture was 10.8%, but only 42.7% of the budget allocation was spent during the period compared to an average expenditure of 63% for all sectors. The actual proportion of the total budget spent for agriculture was 6.6%. Many states engaged in large-scale production of food crops, but results were disappointing. Some fruit and vegetable crop multiplication and production schemes were launched, and some progress was made in tomato production. Rehabilitation of the oil palm- and cocoa-growing activities was achieved. Progress was made in irrigation projects in the northern states, for example, Tiga Dam, which was built to irrigate 5600 hectares. Several tractor-hiring units were established, but these have often not been successful under government management. In general, small-holder production was not influenced much by the Plan, and increasing demand for foods unavailable locally by the affluent who enjoyed increasing earnings from petroleum export resulted in much higher food imports by the end of the Plan in 1974.

THE THIRD DEVELOPMENT PLAN, 1975–1980

This Plan also gave priority to food production and set up definite nutritional goals as a national objective. It stated that "Government will pursue a policy which will lead to the attainment of these minimum requirements by 1979–1980." More concretely, "Government will seek an increase in calorie intake per caput per day to 2200 kcal, and in crude protein consumption of between 60–65 g, as well as an adequate proportionate increase in animal protein relative to protein from other sources." Production of food grains (maize, sorghum, and millet) was to be increased by 8% per annum, rice by 11.5%, roots and tubers by 5–6%, grain legumes and melon by 7.5%, vegetable oils by 9.5%, and vegetables and fruits by 12.8%. The goal was to achieve self-sufficiency by 1985. Other objectives of the Second Development Plan, also embodied in the Third Development Plan, include

> (a) ensuring food supplies in adequate quantity and quality to keep pace with increased population and urbanization, having regard to changing tastes and the need for fair and stable prices; (b) expanding the production of export crops with a view to increasing and further diversifying the country's foreign exchange earnings; (c) significantly increasing the production of agricultural raw materials to support domestic manufacturing activities, especially in the field of agro-based industries in addition to export; (d) creating rural employment opportunities to absorb more of the increasing labor force in the nation, and minimizing the tendency for inadequate and inefficient use of human resources in the rural area generally, and (e) evolving appropriate institutional and administrative apparatus to facilitate a smooth, integrated development of the agricultural potential of the country as a whole.

The Plan also called for integrated policy measures by federal and state governments, including:

- Price incentives to producers.
- Processing involving partnership of federal and state governments.
- Rehabilitation and new planting schemes for tree crops.

- Marketing, involving (1) access-road improvement and construction and (2) grading of stable food crop products and speedy dissemination of marketing information.
- Manpower training to eliminate the manpower shortages that bedeviled the Second Plan.
- Federal and state government participation in direct production, especially of rice, wheat, cotton, and kenaf.
- Expansion of extension services; reduction of the high farmer/extension worker ratio with an increase in contract hours; integration of extension; input supply; supporting services such as marketing and equipment hiring units at the village level as an aspect of the National Accelerated Food Production program (NAFPP); and integrated rural development in the Plan, use of individual farmers in seed multiplication, with farmers' fields serving as demonstration and seed multiplication plots.
- Improvement of input supply and use by state governments; procuring and distributing agricultural inputs through farmers' unions, cooperatives, and extension services.
- Research, with intensification of efforts (1) to improve varieties of industrial and staple food crops and (2) to develop improved, cheap, simple tools and small motor-powered and animal-drawn implements.
- Land use surveys and planning, including those in support of irrigation projects.

The total national capital expenditure for the agricultural programs during the Plan period amounted to $3.5 billion, with $2.6 billion for crops, $550.5 million for livestock, $175.6 million for forestry, and $162.5 million for fisheries.

Through the NAFPP, it was planned to cultivate 24,000 hectares with the participation of 324,000 farmers, resulting in the production of 146,000 tons of rice, 97,400 tons of maize, 40,000 tons of sorghum, 9300 tons of wheat, 3000 tons of soybeans, and 10,700 tons of pigeon peas. Because the NAFPP is the boldest program so far aimed at increasing food production by small farmers, it will be discussed in greater detail below.

PERFORMANCE OF THE THIRD DEVELOPMENT PLAN

It is the practice in Nigeria to evaluate performance of Plans on the basis of the proportion of budget allocations actually spent. While this is also the criterion used here, it must be borne in mind that it is not a very reliable one because quite frequently not all of the amount spent is efficiently utilized, and sometimes it may be spent on activities other than those originally chosen for funding. Moreover, the amount spent on a project does not determine actual success attained. It does, however, give some indication of how far the government has been successful in adhering to commitments in the development program.

Of the revised Plan allocations of $4944 million to the agricultural sector, subsectoral allocation to crops amounted to $2761 million: $1022 million was to be for irrigation, $780 million for livestock, and $163.6 million for fisheries (Table 1). During the first 2 years of the plan, out of a $595.4 million budget allocation to the crop subsector, 21% was actually spent, compared to 24, 13, and 21.7% for irrigation, livestock, and fisheries, respectively. Several companies were engaged in government direct-production activities. These included The National Grains Production Company; the National Root Crops Production Company; the North-East, Western, and National Livestock Production Companies; the Nigerian National Shrimp Company; and the Nigerian National Fish Company.

Some activities of these companies in storage and processing may involve products of small-holders, but, in general, government-directed crop production functioned through the Grains and Root Crops Production Companies, the NAFPP, the River Basin Development Authorities, and Integrated Rural Development Projects, some of which involve small-holders. The National Crop Production Companies initiated seed multiplication, storage, and processing projects. For example, since March 1977, the National Root Crops Production Company has improved traditional gari factories to be supplemented later by Brazilian equipment. These factories, while processing materials from large-scale farms, constitute potential facilities for future food fortification work. To what extent such factories will compete with, or encourage, small-farm production is not yet clear. Ten rural integrated agricultural development projects are to be established during the Plan period, and during the first 2 years three of the projects were completed at Funtua, Gusau, and Gombe. Areas cultivated amounted to 460,000 hectares, 228,000 hectares, and 322,000 hectares at these sites, respectively. Some progress was made in small-holder schemes involving food crops and tree crops. For example, in the Rivers State alone, 17,000 hectares were cultivated to grow cassava (the largest crop), and some maize, yams, and rice. World Bank-assisted projects in Oyo and Ogun States exceeded planned targets by 20 and 60%, respectively.

Other activities involving small-holder production in the Plan include (1) multiplication and distribution of seeds and planting materials for fruits and vegetables; (2) provision of fertilizers at a 50% price subsidy rate; (3) tractor-hiring units that were established by many states but were inefficiently managed, as is often the case with the public-sector-managed projects; (4) expansion of agricultural extension activities at the state level; (5) pest control that resulted in clearing of 25,000 hectares of farmland and the killing of about 25 million Quelea birds; (6) establishment of a National Agricultural Bank that gives loans to farmers but is organized in a way that does not facilitate provision of easy loans to small-holders; (7) formation of River Basin Development Authorities that are at present mainly engaged in feasibility studies; (8) limited progress in livestock programs for small farmers; (9) remarkable progress in tsetse fly eradication, resulting in their extermination in an 8000 km^2 area; and (10) limited progress in the provision of fishing equipment and fish storage and processing facilities for small-holders. In general, a major component of the Third Development Plan involved government-directed production activities and large-scale farms whose performance has so far been disappointing.

Progress in the National Accelerated Food Production Program

The NAFPP may be regarded as the first well-planned and -conceived food crop production program for small-holders in Nigeria. It is one of the projects of the Federal Department of Agriculture that is, among other things, charged with elaboration of integrated national agricultural policy, coordination of projects, and determination of national priorities. Its other activities and units include crop production, agro-service, fertilizer procurement, home economics, farm mechanization, land resources and soil conservation, and pest control and plant quarantine. The Department gives effective support to state governments and is also involved in organizing some joint projects with them.

The NAFPP concept was first formulated and launched in 1972, but pilot projects were only begun in 1974. It aims at making Nigeria self-sufficient in the production of six basic staple food crops—maize, rice, sorghum, millet, wheat, and cassava—by using "Green Revolution" techniques for mass adoption of improved packages of technology for growing these crops. The program involves integration of research extension and agroservice. The NAFPP also involved the *minikit* concept. The minikit has proven to be an effective research and extension tool in nonreplicated trials that give the farmer the opportunity to select the most suitable package of improved crop production technology for his situation. The program, which was planned and coordinated on contract by the International Institute of Tropical Agriculture (IITA), involves activities at three National Crop Centers in

- *Samaru* at the Agricultural Extension Research Liaison Service and Institute of Agricultural Research (AERLS and IAR) for wheat, sorghum, and millet
- *Ibadan* at the National Cereals Research Institute (NCRI) for maize and rice
- *Umudike* at the National Root Crops Research Institute (NRCRI) for cassava

During the first phase, the project was partially supported by USAID with a grant of $2 million.

The Research Component of the NAFPP is located at the above three crop centers, where research and technical work on each crop is carried out and trials are organized for different ecological zones. The extension component gives farmers information and materials on specific crops in the most effective way through training and farm-level trials. These trials use both minikits and production kits. The extension work also involves mass communication campaigns utilizing radio, posters, and other media. The agro-service system consists of Agro-Service centers that provide integrated delivery services to ensure that all the ingredients necessary for adoption of improved technology are available at the farm level. Components of the agro-service include: (1) agricultural inputs (seeds, fertilizers, chemicals, equipment hire, farm supplies); (2) credit for agriculture; (3) marketing (sales site, storage, limited-processing manufacture of simple tools); and (4) an inputs educational program. Agro-service centers are located 10–15 km apart to enable farmers to get to them on bicycles.

The program calls for 2300 agro-service centers, 200 of which are to be built during the first phase. The National Steering Committee under the Director of Agriculture, and State Steering Committees under the Chief Agricultural Officers direct the NAFPP activities. The Crop Centers, State Ministries of Agriculture, and cooperating farmers interact in implementing the program developed in the plans through annual workshops.

During the pilot phase of the program (1974–1977), work was concentrated in eight states (Benue, Plateau, Kano, Anambra, Imo, Oyo, Ogun, and Ondo). During the Second Phase (1977–1980) work on five

TABLE 2. A Comparison of the Number of Minikits Used in
1978 vs. 1977, By Crops[a]

Year	Rice	Maize	Wheat	Sorghum	Millet	Cassava
1978	473	582	58	312	267	217
1977	693	802	52	407	191	219

[a] Source: NAFPP Progress Report (1978).

substations (Ubiaja, Ugwuoba, Dan Hassan, Gashua, and Mokwa)
involved testing of research findings under specific ecological conditions.

ACCOMPLISHMENTS

In 1977, 2364 minikit trials were conducted, and in 1978, 1909 trials
were carried out (Table 2). High-yielding varieties included in the minikit and yields of promising varieties in 1978 are shown in Table 3. The
yields of improved varieties in minikit trials compared to those of local
varieties are shown in Table 4. Minikit trials are visited by means of special tours, and field days are held for farmers. The production kit trials
in 1978 and 1979 are shown in Table 5.

The NAFPP system reduced the interval between introduction and
adoption from 8 to 3 years, and 400,000 farmers are now participating in
the program. Training is a vital component of the program. Some of the
staff involved in in-service training were among the 115 who had had

TABLE 3. Promising Varieties Included in
Minikits and Recorded Yields for 1978[a]

Crop	Variety	Yield (kg/hectare)
Rice		
Upland	TOS 2625	2,625
Swamp	Faro 15	4,626
Maize		
Early	TZE	4,238
White	TZSR	5,139
Cassava	TMS 30211	23,000
	TMS 1525	26,000
	TMS 30568	30,000

[a] Source: NAFPP Progress Report (1978).

TABLE 4. Comparison of Yields for NAFPP Package of
Practices and Local Practices[a]

Crop and State	Local yield (T/hectare)	NAFPP yield (T/hectare)	Potential yield increase
Cassava (Imo)	9.29	15	+60%
Maize (Oyo)	1.3	2.8	+115%
Rice (Oyo)	1.1	2.2	+100%
Sorghum (Kano)	0.65	1.5	+130%
Millet (Kano)	0.65	1.5	+130%
Wheat (Kano)	1.3	3	+130%

[a] Source: Federal Department of Agriculture: Consolidated Report 1971–1978,
Lagos, Nigeria.

specialized training at the International Rice Research Institute, the Center for Improvement of Maize and Wheat in Mexico, and the International Crops Research Institute for the Semi-Arid Tropics.

The year 1978 saw the mass adoption stage at the national crop centers. It was estimated that improved maize varieties were grown on 41,900 hectares, and high-yield rice was planted on 6583 hectares. These resulted in 115,000 extra tons of maize and 16,500 extra tons of rice. Improved cassava varieties were grown on about 22,000 hectares, and resulted in a threefold increase in yield.

In 1978, 187 agro-service centers were started, but only about half of them are still operational.

Some effective feedback was obtained on the program, and revealed the following problems:

1. Improved cassava varieties in Anambra State did not have as high a percentage of starch as was found in local varieties.
2. Improved maize varieties in the southern states were not as suitable as local maize for eating, either boiled or roasted on the cob.
3. Of the upland rice varieties involved in tests, none was preferable to the recommended and widely grown OS-6 variety.

TABLE 5. A Comparison of the Number of Production Kits
for 1978 vs. 1977 by Crops[a]

Year	Rice	Maize	Wheat	Sorghum	Millet	Cassava
1978	211	427	16	145	—	341
1977	134	2,716	14	56	62	2,166

[a] Source: NAFPP Progress Report (1978).

4. Wheat varieties that have good bread-baking qualities were identified, but their potential yields could not be attained because of soil and crop management problems.

In general, although significant progress was made in the NAFPP, achievements have taken longer to be realized than expected. Uneven progress was made in the 19 states of the Federation. Not all states attached equal priority or allocated enough funds to the program. Logistical problems limited extension work and the distribution of inputs. A shortage of high-level manpower and different dates of arrival of those recruited resulted in lack of uniform progress in various aspects of the NAFPP activities. Despite all the progress made in the NAFPP, there was no marked improvement in available food supplies, no reduction of food prices and imports, and no increase in the quantities of cash crops exported (cocoa, palm oil, and groundnuts) from the launching of the Third Development Plan and the NAFPP from 1974 to date.

OPERATION FEED THE NATION

The slow progress made in the NAFPP, the continuing increase in food prices and imports, and a change in the Government of Nigeria ushered in the launching of Operation Feed the Nation (OFN) in 1975. It aimed at getting as many people in Nigeria as possible, including non-farmers, to farm. It was hoped that this would make Nigeria self-sufficient in food crops and even result in surpluses for export, but it only succeeded in the general motivation of people to join in the food-growing campaign. OFN did not contribute significantly to increased food production, to a drop in food prices, or to the reduction of mounting imports, the latter partly caused by changing food habits associated with the oil boom. OFN was more successful as a slogan, and from its inception was doomed to failure because it was begun without up-to-date statistics for planning, with neither a clear definition of responsibilities nor an effective organization. No consideration was given to the shortage of manpower, the logistics for input distribution, or potential problems and the resources needed to provide effective support to all who might decide to participate in the campaign. It did somehow succeed in the elimination of red tape in certain agricultural development and production activities, including the NAFPP. Thus, it ensured timely supply and distribution of fertilizers, machinery, and other inputs. It appears, however, to have had a somewhat disruptive influence on the NAFPP.

RECOMMENDATIONS FOR MINIMIZING PRODUCTION AND NUTRITION
INTERFACE PROBLEMS AND ENHANCING SMALL-HOLDER AGRICULTURAL
PRODUCTION

The Nigerian experience in the planning and execution of agricultural and economic development programs has highlighted several deficiencies that need to be eliminated if rapid progress is to be made and effective small-holder participation in increased agricultural production is to be achieved. Planning by itself is not enough if it is not based on reliable statistics and supporting studies of sufficient scope to ensure that all relevant realities of the situation are taken into account in policy formulation and in determining the strategy to be followed in the execution of the program. This also facilitates early identification of major constraints that may be encountered in the execution that must receive some attention during the planning stage. Recommendations are made in this regard as follows:

1. Food production (and in fact all agricultural production), nutrition, and health should be given priority in national economic development planning as multidisciplinary problems that call for a systems approach. This can best be achieved by ensuring that there is a national body or council that involves all the relevant disciplines in policy formulation and planning for economic development. Such a body should also adopt a systems approach in studies that are used for giving advice and ensuring political commitment to integrated programs in agriculture, nutrition, and health. To be effective, representatives of the various disciplines or ministries should have attained some stature in their areas of specialization and responsibility.

2. The range of factors and disciplines that interact in a complex manner to determine nutritional status requires that effective machinery should be set up for coordination of activities of different individuals often isolated in different ministries (e.g., agriculture, industry, and health).

3. In many developing countries, no significant progress has been made in achieving increased food production on the small farms that dominate the food production industry. This is often because a systems approach to the food production problem is rarely adopted, and existing or traditional farming systems are so neglected that constraints to their improvement and the farmer's whole life-style are not taken into account in determining prior-

ities and strategy in research and generation of technology relevant to the farmer's needs and conditions. It is for this reason that attempts to improve traditional farming systems have often involved wholesale transfer to the tropics of unadaptable technology, materials, and practices developed in temperate regions. Suggested policy guidelines relevant to food production and nutrition are available upon request.

4. Because funds and resources are limited, it is necessary in deciding on the strategy and agricultural development program to give due consideration to alternative strategies that have the highest chance of success in relation to available resources and to the target group that would play the most crucial role in the program. Development programs should be tailored to the executive capacity that is either available or easily attainable, and due allowance should be given to changing world economic conditions. Targets that are realistic on paper are not always easy or even possible to achieve.

5. In economic and agricultural development programs, it is necessary to give priority to the achievement of a reasonable balance or at least meaningful relationships between (a) food crops and industrial crops, (b) agriculture and industry, and (c) rural and urban development.

6. In many developing countries, the perennial problem of an acute shortage of manpower at all levels constitutes a major constraint to success in policy formulation, planning, and execution of development projects. Only through sound and realistic educational programs, and availability of the critical mass of human resources needed in various areas of human endeavor, can success be achieved. Here, cooperation among disciplines, individuals, and institutions at national, regional, and international levels is necessary.

REFERENCES

1. Oyenuga, V. A. From grass to milk: Situation and prospects in Nigeria. *Disc. Nig. Acad. Sci.* 1(1):2-15, 1978.
2. Harlan, J. R., J. M. J. De Wet, and A. B. L. Stemler (Eds.) *Origins of African Plant Domestication.* Mouton Publishers, The Hague, 1976.
3. Ministry of Economic Development. National Development Plan, 1962–1968. Lagos, 1962.
4. Federal Ministry of Information. Second National Development Plan 1970–1974. Lagos, 1970.

5. FMED/CPO. Third National Development Plan 1975–1980. Lagos, 1975.
6. Food and Agriculture Organization. Agricultural Development in Nigeria 1965–1980, FAO, Rome, 1966.
7. Johnson, G. L., O. J. Scoville, G. K. Dike, and C. K. Eicher. Strategies and recommendations for Nigerian rural development. 1969/1985. Consortum for the Study of Nigerian Rural Development and FMED/FMAR/NUC/NISER/EDI, MSU, East Lansing, 1969.
8. FMAR/JPC. Agricultural Development in Nigeria 1973–1985. Joint Planning Committee, Federal Ministry of Agriculture and National Resources, Lagos, 1974.
9. Wells, J. C. Government Agricultural Investment in Nigeria: 1962–1967. Center for Research on Economic Development, University of Michigan/NISER, Ibadan, 1969.
10. FMEDR/CPO. Second Progress Report on the Third Development Plan 1975–1980. Cultural Planning Office, Federal Ministry of Economic Development and Reconstruction, Lagos, 1978.
11. Williams, L. B. NAFPP Progress Report 1978. IITA, Ibadan, 1979.
12. FDA. A Consolidated Report 1971–1978. Federal Department of Agriculture, Lagos, 1979.

Comment

Michael Lipton

Barraclough rightly stresses that a small farm is a relative concept; it is relative to land quality, to the numbers supported by and working on the farm, and to the income required to be generated for nutritional and other needs. Therefore, smallness of farm should really be measured in efficiency units standardized by hectares of land, and allow for the size and composition of the family. I would classify a farm as being small when it provides the operating managers in an average year with enough income to meet food needs, plus perhaps 50–75% additional income to meet non-food needs and to leave a small surplus. In most developing countries that would cover well over half, and in some developing countries, well over two-thirds, of all farm units. In most developing countries, small farm means the same as family farm, i.e., a farm that hires in less labor than it hires out over the year. South Asian farms with such a labor balance are usually below 1.5–2 hectares; in most parts of Africa they are considerably larger, while in Latin America they are somewhere in between, depending on land quality.

Small family farmers have proved remarkably persistent throughout the development process. Specifically, they have proved to be rational (although not necessarily profit-maximizing), price-responsive, responsible, innovative, and generally efficient operators. In many cases they have been shown to be better than large farmers in their use of scarce resources: land, credit, energy. Hence, small farm-base development produces outcomes that result in satisfying nutritional requirements.

But what of the changes in the agricultural sector, characterized by the incorporation of small farmers into commercial agriculture, and the dissolution of self-provisioning agriculture? I think these terms are mis-

Michael Lipton • The Institute for Development Studies, University of Sussex, Brighton, England.

leading. Drastic technical improvement does not as a rule save labor in poor countries unless that technical improvement is artificially helped along, e.g., by tractor subsidies. High-yielding varieties raise labor needs per acre, and, on balance, reduce the farmer's risk. In other words, they tend to favor small farmers rather than large ones. Also, high-yielding varieties tend to be rice and wheat, which are poor people's foods, favorable to the nutrition of the relatively poor, especially if farmed by those who consume their products themselves.

Unfortunately, initial innovation and risk-taking have been in the larger unit that has better access to scarce resources. But there are no economic grounds for suspecting that high-yielding varieties or technical innovation in poor countries disfavors or causes the elimination or absorption of the small farmer. It is not true that the small farm community before innovation (before change) is fairly equal. Nor is it true that increasing polarization between the landless and larger commercial landowners is caused by technical progress.

There are basic technical, techno-economic characteristics of high-yielding varieties and labor-intensive farming that do favor the small farmer, and the initial advantages of access that the larger one has in dealing with these varieties have, in the medium term, been overcome by the economic advantages of relatively small productive units. Even the common fear that, in the wake of high-yielding varieties, the landlords would throw their tenants off the land and resume commerical production themselves has not been at all widely realized. Rents have gone up instead.

If there has been slower adoption by the small farmer, for reasons such as risk aversion, poor water security, and so on, there is growing evidence that once the small farmer does adopt new technology, he does so more intensively, utilizing greater amounts of fertilizers and labor, and even in countries such as Taiwan and Japan, development has not ended subsistence farming. It has not by any means eliminated productive farming for self-provisioning; it has not incorporated and destroyed the microfarmer. On the contrary, it has made such farmers richer, forcing them to become part-time farmers. They farm their land a few days a week and on other days are involved in an urban occupation. Therefore, in the long run, I think there is evidence of the sure survival power of the family farm, although there is a sense in which it ceases to be a small farm.

Given the contention that the peasant method of production has proven extraordinarily durable, it is worthwhile to look at the efficiency of their activities. Land of a given quality cultivated by smaller farmers shows higher output per acre, cropping intensity, and value due to labor intensity. In other words, the crop mix is more valuable, there is more output per acre depending on the crop, and there are more crop seasons on average farmed in a year on the small farm. Moreover, in the slack season, the small farmer is more likely to improve the quality of his land, particularly by water and drainage control, than is the large farmer, mainly because he has more labor per acre. The facts that the small farmer keeps the whole product of his labor, that workers have few other useful things to do, and that family labor needs less supervision also contribute to the finding that the small farmer makes better use of his land, labor, capital, and credit inputs.

As mentioned earlier, recent evidence suggests that high-yielding varieties strengthen this relationship between small-scale and labor-intensive farm use. It is not surprising, therefore, that since high-yielding varieties increase labor requirements per acre, they ought to be more intensively worked by those family farm units with more labor to spare. What is more, smaller farmers show high returns for their credit. In fact, it is a more accurate representation to say that it is the big farmer who defaults because he can get away with it politically. The small farmer knows he is going to have to borrow again, and thus he tends to be very cautious about defaulting. Since in most poor countries land, capital, and credit are scarce and tend to be under priced, while labor is all too plentiful, these considerations add up to a real and substantial efficiency advantage for smaller farmers.

What about nutrition? Are there nutritional implications for the urban poor and rural landless involving the small farmer? If he is an efficient producer of food and resources, the urban poor will benefit, since this will allow for greater transfers of food to the towns. Two points can be made concerning the landless laborers. First, the problem is not quite as enormous as the literature suggests. Second, although the small farmer does rely on members of his own family, he will, on balance, employ more landless labor per acre than do large farmers, which will result in the landless acquiring greater command over food resources.

Given the mass of evidence that the small farmer is a highly price-responsive and efficient operator, which strongly reinforces the case for redistributive land reform, the paradox of small-farm neglect emerges. The small-farm sector, and the small artisan that serves it, are demonstrably efficient in terms of labor-intensive, high return on the use of capital. If you examine investment by sectors, you find that in most of the developing countries the rate of extra GNP per extra unit of capital is much higher in the agricultural sector than in the non-farm sector.

Despite the cautions that economists will wish to make, it appears that agriculture does seem to make more cost-effective use of scarce resources.

Yet Okigbo, looking at the Nigerian data, once more documents the pathetic share of agriculture in total investment: 7% for the 70% of the population in agriculture, and they receive even less than they are supposed to. This is a worldwide phenomenon. As such, the implementation lag in the agricultural sector is attributable to the fact that the agricultural sector generally lacks human resources, administrative resources, vehicles, and offices as well as new investible resources.

Why, then, does the agricultural sector not get the resources it deserves? This observation is not explicable in the terms usually used, which imply that the large, rich, rural farmer is too strong. Except in Latin America intrarural inequality is small relative to that between intraurban and rural–urban. The rural rich share key interests with the rural poor: in good farm prices and a high rural and agricultural share of investment in personnel. It is not a question of the rural rich stubbornly opposing all forms of change that benefit the rural poor. Rather, it is urban–rural relations that count. Barraclough summarizes very neatly what happens: The urban sector (both urban employers and organized urban workers) want cheap food and a high investment share. Hence, they allot small shares of input to agriculture and, in particular, to the small farmer who tends to consume the product of those inputs himself, even if he is more efficient.

Finally, I would like to consider the fact that, in most cases, the Third World countries have maintained a fair amount of growth, but that this has been accompanied by persistent poverty, undernutrition, and low food availability per person. While large increases in farm-oriented rural outlays are a necessary condition for doing something about this, they are not sufficient by themselves. "Spend the money" approaches as the cure-all for rural development, i.e., throwing money at rural poverty with inadequate planning and almost no supervision, will inevitably fail.

Disaggregated target-setting for implementation, advocated by Fiester, is essential, but it will also require local monitoring and feedback on the arrival and distribution of benefits to the rural poor. One needs to know in good time whether a new irrigation system is, in fact, getting through to the small farmer and what its effects are on employment and nutrition of the landless. We have been very weak on developing monitoring schemes. In addition, we require technologies well distributed in space and time, appropriate not just in the sense of being labor-intensive, but also low-risk, locally and easily reparable, and not too dependent on timely delivery of inputs such as fuel and spare parts. The group and personal constraints that operate on the acquisition of appropriate new technologies have to be better understood. But it is indisputable that a rising share of inputs for small farmers, including water and land, will raise total output, income, and hence, nutritional levels. This is the case not only for small farmers, but also for landless laborers and probably the urban poor as well.

Discussion

It was pointed out initially that this session had emphasized "small" not only because "small is beautiful," but more importantly because "small is efficient." In addition, although some participants asserted that every situation in each country is unique, others found it important to create typologies concerning the status of the agricultural sector in various countries in order to formulate appropriate "small-farm" strategies and approaches. Regarding the typologies, it was suggested that future agricultural development should be devoted especially to those countries where a large percentage of the population is engaged in food production.

These represent many of the poorest countries in the world. They are characterized by rapid population growth (2.5–3.5% per year); the rate of increase in the labor force is thereafter commensurate with the growth in population. These countries also do not fit the pattern of rapid industrial growth followed by a rapidly declining labor force in the agricultural sector. Rather, the agricultural labor force continues to grow at a rate similar to the total labor force.

A third salient characteristic of this group of countries, as pointed out in Fiester's paper, is the low volume of agricultural sales, which is attributable to low rural and urban purchasing power. However, given the small size of the urban, commercial sector, the low demand should come as no surprise, despite the fact that production for export does present an important potential growth source. In Africa, for example, many small farmers have taken advantage of the export markets. However, the share of cash earnings on export crops is dominated by a small number of producers operating on the large-scale, highly commercialized plantations.

In order to incorporate the needs of other producers, appropriate technology must be introduced, meeting the following requirements. It should be: (1) scientifically up-to-date, (2) economically viable, (3) labor-intensive and capital-saving, (4) protective of the environment, and, of most importance, (5) capable of reducing poverty and responsive to a community's socioeconomic needs. This demands that a careful "mix" of technologies be employed.

One discussant noted that the great success story of the growth of a dairy organization in India is an illustration of an appropriate technological mix. In that instance, there is hand-milking and daily payment for the milk in accordance with the needs of the small farmer, together with a computerized accounting system and a modern milk processing plant.

The Indian experience represents an instance in which there was a *transfer* of technology based on the socioeconomic needs of the country. This must be clearly distinguished from the *transplant* of whole systems based on a foreign technology, which is unresponsive to the context in which it will be used. Thus, while transfer rather than transplant is important, it is also necessary to devote greater attention to *transformation* of traditional technologies into modern ones.

It was pointed out that, while appropriate technologies in agricultural production often preclude mechanization, it is important not to be too dogmatic about that point. Specifically, it remains necessary to distinguish between the use of tractors in food production and the variety of post-harvest processes for which mechanization may be appropriate. For example, the use of a rubber husker for rice will result in 100% recovery of the grain. Hand-pounding will not have such a high recovery rate. In addition, the rubber husker requires co-operation, as a few farmers must band together to operate the machine and make it economical.

Thus, if technological innovation is a result of the farmer's attempting to be more efficient and encourages people to cooperate, it will inevitably lead to more ingenuity, more skill, and improved capabilities. This, in turn, may result in prospering rural areas and even in expanded rural industrialization, which will broaden employment opportunities.

While the emphasis on how best to assist the small farmers was the basis for much of the discussion, it was also pointed out that the problem if often not *what* to do, but increasing accessibility to the group most difficult to reach. Specifically, the necessity for developing concrete ways of servicing a small farmer within the cost constraints of agricultural extension programs to large and cash crop farmers was suggested.

An illustration of this problem of outreach to small farmers was presented: An extension agent in the United States may work with 200 farmers and may introduce a new technology that will increase profits by $10 an acre. Farmers in the United States have an average of about 200 acres per farm, which means a net increase of $400,000. By contrast, in Central

America, the extension agent may also be working with 200 farmers. He also introduces a $10 increase per acre in farm technology. His farmers, however, have only 2 acres each, so that the net increase in earning from his efforts is $4000. Costs for the extension agent in the United States may be $35,000 to $50,000, including overhead and salary. His efforts result in $400,000 extra income for the aggregate number of farmers. In Central America, the cost for the extension worker would probably be $7000 to $9000; however, he would increase his farmers' income by only $4000. Given these figures, some would argue that it would be better to close the extension service in Central America and just give the money to the farmers.

Clearly, there is a need to find new ways of dealing more effectively with small farmers, using mass communication techniques and the like. Some very interesting research has been carried out recently on mass media communication in Guatemala, Colombia, El Salvador, and other parts of the world. However, to date no one has formulated and documented new approaches and methods of using mass media for farmer extension services. What is needed are ways to change the mind-set and transfer knowledge to small farmers in such a fashion that the information will be accepted and utilized.

VI

Post-Harvest Food Conservation

During the past few years, there has been increasing international discussion of and attention to the most effective means of reducing the substantial portion of developing country agricultural output that is lost between the time of harvest and the point of purchase by the final consumer. Of necessity, such efforts must encompass a broad array of interventions, including improvements in on-farm storage, transportation, processing, distribution, and marketing. Yet, there is a growing consensus that expanded investment in various post-harvest food conservation measures may well represent one of the greatest untapped areas of opportunity in meeting world food problems.

The papers, comments, and discussion in this section provide a sense of both the problems and the potential inherent in such "supply side" interventions. The issue paper by Pariser lays out in comprehensive terms the full scope of the losses now being experienced in developing countries, while the supplemental paper by Guggenheim addresses some of the socioeconomic questions involved in the reduction of these losses. Koga, in his country case study, considers some specific technological problems relating to the post-harvest processing of rice in selected Southeast Asian countries. The dichotomy between technological and socioeconomic considerations is further highlighted in the comments by Parpia and Spitz, as well as in the general workshop discussion that follows.

The editors wish to acknowledge the contribution of Ellen Smith and Margaret Dempsey, who served as rapporteurs for this workshop.

Post-Harvest Food Losses in Developing Countries
A Survey

E. R. PARISER

INTRODUCTION

Efforts have been made since the beginning of agriculture to increase crop yields and to reduce food losses at all stages of the food production and distribution chain. It is only within the past 50 years or so that the world community has been called upon to give systematic attention to the identification, assessment, and reduction of food losses in general, but especially those occurring (for whatever reason) between harvest and consumption.

Shortly after the World Food Conference had convened in Rome over 4 years ago, the President of the United States wrote to the President of the National Academy of Sciences in Washington, asking the Academy to make an assessment of the global problem of hunger and malnutrition and to " . . . develop specific recommendations on how research and development capabilities can best be applied to meet the major challenge." In response to this request, the Academy undertook an in-depth investigation, *The World Food and Nutrition Study* (1). The report issued from this study conjectures that as many as 450 million to one billion persons in the nonindustrialized regions of the world do not receive enough food for their normal growth and development needs, and that this number is bound to increase significantly by the end of the century.

E. R. PARISER • Sea Grant Program, Massachusetts Institute of Technology Cambridge, Massachusetts.

However, in reviewing what had been, and was being, done to cope with this situation, the Academy concluded that, in addition to the traditional strategies that many governments had adopted—attempts to slow population growth and efforts to increase food production—an important avenue had not been sufficiently considered: The reduction of food losses caused by spillage, contamination, and attack by microorganisms, insects, birds, and rodents during and after harvest. Many observers believe, in fact, that a reduction of food losses would greatly lessen, and perhaps even eliminate, some countries' present need to import large quantities of food. In order to encourage such an effort, the Seventh Special Session of the United Nations General Assembly set a 50% reduced global post-harvest food loss as a target to be achieved by 1985, and this decision prompted the U.S. Agency for International Development (AID) to request the National Academy to undertake yet another study, this one of Post-Harvest Food Losses in Developing Countries (2). As far as we are aware, the Academy study is the last of several major efforts to come to grips with the overall problem of post-harvest losses of major food crops in developing countries.

In 1954 and 1956, the U.S. Department of Agriculture (3,4) published what appear to be the only two comprehensive studies—at least in this country—dealing with crop losses. Both reports, entitled "Lessons in Agriculture," concentrated upon pre-harvest (i.e., growing) crop loss reduction, with limited information on post-harvest losses. More recently, of course, the United Nations Food and Agriculture Organization, the Tropical Products Institute in the United Kingdom, and several other organizations have been involved in the specific problem of post-harvest food losses.

DEFINITION OF TERMS AND BOUNDARIES OF THE SURVEY

DEFINITIONS

Just as the production, processing, storage, and distribution of food are location- and culture-specific activities, the perception of what is food and what is food loss and/or food waste is highly subjective. This is especially true in developing countries, where food habits are often more conservative and rigid than those in industrialized countries. In order to minimize misunderstandings likely to arise in addressing topics in a field as diversified and affect-laden as that of food production and loss, it is essential to define certain terms, although such definitions are, of necessity, arbitrary and never quite satisfactory.

Before deciding which definitions to use for the purpose of the following discussion, it may be useful to compare the definitions (or their absence) in different documents.

1. In the *U.S. Comptroller General's Report to Congress (September 1977)*, entitled "Food Waste: An Opportunity to Improve Resource Use" (5), the following simple definition is used:

> For the purpose of this report, loss is defined as the edible portion of any agricultural product no longer usable.

2. In the *FAO Report—AgPP MISC/27 (March 1977)*, entitled "Analysis of an FAO Survey of Post-Harvest Crop Losses in Developing Countries" (6), none of the terms are precisely defined; crop losses are given in per cent weight figures. Cultural considerations are not touched upon.

3. In *Bourne's paper on post-harvest losses* (7), the following definitions are given:

> Post-harvest begins when the process of collecting or separating food of edible quality from its site of immediate production has been completed. It ends when the food enters the mouth.

"Food", in Bourne's paper, means weight of wholesome edible material, measured on a moisture-free basis, that would normally be consumed by humans. "Loss" means any change in the availability, edibility, wholesomeness, or quality of the food that prevents it from being consumed by people.

Food losses may be direct or indirect. A direct loss is disappearance of food by spillage, or consumption by rodents or birds. An indirect loss is the lowering of quality to the point where people refuse to eat it.

This definition is a people-centered definition. "Food" means those commodities that people normally eat and excludes the commodities that people do not normally eat. If the food is consumed by people, it is not lost; if it is not consumed by people for any reason at all, then it is considered a post-harvest food loss.

4. The *NAS Report on Post-Harvest Food Losses in Developing Countries* (2) gives the following definition, which is largely, but not entirely, based upon Bourne's:

> Food is any commodity produced or harvested to be eaten by a particular society. It is measured by the weight of edible material—calculated on a specified moisture basis—that has been harvested, gathered, or caught for human consumption and that is consumed by the population of the area

under consideration. For the purpose of this study, primary attention is focused on the major food crops—cereal grains, grain legumes (the "durables"), and root crops—while secondary "loss" denotes an involuntary state in which one finds oneself—by an act of God, accident, ignorance, clumsiness, but certainly not by design—to be without something that had previously been in one's possession; and where "waste" means a voluntary action by which one spends, discards, utilizes a resource uselessly and destroys it for direct human consumption.

BOUNDARIES

Major emphasis is given in this survey to the major food crops, identified on the basis of estimates of their levels of production in 1976 (8): Cereal grains and grain legumes, nongrain staples, perishables, and fish in rough proportion (60:20:20) to their relative importance and the information believed to be available about post-harvest problems in developing countries.

Commercial food crops, beverages (tea, coffee, cocoa), and other plantation and export crops, such as bananas and sugar cane, are excluded from this survey. All of these commodities are mainly the province of private enterprise; presumably, the entrepreneurs give post-harvest loss appropriate attention, at least by comparison with the nonmarket food crop sector.

Meat and dairy products are also excluded because they pose special kinds of loss problems related to the provision of a storage and distribution system. If such a system exists, it operates more or less efficiently with pasteurization and refrigeration; if it does not, there is little incentive for production beyond immediate, usually modest, needs, and the products are consumed quickly with minimal loss.

Though meat and dairy products are excluded because of their perishable nature (except for cheese) and urgent storage demands, fish is included because of its importance in the world diet (in which it supplies 17% of animal protein consumed) and because losses after harvest are similar to losses in other perishables, e.g., problems of rapid deterioration, selection of preservation and drying technologies, and storage.

NATURE OF THE PROBLEM

GENERAL CONSIDERATIONS

Throughout history man has used some 3000 plant species for food. At least 150 of them have been commercially cultivated to some extent, but over the centuries the tendency has been to concentrate on fewer and fewer. Today, most of the people in the world are fed by about 20 crops: cereals such as wheat, rice, maize, millet, and sorghum; root crops such as potato, sweet potato, and cassava; legumes such as peas, beans, peanuts (groundnuts), and soybeans; and sugar cane, sugar beet, coconuts, and bananas. These plants are the main bulwark between mankind and starvation. It is a very small bastion (9).

Among the hundreds of food crops grown around the world, some two dozen account for approximately 90% of all the food produced. Table 1 shows the reported production of major food crops.

In this survey, two crop groups—the cereal grains and grain legumes, and the perishables—will be discussed because of their overwhelming importance in the world food picture. Post-harvest losses of fish will also be looked at, since this resource represents a very large proportion of the animal protein available to many populations. Although some of the more important terms that are going to be used in this survey have been roughly defined above, the nontechnological, subjective, culture- and society-related dimensions of the post-harvest food loss problem should be stressed once more. It is largely these facets that often make it not only extremely difficult to identify and assess the extent of post-harvest losses in a particular community, but also very hazardous (violation of food habits and systems, possibility of causing further damage to the society) to plan and implement an intervention. If one adds to these cultural and psychological problems those that are directly related to the particular political system dominating a given society and begins to consider food losses induced by, for instance, marketing, taxation, and

TABLE 1. World Vegetable and Animal Protein Production, 1975[a]

	Amount of protein (million tons per year)		
Protein source	Available to man	Fed to livestock	total
Cereals	57	38	95
Legumes	24	6	30
Other vegetables	5	1	6
Livestock	30	3	33
Fish[b]	6	3	9

[a] From Reference 18.
[b] Fish includes all seafoods harvested from the ocean, and for 1975 was estimated at 66 million tons (based on FAO figures), which contained an estimated 14% protein. A reduction from 17.5 to 14% in total fish protein is included for cleaning the fish consumed by man. An estimated 33% of the fish harvest is fed to livestock.

import regulations, the situation becomes even more complicated and intractable.

Perhaps the most striking of the many perplexing aspects that one encounters almost anywhere on examining food losses (however defined) and their causes, effects, and human attitudes toward them are the definitions of what is considered to be food and what is considered to be avoidable food loss, people's attitudes toward the causes of loss, and what people are willing to undertake to reduce these losses. Definitions and attitudes vary wildly and widely from place to place, and from population group to population group. Hardly any edible produce exists that is not utilized as food in one place and considered inedible or abhorrent in another. For some people, only cooked food is "real" food (10). Depending on viewpoint, anything that is moldy or fermented is either delectable or quite inedible.

The same problem of definition applies to what is considered loss of food. Many ethnic groups, for example, offer specially prepared foods to the departed ghosts of friends and relatives (11)—gifts that the living can often ill afford. In the strict sense of the word, that is, of course, a food loss, but such offerings are considered to be so important that the belief is widespread that without these sacrifices, disaster would surely befall a family or community.

The same irrational attitudes exist everywhere toward the agents of loss, for instance toward the animals that people fear and worship very seriously: the vermin that infest and destroy their crops, fish, and cattle. The Estonian peasant was known to protect the weevil and would not kill it because he felt that the more he hurt the beetle, the more it would hurt him (12). The peasant in Central Europe threw a fistful of seeds over his head when he sowed his field, saying "This is for you, sparrows" (13). The rural Germans developed an elaborate system for ridding their gardens of caterpillars: After sunset, the mistress of the house walked around the plot, dragging a broom after her, murmuring: "Good evening, Mother Caterpillar, you shall come with your husband to church," and left the garden gate open for the caterpillar to depart (14).

The existence of such colorful, deeply engrained, and varied attitudes, of course, makes a reasonable estimate of origin and extent of food losses, and the design and implementation of loss reduction measures, extremely difficult. All we know is

1. That huge gaps exist between what is being planted, produced, or harvested as food and what is actually being consumed.
2. That the disappearance of food, its nonutilization, spoilage, and consumption by animals, is regarded by societies in the most varied lights and not necessarily as loss of food.

3. That there is by no means ready and universal willingness to reduce the gap between the harvested and consumed food.
4. That the poor are usually most conservative and not eager to change life-styles and the methods that they have hitherto used to process and treat a particular commodity. After all, this has been the way they and their ancestors have always handled the harvest; it has kept them alive, and they are therefore not ready to rock the boat by trying new ways.
5. That when the willingness exists to protect the harvest by a new strategy, there is hardly ever any assurance that the additional effort that the farmer or fisherman is prepared to make will accrue, at least in part, to his own benefit and not be eroded by the government's or landlord's taking away the increased food.

Loss Estimation Methodology

The production, processing, storage, and distribution of food are highly location-specific and involve a system of movement that is usually very complex and consists of many stages.

The more that loss estimation is analyzed, the more it is clear that there neither is, nor can be, a simple technique, method, or procedure that can be universally applied. The movement and storage of commodities between production and consumption is seldom an easily analyzed flow. Irregular movement and mixing of various batches in post-harvest operations, for instance, make sampling procedures and generalizations difficult.

For these and a variety of other reasons, more techniques have evolved for the estimation of grain losses than for any other major food categories, reflecting the importance of grains as staple foods, their relative physical uniformity, and the comparative ease with which they can be stored.

Grain loss estimation methodology has recently been the subject of a manual prepared by Harris and Lindblad (15) designed to be widely used in developing countries to encourage standardized loss assessment procedures so that results from observations carried out in different locations can be more easily compared.

Overall Assessment

Overall loss assessment is the first, and in many cases the most important, of a series of steps leading to loss estimation and possible loss reduction. Overall assessment of the commodity movement system means a search for the points where the most acute food loss occurs; it implies study of the whole physical, and especially social, system in which the food moves from producer to consumer, and will identify how the commodities are handled (size, number of steps, etc.) and the number of participating middlemen. The objective of this assessment stage is to permit judgments to be made about the possibilities for loss reduction interventions. From the loss assessment and reduction perspective, it might be helpful if a national policy body existed to deal with post-harvest loss problems, to coordinate the efforts of national and international assistance agencies, and to gather and analyze loss information. Relevant loss information can be obtained from a variety of sources: ministries of agriculture, central statistics organizations, university faculties of agriculture and economics, transportation agencies, marketing boards, commercial organizations, and farmers' cooperatives.

Locality- and commodity-specific information is needed to develop a "commodity loss profile" describing the movement of a commodity through the system and highlighting points of potential or actual food loss.

Figure 1 depicts, in cartoon form, the "food pipeline" and the physical and biological ways in which some losses occur. It must be emphasized, however, that the actual movement of food from harvest to consumer almost always involves a much more complex process than a cartoon can represent. Movement can be irregular or can be halted for long periods of time; batches of a commodity can be divided and routed through the system by very different paths and schedules; infusions of a commodity can be brought into the system from different sources.

The real-world "pipeline" is also constructed of a number of different kinds of materials. There are the human and the mechanical parts of the pipeline, the chain of hands, and the line of transport vehicles down which the food passes with greater or lesser efficiency, speed, and ease. The food in the pipeline is propelled by socioeconomic and political forces; regulations and other bureaucratic procedures slow down or accelerate the food's passage from producer to consumer.

Despite the complexities of the system of commodity movement, experienced professionals can make useful estimates of losses and identify possibilities for loss reduction. Simple observation of such visual indices as insects, mold, or leaking roofs may be all that is necessary. Further, information on such things as the use of pesticides or the type of storage facility can provide a knowledgeable person with a basis for judging where losses occur and of what magnitude they are.

The ultimate use of a commodity also bears on loss estimation. Harvested grain may be divided into several lots for different purposes, with each receiving different treatment—some dried and stored for long periods as seed, and some held only for short-term storage and con-

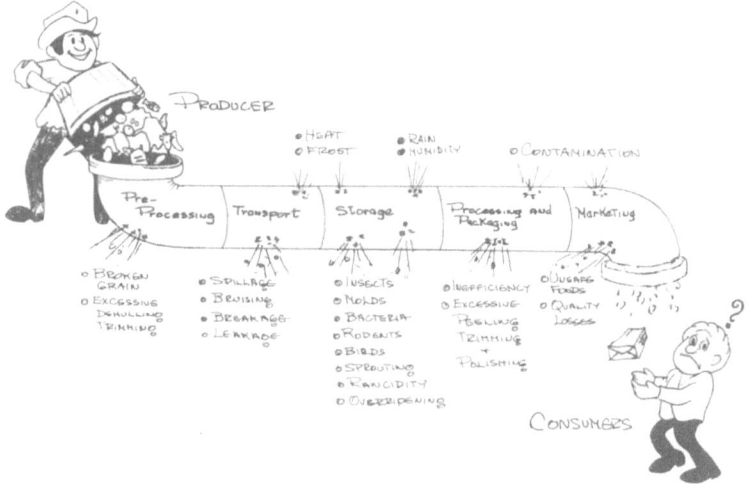

FIGURE 1. The food pipeline.

sumption or movement off the farm. Different levels of risk of loss would be involved for the different uses; farmers frequently consume their low-quality grain first, because it is known to be subject to the most rapid loss.

These observations enable the trained observer to develop a "commodity loss profile" for a particular commodity. Such a profile would indicate the final uses of the commodity, the channels through which it travels to final use, the points at which losses occur, and rough estimates of the relative magnitude of the losses. It should be pointed out that complete information on food-handling is frequently not collected, but that such data—e.g., the number of handling steps involved, the number of middlemen handling the food (with inevitable losses) at each step—are critical. It is only this kind of complete information that will enable the expert to judge with confidence what should be investigated and where priorities are to be assigned.

SPECIFIC CONSIDERATIONS

Cereal Grains and Grain Legumes

The existing knowledge about the nature and extent of post-harvest losses is much more extensive for cereal grains and grain legumes than for other food staples.

There are a number of reasons for this. In most societies, the durable commodities are (or have been) the most important in terms of quantity produced. They are traditionally stored, and security or survival of a community has depended on keen attention to the conservation of these staples. This has been less true in the case of the nongrain food crops. It is easier to protect dormant, dried grain from external attack by insects or rodents than it is to prevent physiological deterioration of or fungal attack on perishables having a high moisture content. Perishables are often seasonal crops that provide a relatively constant supply of (different) fruits and vegetables that are not stored. Many grow with minimum attention; their husbandry is therefore much less important and demanding than that of durable staples.

The bulk of harvested cereal grain and legumes passes through a fairly well-defined series of steps—the post-harvest system. After harvest, the crops are threshed or shelled, dried, stored, and finally processed. This process varies for each commodity, and some commodities require additional steps that enlarge the system (rice parboiling, for example), but there are enough similarities in the flow of durables through the system to enable generalizations about loss problems to be made.

Perishables

The main perishable staples are cassava, yam, sweet potato, white potato, taro, banana and plantain, and breadfruit. In the developing countries these staples and the major vegetables and fruits comprise over 39% of food crops consumed. However, their importance in the diets of many peoples is disproportionately greater than this because they are the major source of carbohydrate and energy, or they supplement otherwise monotonous cereal-based diets with vitamins and minerals.

From the perspective of post-harvest losses, the perishable staples present a very different set of problems than those associated with durable commodities, the cereal grains and legumes. They have relatively high moisture content—from 50% upwards—and are difficult and expensive to dry and hence to store as dry products. Furthermore, the dried product is very different from the fresh and is often less acceptable. Lacking the hard texture of cereal grains, the perishables bruise easily. Although perishables comprise the storage and reproductive parts of plants, even those that are organs of dormancy (such as yams) are metabolically much more active than the seeds of durable staples and seldom have prolonged dormant periods. Roots and tubers continue to respire and metabolize—at a low level compared with the growing plant, but at a much faster rate than in cereals—as they maintain the life of the plant through the nongrowing season. This fact limits their extended storage possibilities.

The edible parts of most fruits and vegetables are not the seeds, which are often discarded, but the fleshy tissues whose natural function is to support the germination and growth of the seed where it falls, or to attract birds or other agents by which the seeds can be spread. The edible tissue is meant to perform these functions when it is ripe, not to serve as a food store in the dry condition, and its storage life may be only days.

The high moisture content seriously affects loss estimation, because it is difficult to express weight loss on a constant moisture basis, and loss of moisture over short periods may be taken to be loss of nutrients. Reports of loss assessment must be meticulous as to the age and state of the commodity.

Fish

Post-harvest loss in the production of fish* is unique among the staples examined in this survey. For no other class of food is there both so much evidence of serious loss at every stage from harvest to consumption and so little precise knowledge of the overall proportion of losses to the potential harvest or to the fish finally consumed.

In this discussion of post-harvest fish losses, attention is focused particularly on artisanal fisheries that are small-scale, poor, dispersed, and unorganized.

In spite of their great importance, two aspects of fishing and fish consumption are not considered here: commercial fishing carried out by large vessels on the high seas and fish meal and fish oil industries.

Previously, we have said that nonutilization or underutilization of commodities not recognized as acceptable food is not loss. However, for fish we need an expanded definition of post-harvest food loss that includes, among other things, nonuse of edible species.

Specifically, post-harvest losses of fish should include fish discarded at sea as by-catch in the harvest of other species such as shrimp. This seems justified not only because the by-catch frequently represents a multiple in weight of the principal—and economically more valuable—harvest, but also because the discarded harvest often contains a large proportion of locally acceptable food fish, and because the loss could be identified and research and development could be applied to reduce this loss.

By extension, the loss definition should include food fish that is

---

*Fish is used here to denote all aquatic animal food produce.

locally unutilized or underutilized for any reason except on religious or ritual grounds, again, not only because this potential food is quantitatively identifiable, but also because an effort should be made to determine, by research, special handling and preservation requirements that might exist for these species.

Because fish harvesting differs in many ways from the land harvests of the other food commodities in this study, an overview of fishing and fish consumption will be helpful as a prelude to further discussion of post-harvest fish losses.

General Aspects of Fish Harvest and Consumption. Fisheries. Fisheries (as opposed to fish farming) involve the greater proportion of worldwide fishing activities, and those on the high seas represent probably the most dangerous and demanding of food-providing occupations.

Although there are significant regional differences, preference on shore and in the marketplace in many, if not most, developing countries is for whole fish. Under the usually prevailing primitive conditions of preservation and distribution, only small harvests can be rapidly disposed of. As a result, most ocean fishing in developing countries is carried out by fleets of many small fishing boats skippered by individualistic, competitive captains, each acting according to his own lights and laws, trying to make the best living he can.

The fishing trade is doubly hazardous: first because of the dangers inherent in harvesting, and then, because of the perishability of a commodity whose consumers demand that it be fresh. The special vulnerability that has forced many fishermen and fish traders to resort to sharp practice in selling their goods has led fish trading to be placed, in many countries, at the very bottom of the hierarchy of desirable professions.

Consumption. Of the 20 to 25,000 species of fish known to exist in salt and fresh waters, only a few dozen species are utilized at present on any large scale.

Experience with toxic species, or those traditionally believed to be poisonous, has compelled consumers, especially in warm climates, to demand that fish remain whole to permit identification of species and inspection for freshness. It has also generated local traditions that only particular fish species are acceptable for human consumption; species that are desirable in one place may, for a number of reasons, be quite unacceptable in others.

If unutilized or underutilized species such as capelin, krill, squid, and other major groups of edible aquatic animals could be economically harvested, processed, distributed, and marketed, the total aquatic food resources would be increased by as much as tenfold (16).

James (17) summarizes the information regarding the costs of expanding existing fisheries to meet the demand, particularly in developing countries. The investment in equipment, manpower, and technical development required simply to double production from the present level would be of the order of 30×10^9, or about $500 per additional ton.

Importance of Fish as Food.   All available evidence indicates that fish has been used as food for man since long before recorded history. At present fish provides about 17% of the world's animal protein intake (Table 1) (18). About 60% of the world's edible fish catch goes directly to consumers in the raw, reflecting their desire to inspect the raw fish carefully for freshness. In countries where Japanese and other Far Eastern fish sausages and sauces are unknown, fish products in which the original identify is not preserved represent only a very small proportion of fish consumed. In certain regions, fish makes up the bulk of a nation's animal protein fare.

It is noteworthy that fish is still largely consumed as it was in ancient times, and, with the exception of canning and mechanical refrigerated freezing, no basic technological advances have been made in its preservation. These observations are significant in that they do not apply to the consumption or preservation of any other staple food, and reflect the general, long-term stubbornness of the consumer intent on dealing with fish in a special way. This pervasive attitude continues to influence the nature of the fishing, fish-processing, and fish-marketing industries. It also affects the possibility of estimating post-harvest losses in developing countries, as fish spoil rapidly and are mainly preserved by drying (with or without salting and smoking).

CAUSES AND LOCI OF LOSS OF MAJOR FOOD CROPS

GENERAL CONSIDERATIONS

Causes

Malcolm Bourne, in his excellent overview paper (7), differentiates between primary and secondary food loss causes. The following is a partial quote from Bourne's publication:

Primary Causes

> *Biological and microbiological.* Consumption or damage by insects, mites, rodents, birds, and large animals and by microbes such as molds and bacteria.

Chemical and biochemical. Undesirable reactions between chemical compounds that are present in the food; enzyme-activated reactions; accidental or deliberate contamination with harmful substances.

Mechanical. Spillages, abrasion, bruising, excessive polishing, peeling or trimming, puncturing of containers, defective seals on cans or other containers.

Physical. Excessive or insufficient heat or cold, improper atmosphere.

Physiological. Sprouting of grains and tubers, senescence in fruits and vegetables, and changes caused by respiration and transpiration.

Some of these losses interact. For example, respiration generates heat that, if not dissipated, will accelerate biochemical and chemical changes. In some cases more than one of these causes may be responsible for food loss. Multiple causes may work simultaneously or sequentially, such as the growth of mold and insects at the same time.

Secondary Causes. Secondary causes are those that lead to conditions in which primary cause of loss can occur:

- Inadequate drying equipment or a poor drying season.
- Inadequate storage facilities to protect the food from insects, rodents, birds, rain, and high humidity.
- Inadequate transportation to get the food to market before it spoils.
- Inadequate refrigeration or cold storage (for perishables).
- An inadequate marketing system.

Legislation.   The presence or absence of legal standards can affect the eventual retention or rejection of a food for human use.

Loci of Food Losses

Losses may occur anywhere from the point where the food has been harvested or gathered up to the point of consumption. For the sake of convenience, the losses can be broken down into the following subheadings:

Preparation. This is the preliminary separation or extraction of edible from nonedible animal and agricultural products, e.g., the dehulling of grain, slaughtering and dressing of animals, extraction of sugar from cane, and peeling of fruits and vegetables. There is some room for improvement here to reduce post-harvest losses, for example, in the dehulling of grain to ensure that grain is not broken or damaged during this process, and in the extraction of sugar to ensure that as much of the sugar as possible is removed from the cane and that the minimum is discarded with the bagasse.

Preservation. This is the prevention of loss and spoilage of foods; for example, the drying of grain or fruit, the refrigeration or canning of vegetables or fish, and the prevention of the onset of rancidity in oil. This is the area where the major emphasis in post-harvest food loss reduction activities must be placed.

Processing. This is the conversion of edible food into another form more acceptable or more convenient to the consumer, e.g., the making of bread from wheat, brewing beer from barley, making sausages from meat, and making instant coffee from coffee beans. The food industry in the developed countries expends its greatest effort in this area because it knows that greater profits can be made by developing some new convenience factor or new flavor to titillate the taste buds of the well-fed than by trying to reduce further an already economically acceptable low level of post-harvest loss.

Processing should not be an area of major emphasis in developing countries where people cannot afford to buy any great quantity of processed food. In these countries food processing occupies a smaller proportion of the total post-harvest food activities than it does in developed countries.

Storage. This is the holding of foods until consumption. For perishable foods such as some fish, meat, and dairy products, the storage life can be very short—a few hours if stored at ambient temperature, up to a week or longer if properly refrigerated. Staple foods such as cereal grains may be stored for several years. Semiperishable foods such as fresh fruits, most tubers, and oil can be stored successfully for periods of one or two weeks to many months if handled correctly.

There is a need for construction of more storage facilities, particularly for durables such as cereals and oilseeds. Large storage warehouses are needed by the big cities and the ports, and many small-scale, on-farm storage facilities are needed for subsistence farmers.

Transportation. Most developing countries need an improved transportation system to reduce the time lag between departure from the site of production and arrival at the market.

Home Preparation. In developed countries there is considerable loss of food in the home. For example, studies in Tucson have shown that the average American household discards approximately 10% of the food that has been purchased (19). It is likely that these in-home losses are low in developing countries because the cost of food accounts for so much of the family budget that food must be of very poor quality to be discarded. In the urban areas of developing countries, the homemaker usually makes frequent trips to the food stores and does not hold any great quantity of food in the house, thus avoiding the risk of losses in stored foods. This area probably requires minor attention in terms of reducing post-harvest food losses in developing countries.

SPECIFIC CONSIDERATIONS

Grain

Causes for Loss

Drying.   Drying is a particularly vital operation in the chain of food handling, because moisture may be the most important factor in determining whether, and to what extent, grain will be liable to deterioration during storage.

In developing countries, the methods available to farmers for drying crops are often limited, usually to a combination of sun- and air-drying, although supplemental heat is frequently employed. In many cases, seed grain may be treated separately from food grains and with greater care. Overdrying—which can easily occur in arid regions or after excessive exposure to sun or other heat—can cause breakage, damage to the seed coat, bleaching, discoloration, loss of germinative power, and nutritional changes. Too-rapid drying of crops with high moisture content also causes damage. For example, bursting (or "case-hardening") causes the surface of the grain to dry out rapidly, sealing moisture within the inner layers. Underdrying or slow drying (a problem in humid regions) results in deterioration caused by fungi and bacteria, and, in extreme cases, leads to total loss.

Storage Losses.   The extent to which deterioration and loss occur in storage depends on physical and production factors, the storage environment, and biological factors. In addition, physical damage to the crop during harvest may also affect storage. Undamaged cowpea pods, groundnut shells, and the husks of paddy grains also afford the crop a noticeable degree of protection from infestation by most insect species, though the space they occupy in the storage bin reduces the volume that can be stored.

Storage Environment.   Storage conditions have much to do with the rate of deterioration. High temperature and humidity encourage mold formation and provide suitable conditions for rapid growth of insect populations. Deterioration is minimal in cool, dry areas; more marked in hot, dry ones; high in cool, damp conditions; and very high in hot, damp climates. Some climates lessen the residual activity of certain pesticides and can reduce the effective life of storage containers and structures. Different structural materials may alter the effectiveness of various formulations of a given insecticide.

Biological Factors.   The principal biological agents of deterioration during storage are insects and mites, fungi, and rodents.

Losses to insects and mites. Insect pests are a greater problem in regions where the relative humidity is high, but temperature is the over-riding factor that influences insect multiplication. At temperatures of about 32°C, the rate of insect development is such that a monthly com-pound increase of 50 times is theoretically possible. Thus, 50 insects at harvest time could multiply to become more than 312 million after four months.

Weight loss is of economic as well as nutritive importance and, in the absence of effective control measures, insect attack on cereal grains and beans can be so severe as to reduce the commodity to empty husks and dust. Large numbers of insects can be expected to produce heavy weight losses, and the resulting contamination by dead and live insects and their excreta can be sufficient to make the commodity completely unpalatable and unacceptable in the market.

Losses to fungi. Fungal attack in storage generally occurs when drying has been inadequate, when large numbers of insects are present, causing a temperature rise in the grain, or when the stored crop is exposed to high humidity or actual wetting. Fungal development does not normally take place when the moisture content of the commodity is below that moisture content in equilibrium with a relative humidity of 70%.

Fungal spoilage is more serious in those regions with a permanent high relative humidity, or where a season of high humidity coincides with the time when grain is being dried or kept in store. Microorganisms may multiply and create heat that can increase in unventilated grain to the point of complete destruction. However, losses due to fungi can be reduced by improvements in drying and storage technology.

Losses to rodents. Rodent damage to stored food can occur in a num-ber of ways. The animals not only consume the food, but also foul a large amount with their excretions (which may carry microorganisms patho-genic to man), destroy containers by gnawing holes that result in leakage and wastage of grain, and paw into and scatter grain while they eat. This scattered grain, along with what leaks from gnawed holes, is subject to contamination and admixture with impurities. Damage to grain stored in bulk may be much less than to grain stored on the head or in bags because rodents are unable to burrow into the bulk.

These problems have recently been reviewed by Hopf *et al.* (20) in a report prepared by the U.K. Centre for Overseas Pest Research and the Tropical Products Institute.

The three main species of rodent are *Rattus norvegicus*, the Norway, common, or brown rat; *Rattus rattus,* the roof, ship, or black rat; and *Mus musculus,* the house mouse. Other species such as the bandicoot rat *(Bandicota bengalensis)* are important pests in particular areas. Locally, other species can assume greater importance.

Losses during Primary Processing. These occur in threshing and milling, in parboiling, and in further processing (baking, brewing, canning, packaging, etc.), which, although important, is outside the focus of this survey.

There is a tendency for processing losses to increase as larger amounts of crop are produced that strain the capacity of the traditional processing system. Maize traditionally shelled by hand, for example, may be placed in sacks and pounded with a stick to detach the grains from the cob. Mechanical processing is generally less efficient than manual processing, both because it is incomplete and because of damage to grains caused by their variation in size or poor adjustment of the machinery. The manual processing efficiency may be used as the standard against which the efficiency of machinery is measured.

Processing losses are generally specific to particular crops. There are, however, some general loss problems resulting from processing. Attitudes toward broken grains vary from society to society, e.g., off-color grain caused by poor parboiling or drying practices may or may not be accepted. In many cases, this simply means that the poorer members of population have the broken grains and dust, or otherwise lower quality grain, and there is little loss. In Pakistan, the Council on Scientific and Industrial Research has experimented with reconstituting "whole" rice grains from broken grain and rice powder with good acceptance.

In many societies, central milling facilities process grain brought in by farmers for a price determined by the initial unmilled volume or weight, and there is thus little incentive to reduce subsequent losses caused by poorly adjusted equipment or leakage and spillage.

Perishables

Preservation and conservation of nongrain staples is very different from drying and storing of durables. In many developing countries there has been no need (because of abundant, cheap supply) or no policy (because of a predominant interest in export, commercial crops, or grain or legumes) for trying to reduce these losses.

The commodities cover a wide range of roots, tubers, fruits, and vegetables, with possibly more differences than similarities among them. There are, however, certain general observations we can make.

Causes for Loss

Mechanical Causes.   Perishables are much more susceptible to injury than are durables because of their shape and structure, the relatively soft texture associated with their high moisture content, and the need for more frequent specialized handling. Injury can occur at almost any point in the post-harvest system and results from poor handling and packaging, from transportation and storage conditions, or from damage in the marketplace.

Physiological Causes.   Physiological losses are the result of endogenous respiration or reduction of moisture content from wilting or transpiration and may be abnormally high if the product is exposed to undue heat, cold, or otherwise unsuitable environmental conditions.

Losses from Disease.   Possibly the greatest single cause of post-harvest loss in perishable produce is decay caused by microorganisms. This usually occurs from initial infection by one or more specific pathogens, which may then be followed by secondary infection by a broad spectrum of biodeteriogens saprophytic on the dead or moribund tissue remaining from the primary attack (21).

Rodents and Insects.   Attacks by rodents or insects in stored products are usually of relatively minor importance in comparison to decay from microorganisms, although these factors may be important in particular instances.

Loss Foci

Storage Problems. Storage deterioration is brought about by endogenous physiological processes or by attack of pathogens (fungi and bacteria), both of which may be aggravated by physical damage to the crop. The main causes of storage loss in perishables are:

- Fungal damage, influenced by the lack of rigidity of perishable crops as compared with grains and the ease with which they are damaged during harvest or handling.
- Sprouting at the end of the natural period of dormancy, which affects roots and tubers.
- Insect damage, usually a relatively minor problem of perishables stores fresh, occurring most frequently while the root is still in the ground, or the fruit or vegetable is still attached to the plant, and relevant mainly in that it aggravates fungal problems by providing additional points of entry.

Remedies and Their Limitations

Cooling and Refrigeration.   Refrigeration is undoubtedly an important means of prolonging the storage life of high-quality, fresh tropical produce, but it has a number of limitations for reducing food losses in developing countries, including:

- Many tropical horticultural products are liable to low-temperature injury—physiological deterioration at temperatures near, but above, freezing.
- Many of the commodities are currently too low in unit cost to support the expense of mechanically refrigerated storage.
- The capital cost—and the not inconsiderable cost and organization of efficient and continuous maintenance of significant amounts of mechanically refrigerated storage facilities—is likely to continue to be a major limitation for the foreseeable future.

Handling and Packaging.   Major reduction in the amount of loss can undoubtedly be accomplished by improved handling and packaging at all stages of the movement of perishables from harvest to consumption. Delicate produce is often handled in the same way as the durable crops are, and the mechanical damage greatly increases the rate and extent of both physiological and microbiological deterioration. Improvements in packaging and handling may also often be accomplished at little cost. They may require nothing more than ensuring that the produce is handled in smaller quantities and put into shallower containers, for instance, in rigid wooden crates or cardboard cartons rather than in sacks or in loose bulk. These improvements are normally so situation-specific that a detailed discussion is beyond the scope of this report. Proper packaging and handling are so important, however, that they should be among the first aspects of food loss to be investigated.

Improved transportation and marketing systems to reduce the time between harvesting and consumption can also greatly reduce loss.

Fish

Serious post-harvest food losses begin immediately after harvest on board ship because of the lack of means to preserve the catch until docking. Important losses are caused by enzymatic spoilage and insect infestation as the catch is landed, is processed on the beach, and awaits transportation to the market. Further heavy losses are caused by primitive methods of handling, preservation, transportation, and exposure at market.

Moreover, the entire marine fisheries industry in developing countries is so fractionated by local customs and cultures, and is controlled by so many individual entrepreneurs from harvest to consumer, that losses occur simply as a consequence of frequent handling and transfer of the variously processed food from one middleman to another. It seems, therefore, fair to say that no reliable figures for overall post-harvest losses are available at present for any one region.

Fresh Fish. The extent of post-harvest losses on board the fishing vessel is likely to be considerable, especially in warm climates because of spoilage due to poor handling and lack of refrigeration. Actual losses are camouflaged, however, because even stale or spoiling raw fish is later processed. This results in economic loss, as the price for fresh and poor-quality dried product is, in many countries, often the same per unit weight. Major losses occur with the traditionally processed products.

Drying. The simplest, and most widely used, technique for preserving fish is sun drying, in which the landed fish are spread on the beach, or on a mat, and allowed to dry in the sun. Under these conditions, the wet fish are subject to attack by blowflies, mainly *Chrysomyia* spp., whose larvae burrow into the fish and cause damage and spoilage. Apart from the physical damage to the fish and the associated enhanced spoilage, the blowflies are a serious source of disease, particularly because the beaches they infest are widely contaminated with human feces as a result of limited public sanitation facilities.

The dried fish is also subject to attack by *Dermestes* beetles. If this infestation is allowed to proceed, the beetles consume the fish.

Salting. Preliminary salting is often used to enhance the quality and acceptability of naturally dried fish. Salting, either by stacking the split fish with dry salt between the layers, or preferably by immersing the fish in brine, serves to speed up the removal of water from the flesh and to reduce the time necessary for air or sun drying. In the case of oily fish, such as sardines, prolonged drying leads to discoloration and rancidity.

Salting is also a chemical method of bacterial and insect control. Flies will not attack fish that has been brined before drying, and the rate of attack by beetles is inversely proportional to salt concentration (17). One of the most difficult problems with salted, dried fish is the control of reabsorption of moisture from a humid atmosphere. Proper packaging is therefore required for this purpose.

Smoking and Smoke Drying. Smoke drying is widely used in West Africa for a variety of foodstuffs, many of which spend some time suspended over cooking fires as a means of deterring insect infestation. In the Lake Chad area, fish may be partially dried in the sun, then covered with grass or papyrus that is set on fire, which scorches and blackens the fish to form a hard, protective outer surface.

These methods, however, offer little defense against insects that deposit their eggs in the flesh before and during drying. During smoking of thick-bodied fish, the insects are deterred by heat and smoke, but the larvae already present in the fish penetrate the deeper parts of the fish where heat and smoke cannot reach. Traditional processing may be responsible for a loss of value as high as 15% (22).

Storage and Distribution. In addition to losses caused by insects, the most important physical and economic losses result from crumbling of the product during storage and distribution. Poorly dried fish is a fragile product, which, if roughly handled or vibrated on overloaded trucks on poor roads, will crumble to a powder.

MAGNITUDE OF FOOD LOSSES IN DEVELOPING COUNTRIES

In this section, we will attempt to summarize what is known about the magnitude of loss in major food crops in developing countries. For this purpose, we will use the figures arrived at by the post-harvest food loss group working under the aegis of the National Academy of Sciences (2) and those compiled by FAO in its worldwide investigation (6).

AVAILABLE GENERAL INFORMATION

Answers to requests by FAO (6) for data on the magnitude of food crop losses in three crop categories provide an instructive overview of the information available in 51 countries in four regions of the globe:

- Durables (cereal grains and grain legumes). Detailed loss estimates were received from 16 countries, or less than one-third of those questioned. Sixteen nations provided no information.
- Fruits and vegetables (perishables). Detailed loss estimates were obtained from only 7 nations, or 14% of those asked. No information was obtained from 29, or 57% of the countries.
- Fish and crustaceans. Detailed loss estimates were received from only one country; 35 (69%) provided no information.

It is clear from these figures that the available body of information is highly deficient.

SPECIFIC QUANTITATIVE INFORMATION

Cereal Grains, Grain Legumes, and Perishables

A considerable effort was made by the NAS Post-Harvest Food Loss Study Group to collect quantitative data from whatever reliable sources could be identified to supplement the loss figures that had been obtained by FAO. Tables 2–4 (23–26) contain information from both sources, together with indications, wherever possible, of where in the food pipeline the losses actually occurred.

We would be inclined to consider the figures for losses of rice, especially, as reasonably accurate; the accuracy of figures given for other cereals, and especially grain legumes, is more difficult to assess.

When we look at the loss data for perishables in Table 4, the very wide range of losses cited, and, in a few cases, the improbably precise, narrow range of losses cited, would suggest the need for caution in accepting these values. The opinions of a group of professionals (2) with long experience with some of the perishable commodities in developing countries produced the following figures as being typical of normal loss ranges:

White potatoes in Chile, Peru, and Venezuela	25–30%
Cassava in Venezuela, Colombia, Ecuador, Dominican Republic and Central America	15–20%
Tomatoes for fresh market in most developing countries	50%
Yams in Nigeria and Ghana	10–20%

Fish

FAO estimates for fisheries in some countries place fish losses among the highest for all commodities. There are very few documented studies to support this; one carried out on Lake Chad indicates that fish losses there may be as high as 50% and sometimes close to 100%.

James (17) roughly estimated losses of dried fish to insect infestation at 3 million tons per year (25% of 12 million tons produced); discarded edible by-catch from shrimping alone at 5 million tons (five times the total shrimp catch); and loss to spoilage at 2 million tons (i.e., 10% estimated spoilage loss of the 46 million tons used for direct human consumption, of which 20 million tons are estimated to be consumed fresh). These rough, conservative approximations give a loss figure of 10 million tons per year—20% of the total catch now going to direct human consumption.

These figures are highly speculative, because there are—with very few exceptions—no reliable data for any developing country on either post-harvest losses or the unregistered harvests caught by unchartered and uncontrolled individual fishermen.

TABLE 2. Cereal Grains and Grain Legumes: Reported Losses of Rice within the Post-Harvest System[a]

Region, country	Total percent weight loss	Reported national production (tons × 10³)	Remarks	Source
West Africa	6–24		Drying 1–2; on-farm storage 2–10; parboiling 1–2; milling 2–10	H. van Ruiten, personal communication (1977)
Sierra Leone	10	580		
Uganda	11	15		
Rwanda	9	5		
Sudan	17	7	Central storage	A. H. Kamel, personal communication (1977)
Egypt	2.5	2,300		
Bangladesh	7	18,500		
India	6	70,500	Unspecified storage	
	3–5.5		Improved traditional storage	Reference 23
Indonesia	6–17	22,950	Drying 2; storage 2–5	
Malaysia	17–25	1,900	Central store 6; threshing 5–13; drying 2; on-farm store 5; handling 6	A. Yunus, personal communication (1977)
Nepal	4–22	2,404	On-farm 3–4; on-farm store 15; central store 1–3	

Pakistan	7	3,942	Unspecified storage 5	
	2–6		Unspecified storage 2	H. A. Qayyum, personal communication (1977)
	5–10		Unspecified storage 5–10	J. H. Greaves, personal communication (1977)
Philippines	9–34	6,439	Drying 1–5; unspecified store 2–6; threshing 2–6	
	up to 30		Handling	Malaysia workshop (reference 24)
	3–10			Reference 25
Sri Lanka	13–40	1,253	Drying 1–5; central store 6.5; threshing 2–6	
	6–18		Drying 1–3; on-farm store 2–6; milling 2–6; parboiling 1–3	J. Ramalingam, personal communication (1977)
Thailand	8–14	14,400	On-farm store 1.5–3.5; central store 1.5–3.5	
	12–25		On-farm store 2–15; handling 10	B. Dhamcheree, personal communication (1977)
Belize	20–30	2	On-farm storage	
Bolivia	16	113	On-farm 2; drying 5; unspecified store 7	J. P. Cal, personal communication (1977)
Brazil	1–30	9,560	Unspecified store 1–30	
Dominican Republic	6.5		On-farm store 3; central store 0.3	

[a]Based on reference 6 figures unless otherwise indicated.

TABLE 3. Cereal Grains and Grain Legumes: Reported Losses of Maize within the Post-Harvest System[a]

Region, country	Total percent weight loss	Reported national production (tons × 10³)	Remarks	Source
Benin	8–9	221	Traditional on-farm storage; 6 months improves storage	Reference 15
Botswana	7–14	62	Insect damage	Reference 26
Ghana	15	395	8 months storage	Reference 27
Ivory Coast	5–10	120	12 months stored on cob	References 27 and 28
Kenya	10–23	1,360	4–6 months central storage	Reference 29
	12		Hybrid maize, hotter regions 6 months	
Malawi	6–14	1,200	Drying 6; on-farm store 8	References 30 and 31
	min. 10		Hybrid	
Nigeria	1–5	1,050	On-farm storage	Reference 32
	5.5–70		6 months on-farm storage	
Rwanda	10–20	60	On-farm storage	

Tanzania	20–100	1,619	Unspecified storage	Reference 33
	9, 14, 67		3, 6, and 9 months	
Togo	5–10	135	6 months central storage	Reference 34
Uganda	4–17	623		
Zambia	9–21	750	On-farm storage	Reference 35
India	6.5–7.5	6,500	Central storage, 7.5	N. S. Agrawal, personal communication (1977)
Indonesia	4	2,532		
Pakistan	2–7	70		
Belize	20–30	20	Traditional on-farm storage	J. P. Cal, personal communication (1977)
Brazil	15–40	17,929	Farm storage	
Dominican Republic	19	49	Farm storage 15; processing 1	
Honduras	20–50	289	Traditional storage, poor facilities	A. B. Balint, personal communication (1977)
Mexico	10–25	8,945		
Nicaragua	15–30	201		
Paraguay	25	290		
Venezuela	10–25	532		J. Martino, personal communication (1977)

ᵃBased on reference 6 figures unless otherwise indicated.

TABLE 4. 1976 Estimates of Minimum Post-Harvest Food Losses in Developing Countries[a]

	Durables	Perishables	Fish
1976 food production (million tons)	420[b]	255[b]	50
Estimated minimum loss percentage	10	20	60
Estimated minimum loss (million tons)	42	51	10[c]
Estimated price/ton (US $)[d]	165	25	225
Estimated loss value (US $ billions)	6.9	1.3	2.3

[a] "Developing Market Economics" according to FAO definition (reference 6).
[b] Production estimates from FAO (8), assuming 79% of durables and 75% of perishables are actually used for food (based on reference 2).
[c] Based on reference 17.
[d] Figures used by the International Food Policy Research Institute (IFPRI), reference 36.

CONCLUSIONS, RECOMMENDATIONS, AND OPEN QUESTIONS

CONCLUSIONS

Overall Picture

From inspection of published information on measurements of actual losses, it is clear that the aggregate quantity of food lost and wasted in developing as well as in industrialized countries is huge, however it is viewed and measured. This fact has only very recently received any attention at all; and because this is a new concern, there are only a few proven assessment methodologies. Also, disagreements exist among experts on how to interpret results and access to reliable facts is often extraordinarily difficult; therefore the overall picture that we have today is so incomplete and so deficient in statistically sound data that conservative expert opinion resists any kind of generalization.

Measurement of Food Losses

Because estimation (and even very rough estimation) methodologies have, until recently, been accorded little critical attention, with a few notable exceptions, and as the value of published information has been reduced by the absence of standard methods and definitions, the available food loss data are questionable at best, and should only be used as order-of-magnitude indicators. Fortunately, this state of affairs has been rectified for the cereal grains with the preparation of the *Manual of Post-Harvest Grain Loss Assessment Methods* by Harris and Lindblad (15). No comparable methodologies, however, exist for perishables and fish, which constitute an area of priority attention.

Causes and Loci of Loss

From the survey it should be clear that we are, by and large, precisely aware of at least the most important primary causes responsible for food loss in developing and industrialized countries. It is also clear that we have a fairly good idea where in the food pipeline between harvest and consumption these losses occur. However, we know very little about many of the nontechnological, nonbiological secondary causes that are responsible for food losses in small communities, by individual subsistence farmers and fishermen, and by individual members of a family. We know very little as yet about the cultural and social factors that are responsible for people's either wasting food, avoiding consumption of certain foods altogether or at certain times, or distributing food within the family in such a manner that certain members are deprived of nutrients, in other words, lose their share of food. We also know only a little about the attitudes of people toward food in general and about their attitudes toward the loss of food. We know, finally, much too little about the effects of political pressures, taxation, and other official and unofficial government regulations and actions about the attitudes of subsistence farmers and fishermen toward the losses they suffer and their willingness as food producers to reduce these losses, knowing that this might involve the possible risk of penalty levied by the power structure. We also have as yet no clear idea of the variety of decision making processes and motivations that make government officials support or prevent the reduction of food losses—wherever, and for whatever reasons, losses may occur. One fact seems clear: Reduction of food losses is unlikely to take place if the local or national power structure does not wish it to.

Magnitude of Losses

Bearing in mind what has been said above, a few words should also be said about loss magnitudes. For planning purposes, experts cite minimal overall losses in developing countries of 10% durable crops and 20% for nongrain staples, perishables and fish, equivalent to 42, 51, and 10 million tons, respectively, of lost food for the year 1976 (Table 4). If weight and value figures in that table are compared to those compiled by the U.S. Comptroller General for losses in the United States during 1974, we obtain a sobering picture: 60 million tons of food valued at $5 billion were lost in the U.S. during harvesting, for instance, and 32 million tons of food, valued at $16.1 billion, were lost in both household and institutional food consumption settings. It is true that, by definition, losses during harvesting and those related to food consumption were excluded from consideration in the present survey dealing primarily with post-harvest losses in developing countries. It is, however, significant that the total tonnage of food lost in the United States exceeds—for whatever reasons and at whatever place in the food pipeline—the total estimated loss of durables, perishables, and fish in all of the developing nations put together. According to Table 4, the total estimated loss in developing countries for 1976 was 103 million tons; the total loss estimated for the U.S. in 1974, 137 million tons!

Technologies for Food Loss Reduction

It seems, finally, also clear that there are technologies known to be capable of reducing food losses caused by the most common and most important biological, environmental, and physical agents. Having said this much, however, is not of much practical assistance because, just as in many other similar food and nutrition-related situations, the existence of technological remedy to resolve a problem is indeed a *conditio sine qua non* for a solution, but is certainly not sufficient in itself to bring it about.

RECOMMENDATIONS

The following are summaries of major recommendations for urgent action, enumerated in no order of importance. I consider these to be necessary actions, but by no means sufficient to bring about a reduction in food losses or hunger.

Education, Training, and Extension

Priority attention must be given to training programs to remedy acute personnel shortages at all levels of the post-harvest food system. Specifically, training efforts are recommended at the following levels:

- Training programs in post-harvest technology for agricultural colleges and similar institutions for extension workers, farm men and women, and others working in agriculture and fisheries. This, the single most important training need, should be accomplished

within the framework of a system of career development and professional opportunity.
- Courses and in-country training programs for other personnel in the post-harvest food system.

Post-Harvest Loss Estimation

More systematic approaches to loss estimation in developing countries must be developed by

- Adoption of standard loss estimation methodology.
- Development of guidelines for loss estimation of perishables.
- Consideration of socioeconomic aspects of food loss.
- Integration of loss estimation with conservation activities.

Nonpolitical National Institutions

The following essential institutional arrangements and mechanisms should be established, as locally appropriate, in developing countries to deal with post-harvest food losses:

- A nonpolitical, nonpartisan, high-level fact-finding body of experts from various disciplines to establish the "lay of the land," i.e., to find out where the greatest needs for, and obstacles to, food loss reduction are, and what the greatest problems for transferring food to those who need it are.
- A national implementing agency or post-harvest food conservation unit especially competent and willing to assist the subsistence farmer and fisherman.
- A mechanism to facilitate communication among planning agencies, decision makers, villagers, subsistence farmers, and fishing people.

International Co-operation Mechanisms

The organizational capacity of the United Nations University should be strengthened to give additional focus to the neglected areas of losses in perishable staples and fish.

Information on Post-Harvest Food Losses

International technical assistance agencies should cooperate to strengthen and expand post-harvest food loss documentation services.

Research

Socioeconomic Research. Substantial refinement of knowledge about economic cost-benefit factors in post-harvest food loss reduction is needed.

General Research and Development Needs. These needs include

- Development of low-cost cooling systems for food preservation in developing countries. For preserving durable crops, current drying and processing technologies and storage structures are adequate under most conditions in developing countries for considerable lengths of time and at reasonable cost. This is not yet true for perishables. The development of cooling technology with low capital and running costs would extend the life of perishables in rural areas and have a dramatic impact on the health, income, and welfare of rural people.
- Research on insecticides, fungicides, and rodenticides, with particular reference to their safety for use on foodstuffs.
- Fundamental research on tropical food crop deterioration and its relationship to environmental conditions.
- Research on storage characteristics, or other qualities of crops that affect their post-harvest fate, as one aspect of breeding and selection programs.
- Socioeconomic studies of the problems of introducing centralized storage in rural areas, with implications for technology design, costs, responsibility, and management essential to facilitate this process. Because wider introduction of centralized storage is probably inevitable, one research consideration should be ways to reduce the number of hands through which commodities pass, thus diminishing losses.
- Adaptive research on small-scale storage technologies, including development of cheap rodent- and insect-resistant containers that are properly ventilated or sealed, as well as resistant to moisture and rainfall.
- Rodent surveys and greater emphasis on rodent control in both agricultural and health extension services.

Commodity-Specific Research Priorities. The following research areas illustrate the kind of work that needs to be done with individual commodities; they do not comprise a full list of priorities.

Rice
- Economic drying of wet-season rice, including particularly natural ventilation methods, and use of preservatives for short-term preservation.

- Improved design of threshing, parboiling, and milling equipment.

Maize
- Improved low-cost drying and storage cribs.
- Improved village-level processing equipment.

Millet and Sorghum
- Improved traditional storage and fumigation methods.
- Improved village-level processing equipment.

Legumes
- Improved milling equipment.
- Ways to avoid loss of cooking quality during storage.

Roots and Tubers
- Determination of optimum storage temperature, humidity, and ventilation for different varieties.
- Better box and clamp design.
- Storage of cassava chips, flour, and pellets.
- Use of sprouting and rot inhibitors.

Fruits and Vegetables
- Low-cost, controlled-environment storage, including waxing, storage under plastic sheeting, gas absorbents, and rot retardants.
- Better low-cost packaging.
- Damage control during storage and movement and in the market.

Fish
- Better drying, smoking, and salting methods.
- Improved on-board storage and use of by-catch.

OPEN QUESTIONS

We are now at the point where we have to air the questions that both the survey and its results elicit, questions that are in part discussed in the compendium chapter by Guggenheim. I am not offering any answers, but it seems that the questions should be raised.

Statements such as the following appear frequently in discussions on post-harvest food losses: "Conservative estimates indicate that a minimum of 103 million tons of food were lost in 1976; the amounts lost in cereal grains and legumes alone would provide more than the annual minimum calorie requirements of 168 million people" (2).

The arithmetic of the above equivalence between loss magnitude and calories is no doubt correct, but how realistic is the statement and what does it really imply? Under what conditions is it fair to say that if losses could be reduced more people could be fed adequately? In attempts to reduce world food shortages, what is the significance of the quantity of food lost and willfully wasted? Assuming that members of a certain community are malnourished because they are unable, for economic or any other reasons, to gain access to, obtain, and consume sufficient food, does the reduction of food losses in that community mean, *ipso facto*, that those in need can obtain more food? What is the connection between reduction of food losses and increased food consumption? In other words: What are the conditions that will make it possible for a food loss reduction in one locality to permit people in that or another locality to consume more food?

It seems reasonable that, even if all food losses are eliminated, undernourished populations will continue to exist unless food distribution is equitable and dictated by people's needs. Initially, it may be worthwhile to address only the problem of the individual subsistence farmer and fisherman. If only they could be reached and their harvests increased and protected so that they and their families have more to eat—and perhaps to sell—a small step could perhaps be made in this tragic matter.

These are the most important questions that, in my opinion, have come out of this discussion, and that must be most earnestly addressed. I conclude, therefore, on a pervasive question that must be answered honestly at all stages: *Cui bene?*—Who benefits?

REFERENCES

1. National Research Council. Study on World Food and Nutrition. National Research Council/National Academy of Sciences, Washington, D.C., 1977.
2. National Research Council, Commission on International Relations, Board on Science and Technology for International Development. Post-Harvest Food Loss in Developing Countries. National Research Council/National Academy of Sciences, Washington, D.C., 1978.
3. U.S. Department of Agriculture, Agricultural Research Service. Losses in Agriculture. USDA/ARS-201, Washington, D.C., 1954.
4. U.S. Department of Agriculture, Agricultural Research Service. Losses in Agriculture. USDA/ARS-291, Washington, D.C., 1956.
5. U.S. General Accounting Office. Report to the Congress by the Comptroller General of the United States: Food Waste: An Opportunity to Improve Resource Use. CED-77-118, Washington, D.C., 1977.
6. Food and Agriculture Organization of the United Nations. Analysis of an FAO Survey of Post-Harvest Crop Losses in Developing Countries (AGPP: MISC/27). Food and Agriculture Association, Rome, 1977.
7. Bourne, M. C. Post-Harvest Food Losses: The Neglected Dimension in Increasing the World Food Supply. Cornell International Agricultural Mimeograph No. 53, Cornell University, Ithaca, New York, 1977.
8. Food and Agriculture Organization of the United Nations. *1976 FAO Production Yearbook*, Vol. 30. Food and Agriculture Organization, Rome, 1977.

9. National Research Council. Under-Exploited Plants with Promising Economic Value. National Research Council/National Academy of Sciences, Washington, D.C., 1975, p. 1.

10. Levi-Straus, C. *The Raw and the Cooked*. Harper Torchbooks, Harper and Row, New York and Evanston, 1969, p. 336.

11. Frazer, J. *The New Golden Bough*. Theodor H. Gaster (Ed.). New American Library, New York, 1959, p. 554.

12. Holzmayer, J. B. Gelehrten Estnischen Ges Zu. Dorpat, 7, ii, 105. In: J. Frazer, *The New Golden Bough*. Theodor H. Gaster (Ed.). New American Library, New York, 1959.

13. Henrich, G. A. Agrarische Sitten und Gebräuche unter den Sachsen-Sieben Bürgens; Hermannstadt, 15f. In: J. Frazer, *The New Golden Bough*. Theodor H. Gaster (Ed.). New American Library, New York, 1959.

14. Krause, E. Zeitschrift F. Ethnologie 15, 93, In: J. Frazer, *The New Golden Bough*. Theodor H. Gaster (Ed.). New American Library, New York, 1959.

15. Harris, K. L., and C. Lindblad. *Post-Harvest Grain Loss Assessment Methods*. American Association of Cereal Chemists, St. Paul, Minnesota, 1978.

16. Bardach, J., and E. R. Pariser. Aquatic proteins. In: *Protein Resources and Technology: Status and Research Needs*. M. Milner, N. S. Scrimshaw, and D. I. C. Wang (Eds.). AVI Publishing Co., Westport, Connecticut. 1978.

17. James D. Post-Harvest Losses of Marine Foods—Problems and Responses. Paper presented to the Institute of Food Technologists, Annual Meeting, Philadelphia, 1977.

18. Pimentel, D., W. Dritschilo, J. Krummel, and J. Kutzman. Energy and land constraints in food protein production. *Science* 190:754–761, 1975.

19. Harrison, G. G., W. L. Rathje, and W. W. Hughes. Food Waste Behavior in an Urban Population. *J. Nutr. Ed.* 7(1):13–16, 1975.

20. Hopf, H. S., G. E. J. Morley, and J. R. P. Humphries. Rodent Damage to Growing Crops and to Farm and Village Storage in Tropical and Subtropical Regions. Centre for Overseas Pest Research and Tropical Products Institute, London, U.K., 1976.

21. Coursey, D. G. Biodeteriorative Losses in Tropical Horticultural Produce. In: A. H. Walters and E. H. Hueck-Van Der Plas (Eds.), *Biodeterioration of Materials*. Wiley, New York, 1972, pp. 464–471.

22. Hoffman A. The effect of processing and storage upon the nutritive value of smoked fish from Africa. *Trop. Sci.* 19(1):41–53, 1977.

23. Boxall, R., and M. Greeley. Indian Storage Project. Paper presented to the Seminar on Post-Harvest Grain Losses, March 13–17, Tropical Products Institute, London, U.K., 1978.

24. Food and Agriculture Organization of the United Nations, in cooperation with the Government of Malaysia and Food for the Hungry, Inc. *Report of the Action-Oriented Field Workshop for Prevention of Post-Harvest Rice Losses*, Kedah, Malaysia, March 12–30, 1977. Food and Agriculture Organization, Bangkok, 1977.

25. Toqero, Z. Assessing Quantitative and Qualitative Losses in Rice Post-Production Systems. Paper presented at the Action-Oriented Field Workshop for Prevention of Post-Harvest Rice Losses, Kedah, Malaysia, March 12–30, 1977. Food and Agriculture Organization in Co-operation with the Government of Malaysia and Food for the Hungry, Inc., Food and Agriculture Organization, Bangkok, 1977.

26. Rawnsley, J. *Ghana Crop Storage* (PL: SG/GHA7), Food and Agriculture Organization of the United Nations, Rome, 1969, 89 pp.

27. Hall, D. N. Handling and Storage of Food Grains in Tropical and Sub-Tropical Areas. Agricultural Development Paper No. 90, Food and Agriculture Organization of the United Nations, Rome, 1970, 350 pp.

28. Vandevenne, R. Note on Crop Loss after Harvesting in the Ivory Coast. Paper pre-

sented to the Seminar on Post-Harvest Grain Losses, March 13–17, Tropical Products Institute, London, U.K., 1978.

29. DeLima, D. P. E. *A Technical Report on 22 Grain Storage Projects at the Subsistence Farmer Level in Kenya.* Report Proj./Res./AG 21. Kenya Department of Agriculture. National Laboratories, Nairobi, Kenya, 1973, 23 pp.

30. Tropical Products Institute. *The Reduction of Losses during Farmer Storage of Cereal and Legume Grains in Commonwealth Africa.* Report to the Commonwealth Secretariat, London, 1977.

31. Schulten, G. G. M. Losses in stored maize in Malawi and work undertaken to prevent them. *Bull. Eur. Mediterr. Plant Protection Org.* 5(2):113–120, 1975.

32. Food and Organization of the United Nations. ECA (United Nations Economic Commission for Africa), 1977.

33. Mushi, A. M. Country Paper: Tanzania. Paper presented to the Seminar on Post-Harvest Grain Losses, March 13–17, Tropical Products Institute, London, U.K., 1978.

34. Tyagi, A. K., and G. K. Girish. Studies on the assessment of storage losses of food grains by insects. *Bull. Grain Technol.* 13(2):84–102, 1975.

35. Adams, J. M., and G. W. Harman. *The Evaluation of Losses in Maize Stored on a Selection of Small Farms in Zambia, with Particular Reference to the Development of Methodology.* Report G-100, Tropical Products Institute, London, U.K., 1977, 149 pp.

36. International Food Policy Research Institute (IFPRI). *Recent and Prospective Developments in Food Consumption. Some Policy Issues.* Research Report No. 2, IFPRI, Washington, D.C., 1977.

Who Is the Loser in Post-Harvest Losses?

Hans Guggenheim

Introduction

Nutrition planning and post-harvest loss interventions are recognized as multidisciplinary endeavors that revolve around two critical questions. From the perspective of the nutrition planner, these are: (1) To what extent do post-harvest losses impact on the nutritional well-being of specific populations? (2) To what degree can the prevention of food losses during the postproduction food cycle improve the nutritional status of those in need?

These two questions are by no means as symmetrical as they appear to be, for there is an asymmetry that is the consequence of aggregate statistics on the one hand, and the consequence of inequities in distribution on the other.

In order to find an answer to these problems, I believe we must turn those questions on their heads as they are traditionally asked by post-harvest loss specialists and begin by focusing on who suffers from the losses rather than on what and how much is lost in aggregate terms. Thus, we have to consider the role and the responsibilities of the social sciences in the assessment of post-harvest losses and their effect on the nutritional status of target populations, and in the formulation of policies and programs for the reduction of food losses, as well as the implementation stage of projects designed to increase food availability by loss prevention.

One social scientist, actively involved in a major research program

Hans Guggenheim • The Wunderman Foundation, Boston, Massachusetts.

on post-harvest losses for the World Bank, stresses the need for socioeconomic studies:

> Improving post-harvest practices to reduce food grain losses through an ill-conceived programme can negate through extra social costs the benefits derived from any reduction in food losses that has been achieved in a loss-reduction programme. A careful evaluation can help to avoid this if that evaluation recognizes the full social and economic effects of the loss-reduction programme. (1)

Yet, while the need for such interventions appears clear, so is the relative lack of attention given to the problem by social scientists. The need for a more cohesive theoretical framework within which specific problems and solutions can be evaluated is real. As Daisy M. Tagliacozzo (2) has pointed out:

> A superficial review of the literature indicates that the topic of post-harvest food losses has not been given systematic attention by social science disciplines.

Tagliacozzo argues that studies that explain ongoing agricultural practices in relation to other facets of the social system, such as division of labor or household organization, may not explain resistance to change or the difficulties attending the use or distribution of aid. Furthermore, the cost in time and effort to conduct such studies, and the difficulty of interpretating the data, may make them of dubious value to decision makers and development agents charged with implementing new programs aimed at reducing postproduction losses or introducing new technologies. Thus, she calls for sensitive observers with the ability to assess the role of specific variables in order to shorten long research methodologies suited more to academic goals. It is clear, however, that such assessments must be viewed with caution and must be evaluated within a larger framework.

A comprehensive set of social and cultural guidelines for postproduction loss assessment has been prepared by Alan Griff and C. C. Reining (3). Reining grouped the major questions into five categories: (1) Social Organization, (2) Domestic Organization, (3) Cultural Factors, (4) Transition and Change, and (5) Individual Factors.

Astonishingly, nutrition is not included, although some of the questions are of interest to nutrition planners. The questions have been prepared for field workers rather than for social scientists, and, whereas they provide a well-structured approach to data gathering, they give few indicators as to how the data would be used or interpreted. Moreover, the questions, even within a particular category, e.g., Social Organization, are on different levels of complexity and thus not strictly comparable.

The problem is raised here not as a critique of the guidelines, but because it illustrates the basic difficulty of social science involvement. The following example should illustrate the point:

> Question (1.2): Describe the levels of wealth, power, and prestige in the community. (Comment: Relations between social classes can have a profound effect on handling basic items such as grain.)

Given the political and social complexity of "relations between social classes" even at the community level, not to mention at the national level, such a demand appears almost naive. Because it provides no value guidelines, it may do more harm than good. A more direct approach in determining priorities for intervention programs is taken by Greeley in a discussion of cost–benefit analysis as opposed to social cost–benefit analysis (1). In his comparison of the relative benefits from labor-intensive and capital-intensive food-saving technology systems, he writes:

> In social cost–benefit analysis (as opposed to cost–benefit analysis) the conversion of market prices into social accounting prices, using international food prices, allows comparison between projects of their potential contribution to long-term aggregate consumption through increased food availability, and explicitly deals with the distribution and timing of the output. Both the measure of output in terms of aggregate consumption, not food saved, and the recognition of timing and distribution implications support labor-intensive technology systems.

> The distribution of the output between different income groups or between the urban and rural sector is weighted in a manner corresponding to the social value of increased consumption among different economic groups. This essentially means (or ought to mean) that food saved and available to the poorest will be more valuable in social terms than in private terms and vice-versa for rich-income groups. Thus, there is a built-in bias favoring projects that physically get more food to the poorest, which is not a feature of private evaluation. (1)

Greeley then concludes his arguments by pointing to the social profitability of investments in the rural nonmarket sector, especially if the investment is labor-intensive.

Such conclusions reached by social scientists do not necessarily solve problems, but can clarify and pose them in new ways for policy planners. Because of the evidence such researchers are likely to collect, as well as the nature of their analysis, they are likely to conflict with the interests of ruling elites and bureaucrats who may prefer safe "technical expertise." For most serious researchers, however, Weber's "value-free" social science is no longer a possible choice. This may be one reason, rather than that of the "relevance of social science research," why anthropologists, economists, and sociologists are not always a part of interdisciplinary field work in sensitive areas.

Clearly, this poses a problem for concerned social scientists, whether they be economists, sociologists, or anthropologists whose patronage comes either from governments or from major agencies whose ability to work in Third World countries may depend on their skill in putting into jargon such truth as might be unpalatable if understood. As Pierre Spitz has pointed out, another consequence of this situation may be that reports that are clear have to be classified by the responsible institutions (4).

There is another unfortunate aspect to this situation. Our request for Third World scientists to come forward and work in analyzing such problems as food losses, food marketing, and consumption patterns in their own societies is to ask for more than a mere professional commitment. In many cases it means asking for high personal risk-taking by individuals who, unprotected by the shelter of an international body, must place themselves in conflict with the rulers of their countries.

RELEVANCE AND BIOLOGICAL RESPONSE

Perhaps the most difficult aspect of interdisciplinary work will be the relationship between a social scientist and a plant-protectionist. Such cooperation is, however, not only feasible, but also necessary. The life cycle of insect pests depends heavily on structures provided by man — the timing of the planting, for example, determines whether the farmer has to fear an attack by the kele-kele before the harvest or by the heavier pigeons after the millet has been cut down. Granaries in Upper Volta are free of *Sitotroga*, but, only a few miles away in Niger, *Sitotroga* constitutes a pest. A foremost specialist on *Sitotroga* believes that it is the climate, but, in fact, the respective climates appear almost identical. Minor variations in rainfall may make a difference, but the handling and storage methods (cultural) are just as important in reducing losses. The presence of *Sitotroga* may account for differences in design of granaries.

THE DIRECT IMPACT OF AGGREGATE LOSSES ON THE NUTRITIONAL STATUS OF SUBSISTENCE FARMERS

As Pariser has noted elsewhere in this volume, aggregate post-harvest food losses do not readily translate into food deprivation at the individual level, and so-called savings will not improve the nutritional status of a population. One exception to this may be noted: post-harvest losses occurring in isolated environments that depend on restricted food supplies with little or no access to additional sources. This is the situation in subsistence villages in the Sahel after, during, or following drought years, when stocks are at a low level, transportation facilities minimal, and production/productivity reduced. Given such a situation, post-harvest losses because of rodent attacks can create local famine conditions, since rats or mice may attack in Biblical numbers. As one *Commandant de Cercle* stated in a Malian village: "The mice in the trees were so many, I thought they were birds whistling in the trees when these were filled with mice. In Lac Faguibine at Tinasha, over 100,000 rats were pulled out of the lake and killed by the population." Even in the absence of a major rodent attack, aggregate losses to rodents can be serious enough to affect directly the nutritional status of a village.

An interesting macro-level FAO study (5) attempts to calculate the nutritional value of food wastes in Nigeria. The authors compute social as well as biological causes and list, among others: waste resulting from careless treatment in harvesting, the poor system of pricing, lack of market information, climatic losses due to moisture and temperature, biological losses to insects and rodents, inadequate transportation, poor and/or primitive storage facilities, inefficient and primitive processing, and nonutilization of by-products. According to the authors, the quantitative assessment is optimistic in the sense that their estimates are considered to be at the lower bounds of actual waste.

Crop wastes are presented in thousands of metric tons in order to assess the nutritional implications, and broken down into crop wastes in kilograms per capita per year and in grams per capita per day. The breakdown of these losses into essential nutrients gives the total losses per capita in calories, protein, and fat as 308 kcal, 7.71 g, and 4.08 g, respectively. The calorie and protein losses reported constitute about 14.78 and 14.32% of available supply reported in the National Food Balance Sheet for the 1968–1969 year base. In addition, the authors present a calculation of the energy costs in cultivating the crops, basing their estimates on Fox's study (6) on energy expenditures for rural activities in Africa. The figures give a total energy cost of 597,962 million kcal, or a per capita value of 9494 kcal per year, for the production of lost food values.

It is evident in the light of Pariser's paper, and of this paper, that the aggregate figures of this study hide as much information as they provide, in part because they are not made relevant to selected segments of the population. Nevertheless, the approach is valuable because the authors develop a language that permits post-harvest loss students and nutritionists to talk together.

RESEARCH AT THE GOVERNMENT OR BUSINESS LEVEL

It is well documented in many developing countries that the highest losses in grain or fish occur, not at the farm level, but in central or peripheral storage, whether managed by parastatals or private entrepreneurs. Such losses can largely be attributed to pests or rodents, but are ultimately the result of human negligence. Such negligence may in turn be the result of economic cost–benefit calculations that deem the losses to be smaller than the cost of prevention, or it may have its roots in cultural values. Whatever the case may be, research on the social cause for losses tends to threaten the interests of an entrenched management and is thus harder to conduct than among the peasantry. The financial advantages of "losses" can be substantial. For example, a 3–5% weight loss in transportation, standardized into procedures for calculating weight at destination, is easily converted into profit. Clearly, this provides little incentive to allow an outside researcher the opportunity to reduce the "loss." The use of double scales also has its advantages to storekeepers. Farmers bring in their grain and suffer a "loss," but the agent who purchases it does not. Again, the biologist investigating the incidence of *Sitotroga* will not be felt as a threat, but the likelihood that an economist or sociologist could discover the basic reasons for the losses may be feared.

Such considerations led African delegates at a recent workshop on nutrition in the Sahel to consider graft the most serious problem facing nutrition planners. It is unfortunate that difficulties in nutrition planning and in crop loss reduction should interface at this point.

TOWARD A SOCIAL DEFINITION OF LOSSES

From the point of view of the sociologist at least, the question of aggregate losses must be related to a particular group who can be shown to lose, that is to say, a group who have less to eat because food that was available, or potentially available, for consumption is no longer accessible. Yet if we define losses in this way, a whole new class of losses appears. As Amartya Sen (7) has pointed out:

> In an exchange economy, whether a family will starve or not will depend on what it has to sell, whether it can sell, and at what prices, and also on the price of food. An economy in a state of comparative tranquility may develop a famine if there is a sudden shake-up of the system of rewards for exchange of labour, commodities and other possessions, even *without* a "sudden, sharp reduction in the food supply."

According to Sen's analysis, it was the change in exchange entitlements that played a large role in putting the necessary food supplies out of the economic reach of particular groups. The populations thus incurred a "loss" of food that was potentially available and they starved, not because of a flood or the activities of pests, but because of political bungling and economic malfeasance.

One could cite other examples—for instance, the forced requisition of stored grains for taxes and/or export in some African countries, which has left the subsistence farmers at the edge of starvation—but the point is clear. Once we bring the loser into the picture, the definition of losses becomes a different and a more deadly serious problem. One has to consider the problem of distribution of all assets, including food. This has been recognized by the FAO Committee on Agriculture (7), which sees in maldistribution, rather than in a lack of production, the prime factor in malnutrition:

> If the present maldistribution remains unaltered, it is estimated that to reduce the prevalence of undernutrition to 5% (from the present 25%) the per caput daily food supply for developing countries would have to increase on an average from the present level of 2200 kcals to 3000 kcals. A modest reduction, on the other hand, in the inequality of distribution—from the present standard deviation of about 700 kcals to one of 600 kcals—would bring about the same reduction in malnutrition.

Thus, FAO doubts that gains in production will solve the problem of malnutrition unless the problem of distribution is solved first.

Unfortunately, the evidence that this will be possible through development programs is not encouraging. Moreover, the problem appears to be closely related to that of inequality of income distribution. (8) Cross-section studies indicate that income inequality increases in the early stages of development, although it seems to diminish after a per capita income of from $500 to $1000 has been reached. Morawetz (9) suggests that, on the basis of historical evidence from developing countries, " . . . it may not be possible to grow first and redistribute later . . . because the structure of growth may largely fit the pattern of distribution, at least until a much higher level of income is approached."

This growth of inequity in income distribution appears to be parallel to the growth of food production and food distribution. Reutlinger and Selowsky (10), for example, estimated that approximately $0.9-1.4 \times 10^9$ additional people received less than the required minimum daily calorie allowance between 1965 and 1975. Even if one does not accept the minimum allowance they postulated, the problem remains the same.

These concerns hold a major implication for food loss reduction programs and raise the question of whether a reduction in post-harvest food losses, even if it contributes to the total amount of food available, will contribute to the nutritional status of the populations at risk, or whether such gains will merely contribute to the increases in inequity.

THE DISTRIBUTION OF LOSSES AND THE REDISTRIBUTION OF GAINS

I should like to examine briefly the problem of distribution and equity discussed above in terms of a possibly unique case of post-harvest millet losses in a West African country.

Research on millet losses in traditional granaries in West Africa has shown that losses at the farm level are relatively light, ranging from 3% to 12% in unusual circumstances, but that losses in intermediate- and central-level storage can be appreciably higher (11). Nevertheless, emphasis has been on reducing losses at central storage levels, where fumigation teams can operate, and where loss reduction programs appear to be more cost-effective.

It is also obvious that loss reduction programs that would help farmers to reduce losses at their level would be of benefit to the farm population. These benefits would be slight yet significant at the farm level and could contribute to the welfare of the subsistence farmer. Loss reduction programs at central-level storage are, however, operating at an aggregate level and could conceivably help the urban population, but these benefits could not be redistributed to the producers. However, as we have seen, the structure of the growth and distribution process is such that it is unlikely that the urban poor will benefit from the savings in grain, and more likely instead that these savings will be passed on to those least in need.

Although I am aware that the argument made here appears too facile and obscure among a number of complex marketing problems, it may well be true that the farther away from the source of production a post-harvest loss program operates, the less likely it will be to help solve the nutritional problems of those most in need.

SOCIAL SCIENCE RESEARCH: THE MICRO LEVEL

As Barbara Harris (12) has pointed out:

> Most research *could* be in the interest of the target groups. The whole point is that whether or not it *is* depends crucially *not* on the topic but on how the research is conducted, disseminated and used.

In most peasant cultures research on storage is particularly sensitive, not only because farmers are reluctant to allow a stranger to see their reserves (he/she might be linked to the government tax collector), but because they are as afraid of letting their neighbors know how much they have in their granaries as we are to inform our friends about our bank accounts. Nonetheless, farmers in Africa and India will show their grain storage to researchers once they have established a level of trust. Since they do not know that the results will eventually go into a computer, many farmers attempt to enter into a dialogue with the researcher—a dialogue that will focus on their personal interest in reducing losses. If their opinions are respected, and if they see their own interests furthered by the interview, villagers will be cooperative. If not, they may fill the questionnaire with data that have little relationship to reality.

The second point raised by Harris, the dissemination of information that can reduce losses, is of equal importance. Perhaps the most difficult task will be the encouragement of traditional techniques of loss prevention that have fallen into disuse as the high prestige of costly, and often ineffectually used and dangerous, pesticides spreads around the world. Extension workers need the help of Third World social scientists in order to accomplish such tasks. The preparation of information for the use of the people for whom it has ostensibly been collected is generally neglected or delegated to others. Perhaps social scientists as well as their colleagues in biology and chemistry should begin to assume the task of preparing their data in a form accessible to the population for whose benefit it was collected.

Last, we come to the question of the use of data. Here social scientists often face the dilemma that sensitive information, e.g., the quantity of grain in storage or of fish on the river banks, can be used against the best interests of the producers in the target population whom they wish to help. The problem concerns all those who are working in development—nutrition planners as well as storage experts—and I do not pretend to have an answer to the dilemma.

THE NEED FOR A THEORETICAL FRAMEWORK

In his introduction, Pariser listed a number of definitions that describe the nature of post-harvest losses and define the circumstances within which these could be investigated. Although there exist certain ambiguities about what losses are, these emphasize what is lost and how, not who is the loser. In consequence, they have, in directed post-harvest studies, led to a monotonous routine of quantitative loss assessment, supported peripherally by some analysis of social and economic causes and consequences, and the listing of intervention strategies to reduce loss levels.

With a few notable exceptions, few economists or sociologists have attempted to develop a coherent theoretical framework within which the growing amount of data could be interpreted and understood. One reason for this may be historical: As long as the hope existed that the world's food problems could be solved by increasing productivity and production, socioeconomic research was directed into supportive efforts. However, with a general shift in perspective toward the preservation and conservation of resources, more theoretical attention may be paid to loss reduction.

I should like to cite, as an example of neglected research concerns, studies on risk aversion by farmers. Although attitudes toward risk-taking have been the object of intensive investigation, emphasis has been placed on risk aversion in the production decision, not on storage or loss avoidance.

In a study representative of this line of research, Hans Binswanger *et al.* (13) raise the question in an appropriate way:

> How should we judge the effectiveness of the farmer's self-insurance and risk diffusion mechanisms (e.g., storage and losses)? The first criterion is goal achievement: Do they stabilize *real* consumption levels, i.e., are farmers in a position to consume essentially the same *quantities* of goods during drought years as in normal years? This, of course, is a fairly strong condition and would indicate perfect self-insurance and risk diffusion. We may, therefore, weaken the criterion successively and ask whether farmers are able to maintain the quantity of food consumption and—as the weakest criterion—whether they are able to maintain their food grain intake (as an indicator of calorie consumption).

In his discussion, Binswanger does not deal directly with the limiting of the impact of losses on self-insurance and risk diffusion mechanisms such as storage, yet he raises the question in an interesting way. Taking and losing become culturally based, individual decisions directly related to the struggle for survival at the level of the individual. We have finally moved away from the unmanageable quantities of aggregate figures and are confronting the problem of the individual in his struggle for existence: Whether he and his family will be able to outwit the threat of famine may depend on more than the ability to calculate the risks—especially where these include wars and social upheavals in addition to the natural catastrophes and the economic forces beyond his control. Nevertheless, if we can begin to understand the individual, we might begin to find solutions to the problems of the masses.

SOME FINAL RECOMMENDATIONS

This chapter has made a radical departure from most post-harvest loss studies by shifting the emphasis from that which is lost to those who suffer from the loss. Serious collaborative efforts by nutrition planners and post-harvest specialists are needed to examine these issues.

One obvious conclusion from this shift in emphasis is that we need more and more theoretically based social analysis in order to plan responsive and responsible intervention programs. The people most qualified are Third World social scientists working in their own countries, yet we have indicated the risks that might befall them.

At the present time, a number of important research projects in countries plagued by post-harvest losses are being designed and implemented. One of these, in India, is being financed by the World Bank; another in the Sahel is being financed by FAO; a third is being planned by AID.

Another group of institutions is ideally placed to do post-harvest studies, but are prevented from doing so by their charter. These are the international agricultural research institutes such as the Center for Improvement of Maize and Wheat (CIMMYT) in Mexico, the International Rice Research Institute in the Philippines (IRRI), and several others, set up to increase yields through the development of new strains of cereals, rice, and maize as well as through the development of so-called synergistic packages of agricultural production techniques. Since reducing losses could help to alleviate hunger and malnutrition, the United Nations University's decision to consider post-harvest losses one of the three subprograms of its World Hunger Programme is logical and welcome.

REFERENCES

1. Greeley, M. Background Paper for: *Postharvest Food Losses in Developing Countries*. Board on Science and Technology for International Development, Commission on International Relations. National Research Council/National Academy of Sciences, Washington, D.C., 1978.
2. Tagliacozzo, D. M. Personal communication.
3. Griff, A. L., and C. C. Reining. Social and cultural guidelines. In: *Post-Harvest Grain Loss Assessment Methods*, K. L. Harris and C. J. Lindblad (Eds.). American Association of Cereal Chemists, Office of Nutrition, U.S. AID, Washington, D.C., 1978.
4. Spitz, P. Silent violence: Famine and inequality. *Int. Soc. Sci. J.* **30** (4):1978.
5. Food and Agriculture Organization of the United Nations. Post-Harvest Crop Losses: The Nigerian Case. FAO, Rome, Italy, 1977.
6. Fox, R. H. A Study of the Energy Expenditure of Africans Engaged in Various Rural Activities. Ph.D. Thesis, University of London, 1973.
7. Sen, A. K. Starvation and Exchange Entitlements: A General Approach and Its Application to the Great Bengal Famine. Food and Agriculture Organization of the United Nations. FAO Committee on Agriculture, 5th Session, Rome, 18–27 April, 1979, W/G9089.

8. Ahluwia, M. Income inequality: Some dimensions of the problem. In: *Redistribution with Growth*, H. Chenery (Ed.), Oxford University Press, London, England, 1974.

9. Morawetz, D. *Twenty-Five Years of Economic Development, 1950–1975*. The World Bank, Washington, D.C., 1977.

10. Reutlinger, S., and M. Selowsky. *The Anatomy of Hunger*. World Bank Staff Occasional Paper, Johns Hopkins University Press, Baltimore, Maryland, 1976.

11. Guggenheim, H. Of millet, mice and men. In: *World Food Losses, Pests, and the Environment*, D. Pimentel (Ed.), Westview Press, Boulder, Colorado, 1978.

12. Harris, B. Relevant and Feasible Research. Economics Program, The International Crops Research Institute for the Semi-Arid Tropics (ICRISAT), Hyderabad, India, 1978.

13. Binswanger, H. P., N. S. Jodha, and B. C. Barah. The nature and significance of risk in the semi-arid tropics. In: *Proceedings of a Workshop on Socioeconomic Constraints to Development of Semi-Arid Tropical Agriculture*, ICRISAT, Hyderabad, India, February, 1979.

Problems in the Post-Harvest Processing of Rice in Southeast Asian Countries

Yasumasa Koga

Introduction

Efforts are being made to improve the post-harvest processing of rice to reduce post-harvest grain losses. Such technical improvements may be realized only when those efforts coincide with those of small rice farmers who are struggling for the improvement of their daily lives. The post-harvest technology for rice in Southeast Asia is closely related to socio-economic relations among rice farmers and rice millers or rice merchants and to government intervention policies. It is most important to understand these interrelations dynamically in order to modify policies in the direction of helping small farmers and the rural poor. Such modifications would be likely to include improved paddy marketing practices, with the introduction of a paddy quality grading system, promotion of farmer cooperatives, and appropriate price policies. Once such measures have been adopted and improvements in post-harvest technology have begun to benefit the farmers and the rural poor, their own efforts will accelerate the changes. This would lead to increased technical ability and a strengthening of the agricultural cooperatives, better socioeconomic status for the farmers, and truly integrated rural development. This would serve to further prevention of post-harvest losses. These issues will be

Yasumasa Koga • Overseas Merchandise Inspection Company, Ltd., Chuo-ku, Tokyo, Japan.

examined in the light of recent developments in post-harvest rice technology in Indonesia (Java), Thailand, Burma, and Japan.

BASIC PROBLEMS IN POST-HARVEST RICE PROCESSING

PREMISES FOR ACTIONS LEADING TO REDUCTION OF POST-HARVEST LOSSES

In many countries, the post-harvest loss of rice from the time of harvest to its arrival in the kitchen amounts to approximately 10–30%. It must be borne in mind, however, that exact figures are not available. Several survey reports exist, but survey methods are not always described, and sometimes the methods are unsuitable. The figures therefore vary greatly in both place and season. Nevertheless, there is no doubt that much preventable loss occurs in the post-harvest stage, and this is why much effort is being devoted to reverse these losses, to help secure a stable world food supply.

Both increased agricultural production and reduction of post-harvest losses are required to meet the demand for food of an increasing world population. Reducing losses is cheaper than increasing production, because the latter requires expansion of cultivated land—an increasingly difficult matter because most of the arable land is already under cultivation, although this situation varies from country to country. It is also more costly to increase crop yields because this requires intensive cultivation and expenditures for improved seed breeding programs, irrigation, drainage, fertilizers, and pesticides. Furthermore, it is not easy to introduce new technology in agricultural production in Southeast Asia because the manner in which small-scale farmers grow crops is closely linked with their traditional way of life. Contrary to this, it is assumed that improvements in post-harvest processes can be achieved easily simply by replacing or by introducing related equipment such as threshers, dryers, storages, and rice mills.

ARE THESE PREMISES CORRECT?

Based upon such premises, with the aim of lessening post-harvest losses and winning farmer acceptance, research has centered on small-scale technology, i.e., to identify, develop, and advocate simple, inexpensive equipment that can easily be used by small farmers and farm cooperatives. Included are simply made threshers, husk-fired or solar-heated paddy dryers, low-cost paddy storage containers, and the like. Small rice mills for cooperatives and rice merchants, better parboiling methods, and improved transport facilities are also included.

Because most grain losses are thought to occur at the farm level, especially between harvest and threshing (1), and during the rainy season, when the harvested paddy is improperly dried, international agencies and governments are seeking methods and equipment that will be suitable for use on the farm. Such efforts must continue and should be strengthened further. But one must ask if post-harvest losses result chiefly from the existing low technological level. Identification and transfer of "appropriate technology" is often mentioned as one solution. Would this really help?

ARE TECHNOLOGIES FOR POST-HARVEST LOSS REDUCTION PROFITABLE?

From the farmers' point of view, post-harvest processing is a step that transforms farm products into food for their own direct consumption or into marketable produce to be sold to merchants or industrialists, who buy paddy for the purpose of turning it into white rice to be sold on the market. This involves drying, storage, and milling. Whether the processing is done commercially or by the farmers themselves, the most ideal technical process to prevent post-harvest losses is not always beneficial to them. It may be argued that even a small saving of grain during post-harvest processing would benefit both farmers and commercial dealers. However, when supplies increase, the unit price of the products often drops, causing an economic loss.

Is there any assurance that improved post-harvest technology alone would lead to socioeconomic well-being? It must be remembered that Southeast Asian farmers and rice dealers cannot introduce new methods when they are so short of funds. They face many other constraints, such as high interest rates on loans, poor housing, unsanitary living conditions, lack of roads and transport vehicles, few recreational opportunities, and inferior education for their children. Some might well prefer to invest in improving their living conditions rather than in augmenting food supplies through prevention of post-harvest losses. If the goal is to be attained, the prospects of its having beneficial effects on other aspects of life must be perceived to be bright, or it will probably not be a priority. Even if money given to subsidize better agricultural implements, fertilizer, or post-harvest machinery is used to purchase pocket radios or bicycles, this is not necessarily wrong if the farmers' daily lives are improved. From their standpoint, this is more desirable than using the subsidy for government-recommended investments.

SOCIOECONOMIC IMPLICATIONS OF POST-HARVEST TECHNOLOGY

There are those who insist that reduction of post-harvest losses will inevitably bring additional income to those who invest in improved technology. It is likened to the goose who lays a golden egg. The matter is not so simple. Farmers are frequently forced into debt by having to take out loans that have interest rates ranging from 40 to 200% per year. If they had any money to invest, it might be far more economical for them to pay up a debt than to reduce post-harvest losses by a few percent. If the harvest itself has to be used to pay off the loan, reducing losses would mean almost nothing to the farmer because he could deal only with the merchant to whom he is indebted. The harvested crop would be out of his possession, and post-harvest processing out of his control.

For these reasons, post-harvest processing is closely interwoven with the daily socioeconomic situation in a farmer's life. It is more closely linked with the traditional way of life than are agricultural production methods. It therefore does not follow that a particular investment will invariably increase income through reduced crop loss. Agricultural practices are intertwined with post-harvest processing. If a farmer is capable of increasing production, he would also be able to apply better post-harvest techniques. Case studies from several countries have borne this out, and will be discussed in more detail later.

DIFFERENCES BETWEEN POST-HARVEST TECHNOLOGY AND AGRICULTURAL PRODUCTION

Agricultural production is an activity undertaken solely by farmers, whereas post-harvest processing is done by both farmers and commercial dealers. This involves the interests of different social classes, and the situation can differ greatly according to the balance of power among these classes. This must be kept in mind.

Farming itself consists of helping plants to grow. Whatever mechanization is used is directed toward providing suitable growing conditions for the crops, but this is limited by environmental factors and the genetic potential of the plants. In contrast, for post-harvest processing, mechanization means both improved work efficiency and better products. Machines are readily applicable to processing paddy grains since they are more or less uniform granules.

Taking the comparison between the use of machines in agricultural production and their use in post-harvest processing a step further, we may note that, except for work efficiency, plant growth is identical whether ploughing is done by manual hoeing, draft animals, or tractors.

However, when it comes to husking the paddy, it makes a great deal of difference in the final product whether the husks are removed by a rubber roller-type husker or by hand with mortar and pestle. The latter method breaks almost all of the rice grains during the process, while the mechanical husker damages very few. Similar conditions prevail for the entire post-harvest process; the quality of the equipment used profoundly affects the end product.

SOCIOECONOMIC LIMITATIONS ON TYPES OF POST-HARVEST TECHNOLOGY

The physical processing of rice includes threshing, cleaning, drying, transportation, milling, and storage. That is why appropriate technology is advocated to renovate machinery and equipment in order to improve post-harvest processing and prevent losses. However, which types of machinery can be used is determined by the socioeconomic background of the individual farmers and processers. Economically feasible, minimum-scale operations could generally be expanded by the use of more advanced machines, but for the scale of farm mangement of the rice growers in Southeast Asia, this is too expensive. It therefore behooves them to buy jointly and share the use of machines in agricultural cooperatives, or to rent them.

The aim of farmers in post-harvest processing is either to produce food for their own consumption or to increase potential profits by providing processed products for sale. Both are influenced by succeeding processes and marketing conditions. For example:

1. When custom rice mills are too far from the growers, or the milling charge is excessive, farmers hand-pound their rice, despite the fact that they know that more grain will be broken and milling recovery will be much lower.

2. If farmers work to improve their paddy but receive no better price for it than do farmers who bring in paddy of lesser quality, their lack of reward discourages them from trying again.

3. When farmers must pay back a high-interest loan, or find themselves short of cash, they are forced to sell paddy immediately after harvest and cannot hold it until prices rise to more profitable levels.

4. In order to bargain to their advantage, farmers need to cooperate with each other when selling their products. This implies such approaches as post-harvest processing in cooperatives to share use of machinery. But in the absence of an objective, equitable system for assessment of paddy quality, as is now the case in Southeast Asia, farmers cannot maintain solidarity when buyers judge all paddy quality willfully. This serves as a disincentive for farmers to cooperate.

5. When rice merchants or industrialists collect paddy from needy farmers at harvest time, they hoard it until prices rise so that they can sell rice for a good profit. They are more disposed to loan money to poor farmers at high interest rates and to stockpile rice than they are to reduce losses in milling and storage by improving rice mills or warehouses. Because people regard them as the "bloodsuckers of farmers," they feel uneasy and refrain from investing in fixed assets and pursue commercial profit even further. Hostility to rice millers creates a vicious circle.

6. Two systems of payment exist in custom rice mills. One is to return all of the rice product to the customers and charge them a certain fee per unit of weight or volume of the material processed, which does not give the rice miller much incentive to improve his milling technology. When the bran and small brokens produced during milling are retained as the milling fee, the lower the milling recovery the better the income is for the miller. The other system is to return some fixed percentage of white rice from the processed paddy to the customers, which encourages the miller to improve milling recovery through better technology.

RELATIONSHIP BETWEEN POST-HARVEST LOSS REDUCTION AND LIVING CONDITIONS

Basically, the socioeconomic circumstances in any area determine what, if any, technical improvements can be made in post-harvest processing. These circumstances are far from static—they may be altered by government action, or the people concerned may have to modify existing conditions. These are the factors that, for all practical purposes, act for or against technological innovation.

Technology to modify conditions cannot exist outside the popular will. Its use depends on human interrelations and behavioral patterns. When such terms as "technology transfer" and "appropriate technology" are used, an illusion may be created that technical development can be attained by simple transfers of things or combinations of things from one place to another, with or without modification. This is often done without any consideration of the cultural context within which the new technology might be perceived by the people themselves. It is as though a horse could be made to drink by offering him juice, soup, or Coca Cola when all he wants is plain water at a time that suits him.

What is urgently required is an understanding of actual living conditions in the place where changes (whether technological or not) are to be introduced. The people's own aspirations are the most basic starting point. However much it may be in the national interest to reduce post-harvest losses by a certain percentage, no program to do so can succeed unless it is perceived locally as being closely linked with the people's own concerns. They are not likely to be interested in accepting a program unless it will improve their living conditions.

Because farmers derive their living from processing and marketing agricultural products, their efforts toward raising their socioeconomic status will eventually include improvement in post-harvest processing, which would obviously give them more and better products to sell once marketing conditions are geared to give them a better profit. When this happens, rural community development may open up with local participation, sharing of ideas, expansion of agricultural capabilities, and mutual cooperation. Such a process would surely result in improved agricultural production and concomitant prevention of grain loss after harvest. Several case studies in Southeast Asia bear this out, as will be seen in the following section.

PRESENT STATUS OF POST-HARVEST RICE PROCESSING AND SOME ASSOCIATED PROBLEMS IN SOUTHEAST ASIA

JAVA

Traditional Rice Processing in Java

Tables 1 and 2 show the predominance of rice in food crop production and consumption in Indonesia (2). Java (including Madura) has a population of about 80 million, and roughly 14 million tons of paddy were produced on 4.5 million hectares in 1976. The average farm house-

TABLE 1. Major Food Crop Production in
Indonesia, 1976[a]

Crop	Quantity (tons $\times 10^3$)
Paddy	23,300
Maize	2,572
Cassava	12,190
Sweet potatoes	3,381
Peanuts	341
Soy beans	522

[a] Source: Biro Pusat Statistik.

TABLE 2. Per Capita Food Consumption in Indonesia (kg/year)[a]

Food	1975 Food demand–supply	1976 Consumption survey
Rice	114.2	117.3
Maize	20.6	19.4
Cassava, etc.	60.7	46.9
Sweet potatoes	16.8	8.4
Fish	8.5	13.1
Beef	1.5	0.7
Mutton, goat	0.2	0.2
Pork	0.3	0.5
Milk	0.3	0.4

[a] Source: Biro Pusat Statistik.

hold has 0.6–0.7 hectare of cultivatable land. More than half of the farmers own less than 0.4 hectare (2, pp. 204–207).

Traditional harvesting and post-harvest rice processing in Java used to be atypical of patterns in other Southeast Asian countries. Rather than using sickles to harvest paddy, a knife called the ani-ani was used to cut panicles one by one. This could be done by any woman who wished to work at harvest time, and usually women from the same village worked in one area. They were allowed to keep a certain portion of the harvest in exchange for working—a mutual assistance custom referred to as gotong royong. Under the gotong royong arrangement, with ani-ani harvesting, the quantity harvested by a worker determined her income, and immature panicles were often overlooked or trampled on. This method of harvesting was not labor-efficient and resulted in considerable waste, but it nevertheless created job opportunities for landless workers and permitted them a share of income. About 70% of the rice produced was consumed by the growers.

The harvested panicles were bundled, dried, and stored as they were. They used to be marketed in panicle form. The rice mills buying them would allow them to dry further and store them until milling. Just before milling, the bundles were opened, and separated panicles were thrown into threshers to extract the paddy grain. Bundled panicles are bulky and are not amenable to machine handling the way paddy grain is. However, for storage purposes, the bundles required no containers and were thus better ventilated and less susceptible than paddy grain to spoilage from fungi or molds.

Husking and milling of rice by hand-pounding used to be done

TABLE 3. Effect of Growing Numbers of Small Rice Mills on Milling Capacity and White Rice Production, Java, 1969–1976[a]

Year	Number of rice mills (A)	Total milling capacity (tons rice × 10³) (B)	White rice production (tons × 10³) (C)	B/C
1969	4,590	2,795	7,355	0.38
1970	5,560	3,380	7,682	0.44
1971	6,793	4,096	7,729	0.53
1972	6,917	4,799	7,861	0.61
1973	10,663	6,460	8,080	0.79
1974	18,391	9,859	9,141	1.07
1975	20,421	10,875	9,142	1.18
1976	21,803	11,607	9,287	1.24

[a] Source: Prdoman Pengdaan dalam Negeri Tahun 1978/79 (BULOG).

largely by rural women. This method was not efficient—it produced much broken rice and overall milling recovery was low—but it was the most important source of employment for women. This system of harvesting and post-harvest processing prevailed in Java until the late 1960s.

Recent Changes

Late in the 1960s and into the early 1970s, these methods changed drastically. Small rice mills began to appear all around Java. In the mid-1960s, 90% of farm-consumed rice was hand-pounded, but by the end of the next decade, all rice was machine-milled. Competition among mills lowered the milling charge sharply, and hand-pounding went out of existence (Table 3)(3,4). Because machine-milling yields a larger recovery with better quality and fewer brokens, a market price could be maintained, and all farmers switched to custom mills. This was a severe blow to women, especially in landless families, who had previously earned at least a partial living by hand-pounding (5).

The second change was a shift in harvesting technique. The sickle began to replace the ani-ani, and by the end of the 1970s, half of all harvesting was done by sickle.* Sickle harvesting is three to five times faster than knife harvesting (6), and, again, this meant that many women were

*Information supplied by the Agricultural Extension Office, Madium. As indirect proof of the transition from ani-ani to sickle harvest (stalk paddy to paddy grain), indication of rice production in agricultural statistics has changed from stalk paddy ("Padi") to paddy grain ("gabah") since 1976.

thrown out of work. Farmers needed only a few workers, and hired them by prearrangement. In contrast to knife harvesting, sickles cut down the whole rice plant, and the harvested rice is threshed right in the paddy field. This lowers the shattering loss, especially with the high-yielding varieties that are prone to shatter.

The villagers who lost income because of changes in rice technology naturally opposed the farmers, who responded by making an arrangement ("tebasan") with merchants to purchase standing paddy in the field just before harvest (7). Farmers contracted to buy back whatever rice they needed for their own consumption.

The third change was that now Indonesian farmers, like their Southeast Asian counterparts, turned to threshing, drying, and cleaning their own paddy grain instead of taking bundled panicles to rice mills. This meant that threshing machines were no longer needed in the mills, and for the past 7 or 8 years, no such machines have been sold, according to agricultural equipment manufacturers.

Paddy grain has a higher bulk density than panicles have, and must therefore be dried with more care. It is important that it not be dried too quickly because sudden drying cracks the separated grains. Sickle-harvested paddy also requires cleaning to remove immature grain, straw, and other foreign matter.

Further Consequences of the Emergence of Rice Mills

What brought about these sudden changes in rice harvesting and processing, and what implications do they have for reducing post-harvest losses and increasing food supplies? The rapid emergence of small mills was a threat to the large rice mills that had previously dealt with large quantities of rice. Many were thrown into bankruptcy. All of these small mills created a demand for machinery, and local manufacturers began to produce impact huskers and Engleberg hullers. Small huskers and whiteners could also be imported from Japan and Taiwan.

The real reason for the rice mill boom was a series of political and economic changes. After the fall of Sukarno and the establishment of the Suharto regime in 1967, the government took steps to check the power of the large mills and the rice merchants, who were mostly Chinese. It wanted to create jobs for Indonesian nationals. The National Logistic Bureau (BULOG) was established and strongly supported to stabilize the price of rice and end the practice of hoarding by large merchants and millers. It also simplified the procedure for obtaining a license to set up small mills so that Indonesians could do so. Agricultural cooperatives (BUUD or KUD) were formed with government support so that each cooperative unit could have its own small mill. Despite the labor surplus in Java, maintaining the inefficient hand-pounding system could not be justified, and when the licensing constraints were removed, small mills sprang up like mushrooms all over Java. Once this simplified procedure for forming small mills was in place, those with extra funds to invest hastily moved into the business of custom milling for farmers.

With the competition among mills, milling charges fell and not only farm paddy but also the marketed paddy that used to be processed in the large mills began to flow into the small ones. No longer able to maintain their monopoly or hoard rice for profit, the large mills closed one by one. In the rice retail shops, hand-pounded, half-milled rice disappeared.

Some have argued that since the large mills have closed, rice technology in Java has declined (8), but this is not the case. To be sure, large mills had more equipment—threshers, paddy cleaners, disk huskers, compartment separators, whitening cones, brokens separators—while small mills have only rubber roller huskers and either air-jet friction whiteners or Englebergs. But what they replaced was not only large mills but, to a far greater extent, hand-pounding. Hand-pounded, cleaned paddy yields 50–60% white rice, whereas paddy processed in a combination of rubber roller husker and friction whitener yields 62–68% white rice. This 10% or more of increased yield must have meant an enormous saving of rice for Java. Hand-pounded rice is only half-milled, while machine-milled rice is thoroughly milled, and though the difference in quantity of rice may not be in that proportion, the digestible portion of the rice grain is much greater after machine milling.

It has often been suggested that less milling would increase both the quantity and the nutritional value of rice. Some countries, such as India,

TABLE 4. Percent Digestibility and Digestible Quantity of Brown and White Rice after Various Degrees of Milling[a]

Degree of milling	Milling recovery (A)	Quantity of bran	When eaten as grain		When eaten powdered	
			Digestible percentage (B)	Digestible quantity (A × B)	Digestible percentage (C)	Digestible quantity (A × C)
Brown rice	100	0	0.90	90	0.94	94
Half-milled	96	4	0.94	90	0.96	92
70%-milled	94	6	0.96	90	0.97	91
White rice	92	8	0.98	90	0.98	90
Over-milled	88	12	0.98	86	0.98	86

[a] Source: Kome no Hinshitsu to Chozo, Riyo. (Quality of rice and storage and utilization of rice), Food Research Institute, Ministry of Agriculture and Forestry, 1969 [in Japanese].

Sri Lanka, and Japan, have taken legislative steps to limit the degree of milling, but when such rice is sold, many consumers have tried to remill it by hand-pounding or have taken it to illegal rice mills for further processing. This is more wasteful in terms of grain, labor, and power use than making proper white rice in the first place, and it is also against the law. However, it may not be wise to force people to eat undermilled rice because of digestibility problems, as evidenced by higher fecal bulk. Table 4 (9) shows the percent digestibility and digestible quantity of brown and white rice after various degrees of milling. Different studies have shown different results, but this table reflects the general picture. It would appear to be more advantageous to mill rice properly and find a way to utilize the bran.*

Implications of Changes in Harvesting Methods

The introduction of new, high-yielding rice varieties in Java was a major reason to adopt the sickle method of harvesting. These varieties are shorter and not suitable for knife harvesting. Their panicles are too small to be picked one by one for bundling. They are more prone to shattering than the traditional semi-*japonica* varieties, so they are sickled and threshed on the spot. In some places, however, the ani-ani is still used, in which case the panicles are not bound but carried in sacks or bags. Traditional varieties are sometimes harvested by sickle, the panicles are bound, and the rest of the straw is cut.

Another, perhaps stronger, factor behind the change to sickle harvesting was the farmers' desire to reduce the amount of the harvest allotted to the harvesters (7). Fewer, more efficient laborers could accomplish this. The share of rice given to ani-ani harvesters amounted to 30–40% of total labor costs, and 20% of the farmers' total production costs (2, pp. 55–56). When farmers encounter resistance to hiring fewer workers, they opt

---

*Apart from its caloric value, well-milled white rice is separated from the nutrient-rich bran and rice germ. People who consume diets made up largely of this rice and who eat little of other foods can become seriously deficient in vitamin B_1. For this reason, Japanese authorities have recommended that rice be only 70% milled but, as explained above, the effect of this recommendation is doubtful. Beyond that, undermilled rice deteriorates quickly, which causes storage problems. Today, a part of the rice is enriched with synthetic vitamin B_1 and added to bulk rice in a proportion of 1:200, bringing the B_1 content up to 0.85 mg/100 g white rice. This practice began in 1954 in Japan, and now such rice comprises one-third of the total amount of rice marketed.

Another recent measure enacted in Japan has been to introduce rice that retains its germ but not the bran. It is processed by special whitening machines and appears and tastes almost exactly like ordinary white rice. About 40–50 thousand tons of this rice are marketed each year.

for the tebasan arrangement described earlier. This represents a conflict of interest between farmers and laborers, since many women have lost their jobs. The ones who can use sickles efficiently are supposedly paid more because there are fewer of them.

Most sickle-harvested paddy is threshed in the field unless the field is poorly drained or under water, in which case the paddy has to be carried to farmyards for threshing. During transport there is a loss of grain from shattering. (Field drainage therefore not only is an important means of preventing the inconvenience of having to transport paddy for threshing elsewhere, but also saves that part of the harvest that would be destroyed during transport. Well-drained fields are also more productive and can be brought under multiple cropping.)

When the number of small mills reached the saturation point, small entrepreneurs went into the transportation business. In the early 1970s, many light trucks (Honda or Colt) were imported from Japan and were modified into small buses. (It might be added that buses have about saturated the market now, and various kinds of people who possess small amounts of funds are looking for other kinds of profitable enterprises.) The buses greatly facilitated local transportation, and as they spread around the country, they introduced a cash economy to the outlying rural areas. This no doubt stimulated changes from archaic farming and processing methods to more efficient production techniques. At the same time, the availability of transportation brought mobility to the labor force and enabled surplus rural workers to migrate to urban centers.

Reasons for Slow Diffusion of Threshers

Once farmers took over the threshing operation, one would have expected that threshing machines would have been supplied rather quickly. This was not the case for several reasons. One was that there were no suitable, cheap, convenient threshing machines for farm-level use. Small-scale agricultural machinery manufacturers are very few in number. In large cities like Bandung, Yogyakarta, Semarang, and Surabaya, there are several medium- and large-scale agricultural machine manufacturers, but small or home industries that make farm equipment in rural towns and villages are almost nonexistent, in contrast to their abundant numbers in other Southeast Asian countries. The few who are in operation make low-quality machines, and there is thus a great lack of decent equipment for farmers. There is little competition among small machine manufacturers and no incentive for higher quality, low-priced implements.

One reason why small-scale industries are few and far between is that there is a stringent licensing system that works against starting even very small manufacturing businesses. This legal requirement (which also involves a considerable unofficial license fee) restricts the development of small or home industries far more than it does large enterprises. Until the licensing system changes, job opportunities and an uplift in the level of rural technology cannot occur. This rural dependence on large manufacturers for simple machinery means high prices and a limited variety of equipment to choose from, because big industry makes few simple implements. Good-quality hand tools like hoes, sickles, hatchets, weeders, and flails are hard to get despite the predominance of small-scale, intensive farming in Java.

There is also a requirement that farmers buy, at considerable cost, permission forms in order to purchase threshers if they are planning to use the machine for custom work. Very few large farmers can afford threshers only for their own use; the ones bought are shared with several other farmers. Naturally, some farmers outwit the system, but the permission regulation hardly encourages farmers to use threshers.

Another factor responsible for the low use of machinery is the absence of a fair, objective system for assessing paddy quality, mentioned earlier. This inhibits the overall advancement of the farmers' technological level. When the better-quality paddy is upgraded to a higher rank and the farmer is paid proportionally for the quality of his paddy, he will be willing to use threshers and dryers to produce the best possible paddy. Suitable paddy threshing would lessen the number of dehusked, damaged grains and prevent contamination by soil. Threshers with built-in winnowers could also remove impurities. Proper dryers dry paddy uniformly, and there is far less cracked grain than is found in sun-dried paddy.

Current assessment of paddy stresses low moisture content, and even this is not accurate. Such factors as impurity content and percentage of immature and damaged grains are largely ignored. There certainly is no incentive for farmers to buy expensive equipment to improve their paddy if their work goes unrewarded. The farmer understandably thinks of implements only in terms of their labor-saving capacity.

Poor-quality paddy can mean not only high moisture content, but also uneven drying, contamination, admixture with foreign material, and damaged or immature grain, all of which lead to high storage losses. The presence of different rice varieties and cracked or unripe grain leads to low milling recovery. These factors increase the amount of broken rice and discolored grains (some are toxic) in white rice.

But waste is not the only result of poor paddy. The farmer's lack of incentive hinders his efforts to improve his socioeconomic status and hampers technological development.

In the Absence of Concern for Quality, Technology is Useless

In spite of an officially set floor price on the paddy market, buyers can judge and price the paddy subjectively. The floor price can be reduced if paddy quality is poor, so the floor price loses meaning. Farmers cooperating to improve paddy prices are discouraged and become divided when buyers price their paddy according to their own judgment of its quality. Small farmers facing unscrupulous or careless buyers cannot maintain a solid front, and there can be no hope of improving their lives.

After a while, if good-quality paddy is consistently priced as though it were poor, farmers cannot comprehend what good quantity and quality paddy is, so why should they care about improving their working methods? They can still *grow* crops without mechanization. As discussed earlier, mechanization becomes important in post-harvest processing. Without incentives, however, farmers are not interested in using mechanical equipment.

International assistance agencies and developed countries have tried to help by giving machines to farmers, and their files are full of instances in which the equipment was never used or was left to rust and then thrown away. The explanation given is that the technologies introduced were too advanced, or that "intermediate" or "appropriate" technologies should have been transferred. These are superficial observations. Technologies, whether appropriate or not, should not be "transferred" at all. They should be created or chosen by the people who want them. Even if technology is brought in from outside, it must appear to the potential users as a "discovery" for them that appeared just as they were looking for a way to solve their own problems. Then they should adapt it for their own use. If people lack the will to solve their problems, no technology can last for long.

The Only Possible Way for the Development of Post-harvest Technology and Its Relation to Rural Society

No matter what technology the government recommends to reduce post-harvest losses in the areas where they are greatest, unless it coincides with the interests of the people producing and processing the crops, it will not be accepted. Post-harvest processing is closely linked with such factors as agricultural production, irrigation and drainage, agricultural cooperatives, farm finances, agricultural machinery production, and marketing practices. If there are no sound policies to back up these activities, it will be impossible to prevent post-harvest losses. The Ministry of Agriculture is making an effort to reduce these losses; the Ministry of Public Works is concerned with irrigation practices; the Ministry of Trade and Cooperatives is trying to set up farm cooperatives; BULOG is attempting to stabilize the price of rice; the Ministry of Industry is involved with farm machinery production; and the Bank Rakyat Indonesia is the center of finance for farming. All of these organizations' activities are limited in scope and they work separately. What is needed is a joint committee representing all of these ministries to deal with post-harvest processing of rice so that the efforts are coordinated. Advocacy and demonstration of this or that technology are fruitless. It is first necessary to motivate farmers to want to undertake technological development. One step would be to set up just paddy quality assessment system. All of the restraints that inhibit production and discourage farmers from trying to work for quality should be removed.

Some have suggested that technical development and mechanization will threaten job opportunities and that mechanization should be selective (10) because rice cultivation in Java relies heavily on hired laborers even for small-scale farms. It is true that more efficient agricultural development through use of less labor-intensive machinery will deprive some people of farming jobs, and part of the labor force will migrate to cities. But if productivity is to be improved, it would be foolish to try to keep workers in rural areas by assuring job opportunities, especially as partial or menial employment is not very rewarding and people earning so little cannot improve their living standards. Even if this situation were maintained artificially, the labor force would continue to leave the farms because of easier access to transportation to the cities, and especially as people become aware that income levels in urban areas are much higher than in the countryside.

Therefore, rather than following the path of selective mechanization to protect rural employment, it is better to improve the techniques of rice harvesting and milling, particularly since the changes that have been introduced in the past decade have interested some farmers in becoming more productive. This attitude must be encouraged by removing the restraints described earlier so that motivated farmers can improve their skills, notice the good results that come from more efficient farming methods, and be encouraged to adopt increasingly better production techniques. This could lead to multiple cropping, local processing of farm products, and the creation of rural industries to supply farmers with more efficient machinery, all of which would require more hands and improve levels of employment. The result of upgrading knowledge and technical standards would elevate rural living standards, and with these would come pride in the production of quality foods, necessarily leading to reduction of post-harvest losses. All of this progress can only be achieved by joint efforts between the concerned ministries and the farmers themselves.

THAILAND

Cultivation and Marketing of Rice in the Central Plain

Rice is the major staple food of Thailand. Annual consumption amounts to an average of 140 to 160 kg/person. Although rice is the predominant crop, the production of commercial crops largely for export, such as maize, cassava, sugar cane, and rubber, has increased remarkably over the past 10 years, and their export value is now comparable to that of rice. Because of this, rice production in the Central Plain has become more commercially oriented. About half of the rice produced in Thailand is consumed by farmers and the rest goes to market. In 1973–1974, the total paddy, including carryover from the previous year, was 15.7 million tons, of which 9.02 million were consumed by farmers, and 7.65 million were sold (11).

In the Central Plain, a greater proportion goes to market because the land is more productive there and farming is done on a large scale. Therefore, the sale of paddy is an important source of income for the farmers in this region. However, 80% of the paddy is sold during January, February, and March, right after harvesting. The reasons for this rapid, concentrated selling are lack of storage facilities, a need to pay back high-interest loans as quickly as possible, and, when farmers have contracted to pay for loans directly with paddy, the necessity of doing so as soon as it is harvested (although this practice is being halted) (11, pp. 96–97).

In 1976, fewer than one-fifth of the farmers (69 of 399 surveyed) in the Central Plain received the official floor price for their paddy—2500 bahts (about US $125)/ton (12). This is because of a buyers' discount based on high moisture content, presence of impurities, brokens, and damaged grain, but the judgment is one-sided and the farmers have no way of confirming it. Almost all buyers are either middlemen or private rice millers. Agricultural cooperatives collect only 1–2% of total marketed paddy (12, p. 79; 13, p. 78).

The collected, marketable paddy is processed in private rice mills that are generally dilapidated. Most paddy is stored in bulk, and the mill walls are full of openings, so chickens peck the grain abundantly spilt through the slats and rats and sparrows can easily go in and out.

Most commercial rice mills are locally manufactured, traditional types fitted out with disk huskers, compartment-type separators, and whitening cones. The buildings are dark and dusty, with paddy and rice scattered all around, and the wooden frame shakes violently when the machinery is operating. Under these conditions it is impossible to maintain and operate the plant efficiently, much less keep reliable books.

Considering the amounts of rice the mills process annually, renovating the mills would save large enough quantities of rice during both storage and milling to repay the cost of restoration. Rarely is any money invested in mill upkeep, and machines can be bought only to replace those beyond repair or for some additional processing capacity. Some rice millers openly admit that their main interest is in buying and selling rice for profit, and that the milling operation itself is only an unavoidable burden.

Thai people in general regard these middlemen as greedy, just as Indonesians view their rice buyers. To protect farmers and consumers from them, the government annually sets an official paddy floor price and puts a ceiling on the price of rice. However, these are often unrealistic and impracticable. For example, the 1976 guaranteed paddy price for producers was 2500 bahts/ton of nonglutinous 5% paddy, and the ceiling price on rice for the consumer was 4.3–5 bahts/kg for 5% white rice. The actual cost of producing a kg of rice is 4.3 bahts, which does not include any margin of profit for millers, wholesalers, or retailers, and does not even cover the cost of transportation (11, p. 121).

If the millers were to stay with this ceiling, they would have to cheat some place along the line to survive. This reinforces the system of one-sided paddy quality assessment. Also, if they were to renovate the rice mills and warehouses sufficiently to reduce processing and storage losses, they would be viewed as too well-to-do, and the price between paddy and finished rice would be narrowed further. Not only would fixed assets be lost, but the millers would become scapegoats in the event of any sociopolitical turbulence, as has happened in some countries. They therefore naturally elect to pay farmers for paddy in advance so that they can collect high interest rates on the loans. Paddy is bought on better terms for the millers in this way, and they are able to increase their stockpiles for speculation on the market.

Because there is no standardized paddy quality grading system, there is no proof that the buyers are deliberately undervaluing the paddy. The merchants' advance payments to farmers reflect a lack of sufficient institutional financing for agriculture. It must be added that there is risk for the moneylenders, too. These Chinese rice merchants do make a great contribution to the economy in their successful exporting of rice and other agricultural products, and in their capacity to distribute products on the domestic market.

On the other hand, as in Indonesia, the merchants' subjective paddy assessment depresses the farmers' efforts to improve the quality of their paddy and inhibits cooperation among farmers. Once a fair, objective paddy grading system is used, farmers can more easily discern the quality of their own paddy and can see, by comparing their product with the standard, what could be done to improve their farming and post-harvest techniques.

The Paddy Grading System and Prospects for the Development of Agricultural Cooperation

In Thailand's Central Plain, photosensitive varieties of rice have been grown for years, with planting timed according to the seasonal flood. The new, high-yielding varieties are nonphotosensitive and these are grown on irrigated land. Areas planted with these varieties have been increasing steadily, and they lend themselves to second cropping; in 1978–1979, production of these varieties reached roughly 1.5 million tons.

Since the second rice crop is often harvested in the rainy season, threshing and drying are difficult and the farmers need both mechanical threshers and dryers. In order to make the most economical use of these expensive implements, operating time must be spread out. To do this, farmers should cooperate in timing their planting, use of irrigation water, and harvesting so that they can take turns using threshers and dryers, either through shared ownership or on a custom basis. If the paddy thus dried were stored in warehouses in agricultural cooperatives and sold at the most advantageous moment, farmers would benefit further. The most serious drawback to the adoption of this system is that farmers here are not accustomed to cooperating because the practice has always been to rely solely on seasonal flooding.

There are some agricultural cooperatives in this area that receive government support, but their activities are largely confined to farm financing. Farmers need low-interest loans, but because the agricultural cooperatives are agents for the agricultural bank and do not interact directly with farmers, they are cooperatives in name only.

With irrigation playing an increasingly important role in rice-growing, there is a great need for cooperation among farmers so that they can reach mutually satisfactory arrangements for distribution of water, the amount and timing of its use, and for shared maintenance of canals. If this could be achieved, mechanical threshers and dryers could be used to great advantage, and if a standard paddy grading system were introduced, their use would be further promoted. Cooperative selling of paddy produced under these conditions would help everyone in that it would be a giant step toward strengthening agricultural cooperatives and technological development.

Once farmers had learned to cooperate in paddy production, processing, and rice marketing, they could proceed to work together to raise dairy cattle, swine, poultry, fruit, and engage together in fish culture and horticulture. This could lead to small local or home industries to utilize the products and by-products of their agricultural activities. Agricultural cooperatives could thus be nuclei for rural community development.

An Example of the Development of a Rural Multifaceted Agro-industrial Complex

A man named Mr. Kamchai has a rice mill located in Pathum Thani in the Central Plain. It can process 20 tons of paddy per hour. He decided to utilize the mill even more efficiently through a recycling system combining rice mills with animal-raising and fish culture. In the compound of his rice mill, he began to raise chickens, pigs, and fish. Bran and small brokens were given to the chickens, the chicken droppings were eaten by the pigs, and pig dung was fed to the fish. This experiment proved successful, so he started an integrated farm complex on about 100 hectares. On this farm, in addition to the chicken and duck cages, the pig sty, and a brick factory, there are many rectangular patches of land, each surrounded by banks. These patches serve alternately as fish ponds and farmland. When the fish are fully grown, the ponds are emptied and used for growing either paddy or sugar cane, the paddy being milled in his own rice mill. Since the ponds and the farmland are adjoining, water from the ponds is used to irrigate the farmland during the dry season and the ponds serve as reservoirs to catch excess water during the rainy season. When the ponds are emptied, the soil is already fertile from the cultivation of fish and algae. Fish farming is more than ten times as profitable as paddy farming over the same area. The fish ponds not only make it possible to obtain three crops a year from the adjacent fields, but also make the fields more fertile.

Many farm roads have been constructed, using the soil excavated when the ponds were dug, and bamboo will be planted along the roadside for shade; the bamboo shoots will be used for food. On the banks, banana trees have been planted to harden the soil; the leaves and stems are used as feed for pigs. Mr. Kamchai is also planning to construct a fish-processing factory. Eventually, the waste products from the factory will also be used as pig feed. A slaughterhouse and cold storage facilities for pork are also planned. This will make sales of pork more profitable, and the by-products of the slaughterhouse can be used as feed.

Since the rice mill processes parboiled rice, the husk produced is used as fuel for parboiling as well as to generate power to operate the mill. The black ash of the husk is mixed with clay from the pond excavation and used for brickmaking. Paddy husk is also used for fuel in the brick factory. The white ash of the husk from the brick factory is used to neutralize acidity in the soil by mixing it into the soil when ploughing ponds. These bricks are being used for the construction of additional pig sties and warehouses.

A bran oil extraction plant was completed in 1978. Since the bran produced in this rice mill is from parboiled rice, the extraction plant can be operated more profitably. The bran cakes obtained after extraction of the oil are excellent feed for chickens. Bran and chicken droppings are not sufficient, in quantity or nutritional quality, to feed chickens and pigs, and a feed mill is used to mix in cassava and maize that have been dried using the same facilities employed for drying parboiled rice.

To service machines and equipment in the rice mill there is a workshop that manufactures artificial dryers and bucket elevators, and it is also used as a maintenance shop for tractors. Recently, manufacturing of air conditioners was begun; the products are sold in Mr. Kamchai's shops in Bangkok. The air conditioners can also be used in the cold storage facilities.

Mr. Kamchai says that this farm is just an example to show the possibility of rotating land and recycling resources, and he expects this type of integrated farm complex to be propagated all over the country. He has set up a small model farmhouse on his farm to teach his method to other people to suit their various land-scales. It is impressive that he does not expect any assistance from either the government or international organizations.

Mr. Kamchai produces odorless, parboiled rice by a hot water soaking method, and the rice can be exported to various parts of the world that will not accept traditional parboiled rice because of its smell. His method of hot water soaking is worth noting. Shovel loaders are used to remove the soaked paddy from the hot-water tanks and load it onto trucks equipped with steam pipes. The trucks reach the steaming point after being loaded, and steam is blown into the pipes. Then the trucks go to the drying yard and dump the paddy while moving, thus spreading bands of paddy on the ground. This method greatly reduces the labor required and therefore the cost, which opens up the possibility of developing parboiling on a larger scale. As is well known, parboiled rice is much lower in brokens, and has a higher milling recovery, even if it is milled with crude, conventional milling equipment. Of course, fuel is required, but husks, which are normally difficult to dispose of, can be used.

In most Southeast Asian countries, including Thailand, parboiled rice is not consumed. However, if it did not have the objectionable smell, it is quite possible that it would be eaten in rice-eating areas of Southeast Asia where *indica* nonglutinous rice is generally consumed. In Europe, America, Australia, and Africa, odorless parboiled rice is widely preferred. Even though all the rice consumed in Asia could not be replaced by parboiled rice, proportionately significant savings of paddy could be realized, amounting to about 5% of total rice and 20–40% of head rice. Reduced storage losses and increased nutritional quality are added advantages. Studies of people's acceptance of parboiled rice and the introduction or development of a good parboiling system are of great importance.

Another recent development by Mr. Kamchai is utilization of waste heat from husk-fired boilers. Flue gas is directly blown into the rotary dryer that dries the parboiled rice. As the exhaust gas from the dryer is already low in temperature and does not cause a draft, a power-operated fan is used to blow the exhaust down onto the surface of the water so as to eliminate fly ash, thus reducing air pollution.

Improvement of a Village Rice Mill

A notable development in the post-harvest processing of rice in Thailand was the invention of a rice huller for use in custom milling at the village level. Except in Java and Malaysia, where rubber roller huskers and friction-type whiteners are widely used, most small-scale rice milling in developing countries is done in Engleberg-type hullers that produce much broken rice and have a low milling recovery. Though many governments discourage use of this kind of huller, it is still commonly used because it is easily manufactured and the operating cost is low.

The new Thai huller is a horizontal abrasive type (14,15) developed by local manufacturers, copied by others, and now used extensively in the Central Plain. All village rice mills surveyed were using it (12, p. 76). The machine is composed of a horizontal, cylindrical abrasive stone and two to four rubber brakes. Its performance is reputed to be far superior to that of the Engleberg huller, yet its manufacture and operation are just as simple and cheap.

Village mills in the Central Plain might have been improved through a payment system for custom milling. The majority of the mills return rice to consumers at 60% of paddy weight, retaining the rest of the white rice as a milling charge. This practice was found in 300 of 399 mills surveyed. Improved milling recovery as a result of the new Thai huller means increased income for rice mill owners.

BURMA

Rice Milling and Marketing in Burma

Before World War II, Burma exported more than 3 million tons of rice annually, exceeding Thailand's exports. After the war, the rate of increased production did not keep pace with rising population growth, and exports decreased steadily, ultimately dropping to a mere 71 thousand tons in 1973–1974 (Fig. 1).

Burma did not diversify its agricultural production, so its rice monoculture always played a sensitive role in foreign currency earning. Depending on the international market price, the income from rice exports fluctuated, but it was always 40–70% of export value. Any decline in rice exports is such a serious problem for Burma that the government intervened to reverse this trend in the early 1970s. The situation began to improve in 1974–1975, and exports rose to 562,000 tons in 1977–1978.

In Burma, rice exporting and the major part of domestic marketing have been nationalized. Rice farmers have to sell paddy to the government according to a quota determined by the amount of land they have and its productivity (16). They may also sell rice to the free market to a limited extent after they have fulfilled the government quota.

As a rule, rice mills are not nationalized, but the government has confiscated some of the private mills. All private mills must be registered. Because any marketed paddy is under government control, all milling is custom; rice mills cannot buy paddy or sell white rice. Commercial milling is nonexistent. This means that rice mills in Burma are really processing plants, in contrast to the merchant-controlled mills in Thailand.

Marketed paddy, purchased by the government agency known as the Agricultural and Food Produce Trade Corporation (AFPTC), comprises about 40% of all the paddy produced in Burma. The paddy is milled in 829 private mills under contract with AFPTC and in 25 other mills that belong to it. Farm-consumed paddy is supposed to be milled in the 829 mills under contract, in 1000 other mills for farmers (called wunza mills), and in about 1200 smaller mills called huller mills (17).

The AFPTC pays a certain milling charge to the mills under contract, based on the variety of paddy and the designated grade of rice per unit of weight. The amount of white rice to be returned to the AFPTC is determined by a test milling of paddy in a mill, and generally almost all of the white rice produced has to revert to AFPTC, plus all of the by-products except the husks (18). Therefore, even if technical improvements in some mills increased the output and quality of white rice, they would receive almost the same payment given to the other mills. Because no

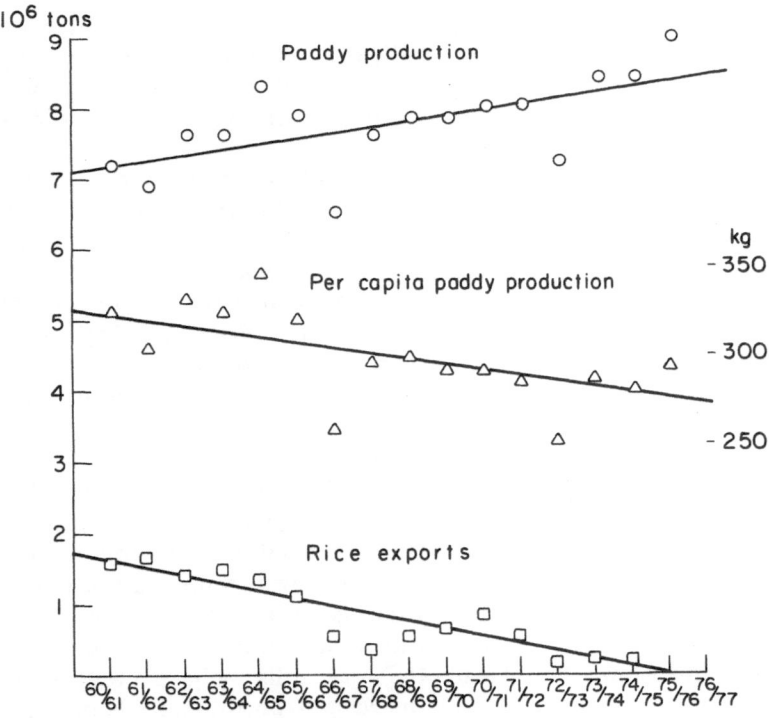

FIGURE 1. Paddy production, per capita paddy production, and rice exports, Burma, 1960–1961 to 1975–1976.

test mill operates according to a standard, mills yielding a higher recovery are not even noticed.

The Consequences of the Village Rice Mill Shortage

In the case of custom milling for farmers, all of the white rice and by-products are returned to them just as they are to the AFPTC. They pay a milling charge based on the amount milled. In contrast to the situation in the Central Plain of Thailand, increasing milling capacity is the major concern of the millers. Farmers recognize that some mills yield more than others when processing a given amount of paddy taken from the same lot. They are supposed to choose the mills that have higher technical efficiency and hence greater output.

In reality, this is not so easily done. There are only about 3000 mills scattered throughout Burma, including all of the different categories of mill. This is in sharp contrast to the 25,000 mills in Thailand and the 20,000 in Java. When Burmese farmers want their paddy milled, they have to take it on either animal carts or barges and wait their turn at the mill gate. Long queues form, and it usually takes 2 or 3 days of waiting before a farmer gets his turn. Under these extreme conditions, farmers can hardly be expected to be selective.

The huller mills use only the Engleberg huller; the rest use conventional types—disk husker, compartment separator, and cone whitener. Huller mills are not officially allowed in the Pegu, Irrawadi, and Rangoon Divisions, the major rice-growing areas in lower Burma. However, because of the mill shortage, a number of huller mills do exist in these divisions, as do unregistered (illegal) ones in other places.

It is reported that the government has banned hand-pounding of rice, and has ordered farmers to turn their paddy over to the mills for processing, but they often have to resort to hand-pounding because of the mill situation. In fact, hand-pounding can be observed in many places. Husking is generally accomplished in clay mills (sold on the market) inlaid with bamboo teeth and the grain is whitened in mortars with foot-operated pestles. The scene was reminiscent of Java 15 years ago.

With the present government control over most of the mills, and the lack of a standard test for mill yields, there is no incentive for technical improvement. Machine parts are very difficult to obtain, and consequently machines have deteriorated badly for lack of repair. Those owned by the AFPTC are in the best condition, followed by those under contract to AFPTC. The wunza mills' equipment is the worst. Many rice mills are over 30 years old; some have been operating 50 years or more, and with the lack of maintenance and neglect of cleaning, many machines are out of order. These poor conditions apply as well to mill buildings and power generators. Most Burmese rice mills use reciprocating steam engines with husk-fired boilers, whose power is transmitted through countershafts. Almost all of these boilers are superannuated, and over 70% are more than 40 years old (19).

The government requires that rice for export be parboiled, but for private millers this is not economically feasible and they avoid parboiling rice even though many of them have the facilities to do so.

Effects of Poor-Quality Paddy

The quality of the paddy collected by the AFPTC is very poor because the government's buying price is much lower than that on the free market, and, even for higher-quality paddy, the government price is not proportionally greater because the buyers have no facility for inspecting the quality of the paddy. After collection, the paddy is often left outdoors and dried unevenly, which increases storage loss. Given these circumstances, plus the poor conditions of the mills, the rice milled from such paddy is poor in quality, whether for export or domestic consumption.

One reason for the poor quality of white rice is the presence of red rice in the paddy and discolored grains. The wasteful milling techniques produce a lot of broken grains. Before the war, the 5% white rice comprised a considerable portion of exported rice, but in 1977–1978 (17), 92% of the rice exported was below the quality of 25% white rice. This, combined with the small quantity available for export, means that the unit price for exported rice is low, which has a negative effect on foreign currency earnings.

The rice supplied by AFPTC to the domestic market is of even poorer quality. Consumers thus prefer the high-quality rice sold on the free market, which pushes up free market prices and widens the gap between the government price for paddy—a vicious circle that lowers still further the quality of paddy processed by the AFPTC.

The government is planning to set up 24 new rice mills and renovate several of the mills belonging to the AFPTC using loans from the Asian Development Bank, Japan, and China. A loan from the IBRD is being used to construct a storage warehouse for 100,000 tons of paddy, also for AFPTC. However, because private rice mills play a much more important role and improvement in paddy quality is urgently needed, measures should be taken to review paddy marketing policies and to arouse the interest of private mill owners in upgrading their technical level.

MECHANIZATION OF RICE CULTIVATION AND POST-HARVEST PROCESSING
IN JAPAN

HISTORY AND PROGRESS

In Japan, 70% of the rice produced is marketed; the post-harvest loss of this marketed rice is estimated to be about 5% (20). The reasons for such a low loss are as follows: (1) Farmers cultivate small land parcels intensively and plan for optimum time of harvest and post-harvest operations with the help of such equipment as reapers, combine harvesters, threshers, and dryers. (2) Since farmers produce clean, selected brown rice by using huskers and grain sorters, the loss in succeeding processes can be reduced. (3) Because there is an official rice-grading system, farmers are motivated to improve the quality of their rice. (4) The method for storing brown rice efficiently has been established. (5) Rice millers make an effort to reduce milling losses because the prices of brown rice and finished product (white rice) are largely controlled. (6) Rice has traditionally been an object of animistic worship, so it is not treated carelessly.

Merely enumerating these factors that have undoubtedly reduced post-harvest losses does not explain their mutual interrelations and the dynamic process of their development. It has often been commented that, with agricultural mechanization in Japan, farmers can sell their rice at five times the international price, and that, therefore, their machines and their technology could not be used economically by farmers in other countries, which is true. Then why is such a high price for rice maintained in Japan? Is the Japanese government especially generous to farmers?

Most governments are currently adopting measures to stabilize the prices of basic agricultural products with the aim of protecting their farmers. In almost all cases, such measures are adopted only when groups of farmers exert pressure on the government. In order to maintain the price of rice in Japan, the farmers had to join forces. This cooperation among Japanese farmers began in the prewar period; it could not have started all of a sudden in the postwar era. Farm mechanization, sometimes alleged to have been the result of high rice prices after the war, also began in the prewar years. It is very important not to misunderstand this point.

Some observers regard farm machinery as "playthings" for Japanese farmers, purchased with their earning from other industries, and point out that the majority of Japanese farmers are no longer farmers but industrial workers who own some cultivatable land. If this is so, how could the farmers have entered other industries so quickly without lowering agricultural productivity? It was possible, of course, only because of the contribution of these very "playthings" and the high level of the farmers' skill. But how were these acquired?

Mechanization of rice farming in Japan dates back to the beginning of the twentieth century—much earlier than the 10-year period during which the number of part-time farmers exceeded more than half of the total number of farmers, and even before the beginning of government intervention in rice prices during the war. However, mechanization was almost exclusively limited to post-harvest processing until the end of the war. Nevertheless, it prepared the fertile soil for the explosive progress of over-all mechanization of rice cultivation in the postwar period under changed agricultural conditions, chiefly as the result of land reform and remarkable advances in technical innovations.

REASONS WHY AGRICULTURAL MECHANIZATION IN JAPAN EMERGED FROM MECHANICAL POST-HARVEST PROCESSING

Why was mechanization of rice farming based on mechanization of post-harvest processing in Japan? First of all, it is absolutely essential to make use of some equipment or machines in post-harvest processing because it is of a purely artificial nature, as explained earlier. Second, the advantage of using machinery for post-harvest processing was decidedly enhanced by the taxation and marketing system for brown rice established before the seventeenth century. Owing to that system, post-harvest processing became as important as the production process itself for farmers, since their function as rice growers was completed only when they had produced brown rice. Long before mechanization (or, more correctly, power-driven mechanization) started, the value of the post-harvesting equipment owned by the average farmer was already as high as 1.5–2 times that of his cultivation equipment.

The importance of the post-harvest process became even greater when the rice grain inspection system was established in the decade beginning in 1910. The remarkable improvements in paddy huskers made during that period are a reflection of that system. On the other hand, the fact that post-harvest processing requires some equipment or machinery means that it also requires a corresponding economic scale of operations determined by the nature of that equipment or machinery. Generally speaking, the required minimum economic scale increases with the transition from manual labor to mechanized labor.

Since the scale of rice cultivation operations in Japan is very small, farmers had to cooperate among themselves when modern post-harvesting machinery was introduced. This was observed in the seventeenth century at the introduction of the clay mill for use in husking in place of the wooden one, and again in the twentieth century when the powered husker was introduced. By the end of the 1930s, almost all husking operations were performed by power huskers, but the overwhelming majority of the machines were cooperatively owned.

The rice whitening stage, as one of a series of post-harvesting processes, could easily be undertaken on a larger scale because it is carried out by commercial rice millers or custom rice millers. It follows that rice whitening could be mechanized much more easily than could the earlier processing stages. In fact, mechanization of the post-harvest process started initially with rice whitening and then proceeded to husking and threshing, in reverse order to the actual sequence of operations.

A phenomenon peculiar to Japan was that the husking operation was not absorbed by the rice milling industry as in other rice-growing countries, but remained the work of the farmers. This fact is of great significance.

EFFECTS OF THE BROWN RICE MARKETING SYSTEM ON THE FARMERS' STANDARD OF LIVING AND ON RURAL SOCIETY

Processing paddy into brown rice is, of course, a burden for farmers, but it has played a significant role in the improvement of their economic and social conditions and in the progress of farm mechanization.

First, it has made farmers recognize the quality and quantity of their own products clearly and precisely. Even before the introduction of the grain quality inspection system, farmers could judge the quality of brown rice visually, which is not the case with paddy. Such qualities of brown rice as the maturation condition, the content of inferior grains, and cleanness are direct results of their farming and post-harvest operations. Farmers can perceive what to improve in their operations by looking at the condition of their brown rice. This was an essential factor in improving farming and post-harvest technology in Japan, in contrast to the situation in other rice-growing countries.

Second, easy assessment of grain quality in brown rice made farmers less susceptible to unreasonable bargaining by buyers. Even though it is difficult to determine the exact grade of a given brown rice in the absence of grain quality standards, comparative differences can easily be judged and farmers need not be fooled by buyers or landlords. Easy judgment of quality also paved the way for the introduction of the grain quality grading system, which, of course, improved the farmers' situation still further.

Third, farmers put considerable effort into the improvement of grain quality because it was in their own interest, particularly after the introduction of the grading system. They became eager to introduce advanced machines on a cooperative basis. Japanese farmers have been used to cooperating in the construction and utilization of irrigation and drainage facilities for rice cultivation for hundreds of years, and this habit helped to ease the difficulties involved in their cooperation in the purchase and utilization of post-harvest processing machinery. When such cooperation in post-harvest operations was developed to the point of marketing their products, then the time was almost ripe for agricultural cooperatives.

Fourth, the resulting improved quality of brown rice made it practicable to adopt advanced whitening technology in the rice mills, which reduced grain loss in storage and milling. For example, since the brown rice produced by farmers is pure and the paddy content is very low (in the case of Third Grade Brown Rice, below 0.3%), rice mills can employ low-pressure whitening machines, whereas in the U.S. the average paddy content in brown rice is about 1%. Such machines are difficult to use in the U.S., despite the fact that it is even more desirable to use them there than in Japan, because medium- and long-grain varieties comprise most of the rice grown in the U.S.

Beyond that, since rice millers have to buy brown rice in accurate quantities and of standard quality, which is not the case with paddy buying in most countries in Southeast Asia, they had no other choice but to reduce storage and milling loss in order to secure their profit.

Fifth, when farmer's cooperation in post-harvest processing was expanded to include wider utilization of power threshers, they could easily grow and thresh harder-shattering varieties with less field grain loss than before. Originally, *japonica* varieties grown in Japan were harder-shattering than was *indica*, but the degree of hardness has been increased more and more. Thus, unless corresponding threshing methods had been introduced, the unthreshed grain loss would have increased, and labor efficiency would have been reduced.

Sixth, since, after the establishment of the grading system, farmers produced and sold brown rice of common grades and varieties, their interests also became common and they could therefore be united in a nationwide organization able to bring pressure to bear on the government or on other rice buyers to raise the selling price of rice, or on the suppliers of fertilizers, agricultural machinery, and other required commodities.

Such an increased scale of cooperation among farmers also enabled great progress to be made in the standardization of post-harvest processing. So-called "rice centers," "country elevators," and other processing factories have improved the efficiency of small-scale operations and helped to keep the labor required to a minimum. Surely, there have been subsidies from the government for these facilities, but the most decisive factor to lead them to success was the accumulation of experience in cooperative operations by the farmers themselves.

Last, but not least, Japanese farmers have become accustomed to using their own ingenuity in various operations because of their involvement in both the natural process of crop production and the artificial process of post-harvest operations. Their engineering capability had long been exercised through their efforts at irrigation and land reclamation, and was further elaborated in post-harvest operations. Many of the inventions and innovations in post-harvest technology came from the farmers themselves. Rapid diffusion of agricultural machinery and the ready application of farm labor techniques to other industries are partly attributable to such qualities in Japanese farmers.

For whitening of farm-consumed rice, in the beginning farmers used to bring brown rice to custom rice mills or they hand-pounded it. Later they came to use cooperatively-owned rice mills, and finally each farm household had its own whitening machine. This meant that farmers could command not only the natural process of plant growing, but also all of the rice post-harvest processing until it reached the kitchen, which enabled them to achieve success in both growing and processing in the light of quality of the final product. Here they could take steps to make progress in many farm-related engineering technologies and thus improve daily life in the surrounding rural community. This can be observed in the innumerable varieties of tools and implements that they have developed, such as those for straw processing, mushroom culture, sericulture, fish culture, spinning and weaving, poultry raising, fruit processing, and making machinery that will manufacture many farm tools.

The development of agricultural technology, specifically that for post-harvest processing, has been brought about through the accumulation and refinement of farmers' experiences. Inventions and devices have mostly been the products of diligent farmers or carpenters and blacksmiths in rural villages. Only after the emergence of metal equipment and machine-driven power other than water wheels did foundries and machine manufacturers come into existence. Many of the present agricultural machinery manufacturing firms originated from such farmers and craftsmen in rural areas.

Farm implements and tools were largely supplied by rural craftsmen or by home industries, not by large industries in the cities. Internal combustion engines for farm use were also manufactured by small machine shops that were located in every small rural town until after the war.

Today, agricultural machinery manufacturers and farmers are distinctly separate. Many of the machines are designed under the assumption that the user will have considerable engineering knowledge—and most of these farmers do. They gained it not only from school education, but also through their practice of post-harvest technology. This has undoubtedly contributed to increased agricultural production, the diversification of agriculture, improvement of living conditions, and the formation of a capability readily applicable to industrial work as well as farming.

REFERENCES

1. Toquero, Z. An Empirical Assessment of Alternate Field Level Rice Post-Production Systems. International Rice Research Institute (IRRI), Los Banos, Philippines, 1977.
2. *Statistical Yearbook of Indonesia*, Biro Pusat Statistic, Jakarta, 1976, p. 336.
3. Prdoman Pengdaan dalam Negeri Tahun, 1978–1979, BULOG, Indonesia.
4. Mears, L. A. Rice Marketing in the Republic of Indonesia. The Institute for Economic and Social Research, Jakarta, 1961, p. 74.
5. Timmer, C. P. Choice of Technique in Rice Milling on Java. Research and Training Network, Agricultural Development Council (New York), Reprint Series, September 1974, pp. 1–20.
6. Koga, Y. Noson Shakai Hatten to Gijutsu—Indonesia Ni okeru Kome Shukakugo Shorikatei wo Megutte [Rural Community Development and Technology—on Rice Post-Harvest Process in Indonesia]. Institute of Developing Economy, 1979, pp. 13, 30 [In Japanese].
7. Collier, W. L., and G. W. Soentoro. Recent changes in rice harvesting in Indonesia: Some serious social implications. *Bull. Indonesian Econ. Stud.*, July 1973.
8. Food and Agriculture Organization of the United Nations. Task Force for Rice Grading, Storage and Processing in Indonesia. FAO, Rome, 1974, p. 53.
9. Food Research Institute, Ministry of Agriculture and Forestry. Kome no Hinshitsu to Chozo, Riyo [Quality of Rice and Storage and Utilization of Rice], 1969 [In Japanese].
10. Strout, A. M. Agricultural growth, employment and income distribution: Dilemmas for Indonesia's next five year plan. *Ekonomi Dan Keuangan Indonesia* **25** (4), 1977 [In Indonesian].
11. Murashima, E. Nenji Keizai Hokoku: Thai 1978 [Annual Economic Report: Thailand, 1978]. Institute of Developing Economy, 1979, p. 90.
12. Maitre, T. Survey on Post-Harvest Practices in Thailand, 1976. Department of Agriculture, Ministry of Agriculture and Cooperatives, 1979, p. 78.
13. Quantity of Paddy Collected by Agricultural Cooperatives, 1976. Ministry of Agriculture and Cooperatives, unpublished [In Thai].
14. Maitre, T. Small Scale Rice Milling Unit. Division of Agriculture and Engineering, 1978.
15. Nopmance, S. Rice Milling Technology and Some Economic Implications; The Case of Nakorn Pattrom, Thailand. Kasetsart University, Bangkok, Thailand, 1974.
16. Saito, T. Biruma no Momi Kyoshutsu Seido to Nohka Keizai [Paddy Quota System and Farm Economy]. *Ajia Keizai [Asian Economy]*, June, 1979.

17. Overseas Merchandise Inspection Co., Ltd. (OMIC): Feasibility Survey Report of Rice Mill Construction Project in the Socialist Republic of Burma. Japan International Cooperation Agency, 1979.
18. Koga, Y. Preliminary Survey of Post-Harvest Rice Processing in Burma. ESCAP, 1978, pp. 5–6.
19. *Annual Report on the Administration of the Boilers Act in Burma for the Year 1968–1969.*
20. Koga, Y. Rice Post-Harvest Process in Japan. In: Food and Agriculture Organization of the United Nations, in Co-operation with the Government of Malaysia and Food for the Hungry, Inc., *Report of the Action-Oriented Field Workshop for Prevention of Post-Harvest Rice Losses*, Kedah, Malaysia, March 12–30, 1977. FAO, Bangkok, 1977, p. 8.

Comment

H. A. B. Parpia

One issue that was touched upon but not addressed directly in a previous chapter should be noted: the utilization of rice bran, from which oil and rice husks represent important products. For example, in India alone, nearly 3.5 million tons of rice bran are available, which can supply almost 300,000 tons of edible bran oil. Only about half of the bran is now being used.

Rice husks also not only provide a good source of energy, but also can be processed into high-quality white ash for the manufacture of refractory brick, cleansing compounds, and many other things. Activated carbon can also be manufactured from the husks. What this suggests is that loss is not an isolated factor in the food chain, but must be considered in the context of the entire system of resource utilization.

As another example of post-harvest loss viewed in the broader perspective, the problem of employment and the issue of economic development are closely linked with food production and conservation strategies. In many heavily populated countries of the world, where 80–90% of the people live in rural areas, agriculture as an employment resource is reaching a saturation point, and alternative means of employment need to be created urgently to make proper use of human resources. The development of post-harvest conservation and processing industries, which are known to generate the largest chain of employment per unit of investment, can make a valuable contribution in this direction.

This broader perspective on post-harvest losses suggests the need to transfer useful and appropriate technology to developing countries. This is to be contrasted with traditional emphasis on developing capital-inten-

H. A. B. Parpia • Research and Development Centre, Agriculture Department, Food and Agriculture Organization, Rome, Italy.

sive, high-energy technologies that serve the needs of advanced countries. Post-harvest technologies must be different scientifically, socially, and economically, and training in entrepreneurship should also constitute a part of the package. Finally, cooperation among developing countries for transferring technology would be of great value.

Comment

PIERRE SPITZ

The first issue that I would like to address concerns the often-heard asser-tion that there is a causal relation between food loss and hunger. If we prevent the losses, it is argued, people will be fed. However, making more grain available does not necessarily mean that the nutritional status of the poor will improve; the whole complex of socioeconomic factors must be considered. That is why I believe that the post-harvest issue has been used as an escape, in lieu of dealing with socioeconomic reforms. It merely represents another example of a technological fix.

A second point is that I disagree with Pariser's suggestion that we facilitate the utilization of central storage systems. I think that this is a dangerous issue, because the small farmer's capacity to retain his own food for self-provisioning is very important. To take food out of his hand, when his major struggle is to retain it, would be tragic. In addition, cen-tralized systems are very inefficient in processing and milling.

PIERRE SPITZ • United Nations Research Institute for Social Development, Geneva, Swit-zerland.

Comment

HANS GUGGENHEIM

It seems that the crucial questions being addressed are: (1) To what extent do post-harvest losses impact on the nutritional well-being of specific populations? (2) To what degree can the prevention of food losses during the postproduction food cycles improve the nutritional status of those in need? If we begin with those kinds of questions, we come to a very different definition of what post-harvest losses are. The reason is that if we are talking about hungry people, we must consider what it is that these people lose. For example, I think we have to include the entire range of losses that a population experiences through changes in exchange entitlements, taxation, and fiscal policy. By doing so, the range of considerations becomes very different, and the problem of redistribution becomes paramount.

The fact is that gains in production will not solve the problem of malnutrition unless the problem of distribution is solved first. The question is: Suppose we utilize all the technology available and *save* all the food now being lost, will that reduce maldistribution or is it going to add to the inequality of distribution? Unfortunately, the evidence that the distribution mechanisms will be improved is very limited.

Cross-section studies indicate that income inequality increases in the early stages of development, although it seems to be diminished—according to some studies—after a certain plateau has been reached. The World Bank has suggested, however, that it may not be possible to grow first and redistribute later, because the structure of growth may largely fit the inequitable pattern of distribution, at least until a much higher level of income is approached. This has a profound implication for food loss reduction programs and raises the question whether reduction of

HANS GUGGENHEIM • The Wunderman Foundation, Boston, Massachusetts.

post-harvest losses, even if it contributes to the total amount of food available, will improve the nutritional status of the populations at risk, or whether such gains will merely contribute to the rise in inequality.

I would like to examine briefly the problem of distribution and equity in terms of millet in West Africa. Research on millet losses in traditional granaries, for instance in Mali and in the Saharian countries, shows that losses at the farm level are relatively small, ranging from 3 to 12% under usual circumstances. Losses in intermediate- and central-level storage, however, can be appreciably higher. Thus, emphasis has been put on reducing losses at central storage levels where fumigation teams can operate and where loss reduction programs appear to be cost-effective.

It could be argued, however, that if loss reduction programs focused on the farm level, it would benefit the farm population. This point supports the contentions of Spitz that, if farmers can retain the food they grow in sufficient quantities, there will be a measurable gain in their families' diets. Loss reduction programs operated at the central storage level can conceivably help the urban population, although there is no way in which the benefits can be redistributed to the rural poor. Furthermore, given the structure of the growth and distribution process in general, it remains unlikely that even the urban poor could benefit from the savings in grain; any savings would probably be passed on to the least needy.

Comment

MICHAEL LIPTON

I begin my comments by expressing disagreement with those who have suggested that post-harvest technology has received too much attention and has been overresearched. Quite to the contrary, it is really underresearched, especially in comparison to pre-harvest technology.

The case for emphasizing research and implementation of on-farm post-harvest technology (PHT) is illustrated by Bangladesh, where 25% of the value of purchased rice comprises value added after harvest; yet probably below 5% of research or extension outlays on rice have been on post-harvest matters. It is likely that we have a "bargain sector" here.

On-farm PHT is the priority. In most poor countries, 60–70% of grain never leaves the village of origin, and 40–50% is stored on the farm household that grew it until it is sold, eaten, or sown. Moreover, permanent, hard-walled, large-scale stores (and ancillary processing devices) are not likely to be inefficient. Massive losses in glut years do occur in public and merchant storage, but this is not due to failures in permanent storage. It is because temporary, hastily constructed, and bad facilities have to "make do"—involving costly cross-haulage—for want of expandible on-farm storage.

On-farm PHT, too, has the most scope for improving the nutrition of the poorest. If their grain runs out a bit later (because of reduced losses in storage, threshing, or milling), they are less driven to borrow when credit and grain are both at their dearest. Moreover, grain saved by improved on-farm PHT belongs to the storer, and is not shared with his landlord or lender.

But the case for better PHT will not be improved, nor its allocation

MICHAEL LIPTON • The Institute for Development Studies, University of Sussex, Brighton, England.

rationalized, by too-high expectations, based on doubtful estimates of post-harvest losses, and/or on neglect of the costs of preventing such losses. It is very unlikely that farm families, who are hungry and who work hard to reap their grain, will stupidly waste it afterwards. The prevailing high estimates of post-harvest losses are largely based on guesses (often averaged!), or else on the inspection of *residual* grain, e.g., in the bottom of a store, when and where damage is exceptionally high. Scientific estimates, based on careful dry-weighing of grain (and deductions for qualitative loss and insect frass) into and out of store, have been made for maize in Central Africa (Miracle), wheat in the Punjab (Wilson), maize and guinea-corn in Nigeria (Anthonio and Upton), and, most recently, by my Institute for paddy in Andhra Pradesh (1). The proportion of harvested grain lost in store is in all cases 4–8%, as against the much higher figures often alleged.

Nevertheless, the Andhra study showed that improved on-farm storage was a good investment privately and socially. Acquisition of simple, cheap, *locally made* improvements to outdoor storage for paddy showed a private rate of return of over 20% and social rates of return of over 25%, although the value of quantitative and qualitative paddy losses in farm household stores (in 18 villages, based on regular grain weighing into and out of store) averaged below 5% of stored grain over five seasons. Costlier, town-made metal bins were much more dubious propositions, and there was no clear-cut, paying proposition to improve indoor storage. Better PHT can help many of the poorest farmers to eat better at critical seasons, but these people are *not* wasting grain.

The work in Andhra revealed the need to set gains from better PHT against costs of improvement. But it also suggested that benefit–cost analysis of storage, in isolation, gives insufficient information to select PHT strategies to help the most nutritionally deprived groups for two reasons. First, the various PHT processes interact; for instance, the quality of drying vitally affects the vulnerability of stored grain to molds. Second, specific undernourished groups rely heavily on direct income from PHT.

Bangladesh illustrates both problems: Rural women often have few alternative sources of cash earnings apart from PHT that are acceptable in Islamic society, and wet harvesting conditions, especially after the early monsoon (aus) harvest, create special difficulties for sun-drying. Hence, IDS, with the Bangladesh Industrial Research Council, is undertaking intensive work (2–4) in eight villages, representing the agro-climatic conditions and cropping patterns of Bangladesh, to estimate size and distribution of grain losses and potential savings in alternative PHT *systems:* threshing, drying, storing, and milling. It is clear that, for both threshing and milling, economically genuine improvements—saving grain, capital, and also (unfortunately) labor per unit of throughput—are coming on-stream. But these improvements tend to displace the impoverished women, especially landless widows and divorcees, who have hitherto relied on custom-threshing and hulling (with traditional microequipment) for access to food. New income sources or (much more plausibly) access to *joint* ownership of pedal threshers and small backpack hullers is essential if better nutrition and economic PHT innovation are not to spell starvation for the hungriest in Bangladesh.

REFERENCES

1. Boxall, R. A., M. Greeley, D. Tyagi, J. Neelakantha, and M. Lipton. *The Prevention of Farm-Level Food Grain Storage Losses in India: A Social Cost-Benefit Analysis.* Institute of Development Studies, Brighton, U.K., 1978.
2. Begum, S., and M. Greeley. Women in the rural labour market: An empirical study. *Bangladesh J. Agric. Econ.* **4,** 1979.
3. Haque, F., and M. Greeley. On-Farm Losses in Five Post-Harvest Operations. SEARCA Conference, Kulala Lumpur, Malaysia, 1980.
4. Greeley, M. Appropriate technology: Recent Indian experience with farm-level food-grain research. *Food Policy* **3** (1), 1978.

Comment

RICARDO BRESSANI

Post-harvest losses of food are a real problem in developing countries, even though actual figures representing these losses are not readily available or are not reliable. The losses are probably low for small farmers who tend to produce enough for their own consumption, plus small additional amounts for marketing. The reason for this is that farmers are aware of the losses they may sustain if they produce more than they can easily market or sell. In this situation, it becomes necessary to upgrade the preservation systems that they have developed or inherited.

Losses can become significantly higher when food crops enter marketing channels. In this case, to make it worthwhile, more land is planted for greater production, and to facilitate marketing, mechanization is introduced. The equipment used in many instances was developed according to the specific characteristics of the crop. For example, corn shelling machines were developed for hybrid corn that has a shape different from that of the common corn varieties planted in many developing countries. This is another area where development of appropriate machinery to avoid losses is needed.

Although the definition or the frame of reference is important in defining or identifying the problem, the important point, keeping in mind that loss should not be confused with waste and that exact figures are not available, is to identify the factors responsible for losses and develop methods to reduce them.

Besides the quantitative loss that takes place, improper preservation also causes losses in nutritional value and has indirect economic implications. An example of the first result is the nutritional loss in quality

RICARDO BRESSANI • Division of Agricultural and Food Sciences, Institute of Nutrition of Central America and Panama, Guatemala City, Guatemala.

resulting when rats attack corn. These animals always consume the germ first, probably because this fraction is softer and of better nutritional value than the endosperm. People who depend on corn to feed themselves will not discard corn partially eaten by rats, and it is processed for consumption, with a corresponding loss in nutritive value since endosperm protein quality is very poor.

An example of the second consequence is represented by bean-hardening. Hard beans are very difficult to cook and the factors responsible for their hardening are not known. They could be genetic, environmental, or the result of poor after-harvest processing and preservation. Common bean losses in Central America during 1978 were estimated to be close to $12 million. However, due to their importance as a protein source for complementing cereal grains and as major dietary components, beans must be consumed. Before consumption, however, these foods must be cooked; recently harvested beans take about 2–2.5 hr to cook at atmospheric pressure, and in Guatemala it has been estimated that they require the energy from 2.5 kg of wood. The same quantity of hard beans under equal cooking conditions was not soft even after 6 hr of cooking, and had consumed the energy derived from 6.7 kg of wood. This difference in wood expenditure represents an additional cost in consuming an already high-priced food. Because of the high price paid for beans, cooking is continued even if they are hard; as a result, nutritive value begins to decrease due to the well-recognized effects of prolonged cooking on protein content.

Other examples come to mind. Moist corn deteriorates rapidly, because of both biochemical reactions taking place in the grain and fungal infestation. In Guatemala, for example, such materials are not discarded and people have learned how to process them. Processing conditions, however, are extreme, resulting in losses of vitamins and other nutrients.

Although not included within the usually accepted definition of post-harvest loss, there are other important losses that can be prevented. An example is the low digestibility of protein in common beans. This may be of genetic origin, or it may be due to poor after-harvest processing. In humans, protein digestibility in beans is of the order of about 60–65%. This means that of 22% protein in common beans, only about 13–14 g are absorbed and 8–9 g are excreted in feces. These 8–9 g of protein correspond to 37 g of beans, which not only have a high value but more or less represent the average daily intake per person. This loss also represents a very low efficiency in land utilization. The same argument applies to corn. Because of its low protein quality, of the 9 g of protein it contains, only 3–4 g are utilized. The difference could serve a more useful purpose if the quality were improved.

Finally, the concept of post-harvest loss should be amplified in developing countries. Our point of view is that of increasing the efficiency of utilization of the energy that has been introduced to produce a crop for the benefit of man. This means that efforts should be made to utilize, through appropriate processing, the energy left in the fields as stalks and leaves. These materials can very well serve to improve the production of ruminants or of products derived from ruminants. Food and nutrition policies should not concentrate on nutrition interventions *per se*, particularly for rural areas, where the main motivation should be to make land more productive for the family and the country.

Discussion

A fundamental theme throughout the discussion of food conservation was that food losses are context-specific (i.e., dependent upon the country, social customs, economic status), and can be considered at different levels (household, community, regional storage). It was emphasized that there is cultural variation with respect to defining food wastage. For example, there is a deeply-rooted Thai custom whereby it is considered improper for a guest to consume all of the food on the table. Therefore, in order to address the issue of food loss, social customs will have to be recognized, as well as technical causes.

In a similar vein, "open food dating" in the United States has become a societal custom or law that encourages high food wastage. Under this system, a product must be sold before a specific date, after which it is removed from the market shelf, even though it may not have begun to deteriorate.

It was also pointed out that another tangential reason for food loss figures being so high in the U.S. is the effort to incorporate losses that occur within the confines of the home into overall food loss estimates, a measurement often excluded from figures in other countries.

The need to focus on post-harvest food conservation efforts at the household and village level was emphasized throughout the discussion. This point is especially germane when one considers that in countries such as India, not more than 30% of the grain enters commercial channels. A logical conclusion of concentrating efforts in rural grain storage is the need to train people within countries to identify technology appropriate in the local setting. Indigenous experience and expertise are essential.

The importance of developing technologies that address post-harvest food losses at the local level was illustrated in reference to large government warehouses that store food grain. Generally, losses in these

facilities are high. Conversely, smaller, private warehouses are traditionally more successful in preventing loss. Thus, a reasonable solution is to
improve technology available to the local villager, rather than to develop
sophisticated new technologies for large-scale storage.

Interestingly, it was noted that the local, low-technology post-harvest treatment of food is largely the responsibility of women. Whether it
be to improve threshing or transport of grains, milling corn, or carrying
water, innovations that alleviate some of the arduous burdens of village
women are badly needed. Where technology such as the mechanized
milling of corn has been introduced, women have been able to enter the
mainstream of the economy. Small marketing and entrepreneurial enterprises can be formed as a result of the greater productivity afforded by
small-scale technology.

It has been argued that technological innovation may result in a loss
of employment for manual laborers, especially women. It is equally con-
ceivable, however, that a more rational and profitable post-harvest technology will increase the quantity, and especially the quality, of opportunities for women. It should be recognized, however, that women, like
men, are distributed among different social groups; thus, helping some
through new opportunities may be to the detriment of others.

Finally, the discussion stressed the need to provide economic incentives for changes in post-harvest technology. If farmers and millers are
convinced that it is in their best economic interest to improve harvesting
and processing procedures, more rapid reductions in post-harvest losses
will soon follow.

VII

Food Price Controls and Consumer Subsidies

Some of the most innovative food and nutrition policy initiatives during the last decade have been directed not so much at increasing the supply of food reaching those at risk of malnutrition as at expanding the effective economic demand of "at-risk" populations to purchase food in the marketplace. The two most common manifestations of such "demand-side" policies have been either to segregate low-income consumers in order to control the prices of the staples they purchase or to subsidize consumers directly (e.g., through food stamps) in order to expand their ability to obtain nutritious food commodities. While both approaches have shown substantial promise in both the developed and the developing world, each is also problematic in that it often requires considerable capital subsidies over long periods of time, either by governments or by external agencies.

In his issue paper, Timmer presents a penetrating analysis of the usefulness of "demand-side" intervention as a nutrition policy instrument. Country case experience with consumer subsidies is then presented for Pakistan by Rogers, for Egypt by Taylor, and for Mexico by Austin. In his discussant's comments, Carvalho da Silva also draws upon similar program experience from Brazil. The final discussion for this section examines both general and specific questions regarding the effectiveness of consumer price subsidies as a nutrition policy initiative.

22

Food Prices as a Nutrition Policy Instrument

C. Peter Timmer

Introduction

Most neoclassical economists are reluctant to encourage governments to intervene actively in the formation of prices for agricultural products. The markets for agricultural and food commodities tend to be competitive and efficient, even in much of the Third World. From the perspective of a Pareto Optimum, government interventions in such markets are likely to make matters worse rather than better, no matter what the motivation for intervention. The constant advice of economists to governments to "get prices right" is usually directed at government interventions that "make prices wrong." T. W. Schultz's latest book, *Distortions of Agricultural Incentives* (1), for example, provides an impressively long list of ways in which Third World governments intervene in agricultural input and output price formation, usually to the detriment of agricultural productivity and rural welfare.

This neoclassical perspective relies on an accumulating body of empirical evidence that demonstrates a positive and frequently enthusiastic response of Third World farmers to agricultural price incentives. Early evidence is summarized by Krishna (2), and more recently cross-country experience has been examined for long-run response patterns by Hayami and Ruttan (3), Timmer and Falcon (4,5), Thompson (6), and Peterson (7). The policy significance of this research has been the consistent message that agricultural price incentives will spur agricultural productivity growth so long as the incentives are positive rather than neg-

C. Peter Timmer • Harvard Business School, Boston, Massachusetts.

ative. And yet the same research has consistently shown that the poorest countries in greatest need of agricultural productivity growth have usually been those with the most *negative* farm price incentives.

Why? Schultz (1) attributes this strong tendency to weak politicians currying favor with the urban masses who clamor for cheap food, and to their in-house economic advisors who " . . . become 'yes-men' in the halls of political economy" (1, p. 9). But there is a more fundamental, and legitimate, reason as well. Although poorly understood empirically by economists, food prices play a major role in determining the protein–calorie intake of poor people. Whatever reason politicians think they have for attempting to keep cheap food readily available, to the extent they are successful they are also improving the short-run nutritional status of the poor. Such a price impact is not easily translatable into Pareto-type welfare discussions because of the explicit income redistribution consequences, but many societies are increasingly valuing nutritional improvements. Indeed, given the many problems involved with the implementation of specific target-oriented nutrition *programs* designed to cope with malnutrition among the poor, much interest now exists in the potential of nutrition-oriented food *policies* to reach this group more effectively and more cheaply.

A fairly obvious dilemma is set up by the dual potential of food price policy to achieve important social goals. Higher prices can help foster much-needed agricultural productivity growth. Lower prices improve the access of the poor to their basic calorie source. Only massive subsidies permit both policies to be pursued simultaneously, and few poor countries can follow this road for long. How does a government resolve this fundamental dilemma of modern political economies? Perhaps it is an academic response to argue that an understanding of the impact of food prices on production and consumption is an essential first step to a rational process of decision, but it is the only response an academic can make.

The effect of price on the production sector is much better understood than its effect on consumption, partly because it is easier to model the production decision empirically based on variants of profit maximization than to model consumer behavior empirically on the basis of utility maximization. The issues and evidence are reviewed elsewhere (8) and are not treated further here.

The process of tracing the impact of food price policy through food consumption to nutritional status draws its impetus from economic planners concerned about guaranteeing basic needs and from nutritionists concerned about the nutritional status of populations at risk. Several diverse threads of research have been reported, including those by Pinstrup-Andersen *et al.* (9,10), attempting to measure the consumption impact of neutral supply shifts by commodity and urban income class, or of shifts in income distribution; those of McCarthy and Taylor (11) and Taylor (12), who attempt to incorporate a food grain sector explicitly in a consistent macro-planning model disaggregated into three urban and three rural income strata; my own model (13) of the impact of food grain prices on the size of the calorie deficit in a Reutlinger–Selowsky (14) type of analysis; and attempts to estimate the parameters needed for this analysis (15,16).

TRACING FOOD PRICE POLICY IMPACT ON NUTRIENT INTAKE

The impact of food price changes is felt through one of three mechanisms: direct price effects on food consumption, exogenous income effects, and endogenous income effects (on farmers). The impact of a shift in food supply curves that lowers food prices on the calorie and protein intake of various income strata of urban households in Cali, Colombia, has already been examined by Pinstrup-Andersen *et al.* (9). This is the simplest of all possible policy effects to trace out because there is a single chain of causation from food supply policy through price effects to nutrition (i.e., consumption) impacting on the urban households. Even so, the methodology requires a full own- and cross-price elasticity matrix by income strata to translate food price changes into income strata-specific consumption changes, and a full set of market equations is required to translate neutral supply shifts into price changes.

Extending the analysis to other vulnerable groups—the landless rural poor or subsistence-oriented small farmers—adds an entirely new dimension to the complexity of the impact. Exogenous income effects via changed employment patterns and opportunities, and endogenous income effects for farmers because of output and price changes, must be added to the direct price effects. Income strata-specific income elasticities are needed to translate the income changes into consumption changes. Much more difficult are the corresponding functional relationships that translate the policy changes into income strata-specific income changes.

The translation of policy change into resulting effects on prices and incomes must be done in the specific political, social, and economic context of the change itself. For instance, any price changes caused by a shift in supply will depend on whether the country is an importer or exporter, the state of the marketing sector, and existing institutional mechanisms of price formation. Similarly, the indirect income effects of a price change will depend on the extent of open or disguised unemployment, the choice of technique in processing and distribution, and mechanisms of wage formation. It is difficult to generalize about these in the absence of a significant number of reliable agricultural sector models capable of tracing through price and income effects by income class. No such models exist at present, although several models are able to trace these effects without disaggregating income.

OBTAINING THE CONSUMPTION PARAMETERS

Regardless of the subgroup or type of policy being considered, at the heart of the analysis is a matrix of price and income elasticities that must be income strata-specific. Obtaining this matrix for aggregated income classes requires a blend of complex theory and sophisticated data analysis that is only possible with restrictive assumptions about the separability of the impact of price changes for one commodity class on changes in demand for other commodity groups (17).

The separability assumptions are quite restrictive, even in the context of such highly aggregated commodities such as food, housing, and clothing. But when important nutrition effects occur because one quality of wheat is substituted for another, or cassava is substituted for rice, then the level of commodity detail needed to reproduce the impact of relative price changes accurately forecloses the "econometric" approach even for combined income classes. Obtaining the necessary price and income elasticity for disaggregated income classes requires innovations in modeling consumer reactions to price and income changes.

One approach is direct empirical investigation via commodity-by-commodity estimation of income-class-specific parameters for both income and price changes, using highly detailed cross-section household food expenditure surveys. However, such research should not be seeking "the" correct set of income and price coefficients for each commodity for each income class so much as the functional relationships behind each of the parameters in the Slutsky equation:

$$e_{ij}^h = \epsilon_{ij}^h - \alpha_j^h E_i^h$$

where e_{ij}^h is the total demand elasticity for commodity i when commodity j price changes, for the hth household (or hth income group); ϵ_{ij}^h is the compensated (Slutsky) demand elasticity for i,j as above; α_j^h is the budget share of commodity j for household h (or income group h); and E_i^h is the Engel (income) elasticity for commodity i for household h (or income group h).* Income appears to be the most powerful variable in functional specification of systematic variation in e_{ij}^h and E_i^h, but other economic, social, and cultural variables are also likely to be significant. For example, the Engel elasticity for rice will of course depend on the household income, but also on the traditional role of rice in the diet of the region and the availability of other basic foods such as cassava and maize. Empirical results surveyed so far indicate that this is a promising avenue of research (18).

PRICE INTERVENTIONS WITH NUTRITIONAL GOALS

The first step in a solution to global malnutrition lies in increasing the food intake of the poor. Most village-level nutritional surveys have found that where energy intake is adequate, then protein needs are also satisfied. The possible exceptions are areas where bulky root crops provide the basic energy source, but even in such environments increasing food availability among the poor, including more food from roots and, their dietary accompaniments, is likely to improve rather than to impair nutritional status (19).

The means to increase food intake include food fortification, institutional feeding, nutrition education, and, most importantly, nutrition-oriented food policies. The policy approach aims at guaranteeing to the poor access to an adequate food package by keeping the cost low. The important issue is whether social costs can also be kept low, or whether large and expensive subsidies will be necessary to guarantee adequate food intake by the poor.

Empirical evidence of the sort now available for Indonesia (15,16) is demonstrating that the poor are quite sensitive to calorie prices in determining how much food they consume. This is not surprising in terms of the large share of their budgets devoted to purchasing (or growing) food. The notion that much hunger and malnutrition are attributable to inefficient allocation of household resources is probably not generally true for the very poor. However, two areas do exist where improved household decision making could lead to improved nutritional status without substantial increments in household financial resources.

First, as their incomes increase, the poor may increase calorie intake,

---

*The notation used here is identical to that used in Timmer (18). Partly on the basis of Indonesian results, that paper demonstrates the likelihood of a functional relationship between e_{ij}^h and E_i^h, both as a function of log a^h, i.e., of the logarithm of total household expenditures or income.

but they also tend to purchase higher-quality (i.e., higher-priced) calories. In the case of Brazil, World Bank research indicates that increases in the purchasing power of the poor in urban centers did not seem to cause increased caloric intake, but rather led almost entirely to the purchase of higher-priced calories. Although the nutritional (and social) value of such higher-quality energy sources may be better—rice rather than cassava, wheat instead of millet—if energy intakes remain relatively less adequate than protein intakes, which is typically the case, then nutritional status will not improve as rapidly per dollar of increased income as it would if the original food patterns were merely extended in quantity. The role here for appropriate nutrition education is obvious, but what should be conveyed is that the composition of poor people's diets is good and that emphasis within the household and within the planning agency should be on magnifying quantities consumed by the poor. Where such diets contain low-status foods such as roots and coarse grains, this advice runs counter to deeply held prejudices in both the nutrition and planning community.

The second source of inefficient household decision making is in the distribution of foods within a household. A pattern of withholding food from children in order to feed working adults better is not likely to be efficient from a social point of view, and any educational input into households with serious constraints on food availability should be aimed at redirecting some food resources to pregnant and lactating mothers and to weaning-age and toddler children.

The Nutrition and Basic Needs paper of the World Bank (20) argues that poverty-linked hunger and malnutrition are: (1) not just a function of low average per capita incomes in a country, nor (2) likely to disappear in the course of the economic growth expected to occur over the next generation in the absence of very substantial structural and policy changes that would drastically alter the role of the poor in the production process. Because most countries are reluctant or unable to make such substantial changes, the search for ways to eliminate malnutrition within two or three decades must focus on the causes of the wide variation observed in nutritional status among quite poor countries and regions. The result is a scramble to understand how Kerala, Sri Lanka, China, Cuba, Taiwan, South Korea, and a few other countries have managed to achieve low rates of infant mortality and high life expectancy—proxies for good nutritional status among the poor—at low per capita income levels.

Two general patterns emerge. In both a relatively "good" pattern of income distribution exists. In the first pattern, such incomes are rising rapidly, and access to food is maintained by careful supply management of macro food markets with little effort made to make food a public rather than a private good. Thus, well-distributed and rapidly rising incomes, plus attention to the macro food situation, seem sufficient to eliminate most hunger and malnutrition, as the cases of Taiwan and South Korea indicate.

In the second pattern, incomes are also relatively evenly distributed, but they are not growing rapidly. In this situation it has been necessary for the governments to manage food distribution in a much more activist fashion, thus converting food into a near-public good. Programs take the form of free or subsidized direct distribution (Sri Lanka), or differential access to ration shops where basic foods are highly subsidized for the poor (Kerala in India, Cuba). China seems to be an intermediate case, where urban rationing in recent years serves more to control mobility and provide control of macro food supplies than to serve the poor directly.*

These two patterns demonstrate the dilemma of eliminating malnutrition without major structural and policy changes in a society. For those societies (of which Korea and Taiwan are examples) where the incomes of the poor will grow rapidly and where reasonably competent supply management is undertaken, the problem will take care of itself. But there are very few such countries. For those countries where growth has been slow or where the poor have been, and are likely to continue to be, excluded from the benefits of the growth process (or will participate at no more than the average rate), activist food policies and distribution programs will be required. However, the evidence so far is that these programs are quite expensive, are difficult to manage and administer, and may divert sufficient resources and distort farm incentives so that the growth process is seriously impaired. The dilemma posed by subsidized food consumption for the poor, while attempts are made to maintain adequate price incentives for food producers, is especially difficult in a single-staple food economy attempting efficient budgetary management. The temptation to use imports, especially if available on concessionary terms, to cover shortages and to use low farm prices as a means of controlling budgetary costs is frequently irresistible.

It is here that a nutrition-oriented food policy perspective may

---

*Although relatively little research has been directed to the nutritional impact of these different food price subsidy schemes, a start has been made, primarily at the International Food Policy Research Institute (IFPRI) and the World Bank. For sources that deal with the question at least indirectly, see references 21–27.

reveal greater degrees of freedom for policy intervention by focusing on actual consumption patterns of the poor. In nearly all poor countries that are not significant grain exporters, the poor consume different staple foods from those consumed by the middle class and the rich. Attention to biological research, production, and marketing of these staples may offer the opportunity for self-targeting food programs that reach primarily the poor at little enforcement cost.

Even where this is true, however, subsidies may still be essential if the poor are to increase their food intake significantly. Reducing enforcement costs by using self-targeting foodstuffs addresses only half the problem of targeted deliveries to the poor. The other half of the problem is the sheer lack of income that requires subsidies if the goods and services are to reach the truly poor in sufficient quantities to have a meaningful welfare impact. Clearly, by subsidizing commodities only the poor wish to consume, the overall fiscal burden will be smaller than it would be if more popular commodities were chosen and freely available at the subsidized price. Correspondingly, the policy base of support for such a program will also be substantially narrowed. Keeping rice prices cheap in Indonesia is enormously popular and it does help the poor. Subsidizing maize and cassava prices while allowing rice prices to rise substantially will not be popular even if it does help the poor more. Eliminating the direct rice distribution program for the military and civil servants (a program that is in addition to keeping the general rice price level below international levels) will be equally unpopular with an important political constituency and will help satisfy the basic needs of the poor only indirectly (through differential availability of budget resources).

Cross-subsidy programs can probably work effectively in the food area. Because of substantially different income and price elasticities by income class for important foodstuffs and different qualities of those foodstuffs, the opportunity exists to subsidize, for example, low-quality broken rice while extracting a premium on higher quality rice or for preferred varieties. The same cross-subsidy could also be used across foodstuffs, e.g., by subsidizing cassava from proceeds of high-priced wheat or rice. It must be emphasized, however, that there is very little positive concrete country experience from which to learn in this area of food price subsidies. The existing record is not encouraging, as subsidies typically accrue primarily to urban middle classes, or low urban prices are enforced uniformly at the expense of adequate farm incentives. The real social costs of a cheap food policy can be significant if the poor do not participate adequately in the benefits of increased consumption. If they do, then redesigning the food policy to ensure both adequate incentives and adequate food intake is a complicated undertaking not to be rushed under the flag of "getting prices right."

IMPLEMENTATION ISSUES

Food prices are a blunt instrument for improving nutrient intake. When food prices work *against* the objective of greater food consumption by the poor, sectoral programs and targeted delivery schemes with the same goals are likely to be ineffective or costly in their effectiveness. Similarly, however, the more precise instruments are likely to gain measurably in effectiveness and efficiency in the context of a conducive price policy. As a matter of *strategy*, then, implementation of food price policy interventions should be coordinated with planned interventions at other levels of the problem. The strategic discussions must deal with four basic requirements for a successful intervention to improve nutritional status: (1) the demand requirement, (2) the supply requirement, (3) the delivery requirement, and (4) the sustainability requirement. Intersecting these four program requirements are four levels of strategic design:

- Structural changes leading to significant asset redistribution and to more equitable functional income distribution, thus providing the poor with better access to food because of long-term improvements in real purchasing power.
- Policy changes in the macro-environment that affect the rate of economic growth, the degree of participation of the poor in that growth, and further improvements in real purchasing power.
- Sectoral interventions designed specifically to improve the access of the poor to basic goods and services, such as a well-designed and managed rural health program or agricultural development program designed for small farmers.
- Targeted delivery systems for either single commodities or integrated basic needs packages focused on the needs of the poor.

The essence of a package-oriented targeted delivery strategy of meeting the needs of the poor is that the first three requirements are intimately interlinked. At its simplest, such a strategy succeeds because delivered supply creates its own demand. However, the welfare-oriented, transfer nature of this simple strategy has raised justifiable concerns in poor countries over its impact on economic growth and over the long-run sustainability of the recurring fiscal burden. Hence, the problem of meeting all four requirements simultaneously directs the discussion to the four levels of the strategy ladder. How far up that ladder is a society willing to climb to ensure that the nutrient needs of all citizens are met?

Higher levels of strategic design should subsume the lower-level issues and strategies, not vice versa. It is perfectly feasible (at least in the short run) to pursue a package approach at the village level without any broader concerns for sectoral strategy, policy setting, or asset redistribution and functional changes in income distribution. Efficient sectoral interventions are likely to require integration with package approaches if the poor are actually to be reached and benefited, but such sectoral/package strategies can be implemented without macro-policy or income distribution changes. Similarly, a nutrition-oriented macro-policy set will require appropriate sectoral and package interventions to be effective. Also, income redistribution, especially through asset redistributions such as land reform, is unlikely to have a lasting or even short-run impact on the poor without simultaneous attention to policy, sectoral, and packaging/delivery issues.

A package approach alone is widely seen as a purely palliative attempt to help the poor without disturbing any of the basic mechanisms that cause poverty in the first place. However, in many situations, palliatives are the very best that can be achieved, and the alternative is not more effective structural or policy reforms but doing nothing at all for the poor. Efficient palliatives in the form of well-designed and -delivered packages of basic food and health services can be justified on welfare grounds alone, but the sustainability issue is serious if satisfying the needs of the poor does not have a longer-run productivity effect through the creation of human capital.

This productivity effect depends critically on the policy (and possibly on the structural) context of the sectoral and package programs that supply basic needs to the poor. In the right macro-policy environment, investment by society and by the poor themselves in the development of human capital for the poor will be repaid by productive opportunities to find remunerative employment. With the wrong macro-policy environment, not only will the labor power of the poor be largely redundant in a remunerative sense, but so also will their new skills and productivity potential. In such a context, the long-run sustainability of the simple palliative approach is highly dubious.

On the other hand, such an approach does not require drastic changes at a structural level as a precursor to meeting nutritional goals. The strategy is appealing for those societies with genuine concern for the welfare of the poor, but without either the political commitment or administrative and analytical capacity to carry out meaningful redistribution leading to new functional income distributions. This bottom-up, gradualist approach to pulling the poor back into the mainstream of society is very appealing to outside donors and to the personnel in the planning agencies of most countries where gradualist (marginal) thinking is deeply instilled by the nature of their academic preparation.

The other basic strategic approach is from the top down via significant changes in asset redistribution as the first step. Apart from the political difficulties with such an approach (both internally and from the point of view of outside donors), Griffin and James (28) argue quite forcibly that the supply management of the public and private goods, especially food, in any basic needs package will be extremely difficult in the face of significant income redistribution.

This does not argue that asset redistribution or other mechanisms for changing income distribution will fail to improve the status of the poor. On the contrary, such structural changes, in combination with coordinated policy, sectoral, and package approaches, are the only fairly certain road to meeting basic consumption needs for all elements of a society. To say this, however, is to say merely that Utopia is Utopia. Donors and governments have precious little experience in these matters.

DELIVERY ISSUES

The delivery issues can be treated in parallel with implementation issues as a sequence of topics that start with macro-strategic concerns and end with very micro-target focus issues. At the top, the primary issue is the appropriate mix of public sector versus private sector interventions, and a major strategic question is whether food should become more of a public good. In other related sectors, delivery of health, water, sanitation, and education interventions might be more effective if the private sector were more involved than has traditionally been the case.

Two issues are important. First, if *public* delivery to the poor of food and other basic-need goods and services is to be expanded, then major efforts at building the public institutions charged with this responsibility will be needed. This will mean building a new direction and mission into these public institutions. Reaching the poor has not been the strong suit of many Third World public agencies (or of their supporting donors), and institution-building with a focus on reaching the poor will not be easy, and will almost certainly not be achieved by legislative mandate.

The importance of participatory involvement of the beneficiaries themselves at various levels of the identification, planning, and implementation stages of the basic needs program should not be overlooked.

In fact, positive efforts to ensure such participation have resulted in success in many programs, whereas the absence of such participation has been credited with the failure of other programs.

Second, to the extent that private markets will be used as the most efficient vehicles for delivery, the primary public responsibility will be to ensure careful supply management on the macro side. Thus, both short-run and long-run planning of food supplies in the market place will be essential if direct public food deliveries to the poor are not contemplated. Such reliance on the private market for distribution will also mean a public responsibility for micro-demand management, which obviously implies an effective government concern for generating basic purchasing power for the poor. The obvious link between the macro-planning needed on the supply side and the micro-effective-demand management will be the prices of the various commodities.

Balancing the need for price incentives against impact on demand by the poor may require price subsidies. Subsidy schemes for consumption goods have a justifiably bad reputation for not reaching the poor, with most benefits going to the urban middle class. Using public subsidies to meet the food needs of the poor will require either much more carefully targeted distribution schemes, with their attendant high enforcement and administration costs, or more careful choice of what will be subsidized.

This choice has three major components: (1) What products should be offered to the poor, what should their "quality" be, and what standards of "acceptability" should be used to make the choice? (2) How should the products be produced, processed, and distributed, and how can program design ensure that appropriate technology will be used? (3) What kinds of institutions will be needed to implement strategies that contain both appropriate products for the poor and appropriate techniques for production? This third question encompasses the first two and raises directly the issues of the availability of technical assistance capable of providing appropriate rather than inappropriate solutions, as well as training programs that will have the same effect.

The appropriate technology movement has centered on these issues as the essence of the bias against reaching the poor inherent in most current development efforts. There can be no doubt that enormous biases exist in Third World planning agencies and in the donor community that work against both the products the poor consume and the labor-intensive, participative techniques that are likely to be the most appropriate way to produce them. Enforcing middle-class or elite standards of acceptance on the food, health care, shelter, education, and sanitation standards "permissible" for the poor to consume in greater quantities is perhaps the single greatest factor preventing the poor from enlarging their consumption share.

Breaking out of this pattern will require much more sensitive attention to the actual consumption patterns of the poor and to the degree to which these patterns change when the causal variables—income, prices, knowledge, household location—change. In addition to understanding in greater detail what the poor consume, it will be important to determine the sources of their incomes in functional terms. It is likely that much of the income the poor earn will be from activities that are highly sensitive to displacement by less labor-intensive techniques or products. Lack of attention to which techniques or products the society will produce, even as basic needs for the poor themselves, can easily undo, from the income-generation side, all the good being done on the supply management side.

Three levels of important linkages exist among sectoral programs designed to improve the delivery of food to the poor: (1) the planning level, (2) program coordination, and (3) field integration.

Macroeconomic and social planning has four major responsibilities in this context: management of aggregate economic output via the macro-production function; an interactive relationship with sectoral planners; a joint concern with sectoral planners for macro-supply management, implemented partially via pricing mechanisms; and an input into micro-demand management for food and those other "basic needs" sectors where private markets are an important component of the delivery system. Here the input is partially direct, through management of the macro-production function and influences over prices, and quite roundabout, via sectoral and field-level interventions.

Sectoral program coordination requires that each sectoral plan be made in the context of all other sectoral plans to enable two important kinds of synergistic effects to be captured. First, locating and functionally identifying the poor in need of assistance can be quite difficult and expensive. There is little rationale for separate studies by sectoral planning offices when the likely result will be a common target group. Second, the coordination required among all the basic needs sectors for field interventions to be effective can only be instigated at the sectoral planning level.

Integration of field delivery programs is the third level where program linkages are important. Little empirical evidence exists that there are major economies of scale, but this may be because few programs have successfully reached the poor with an entire bundle of basic needs, goods, and services. To have done so *without* field-level integration of staff and facilities is likely to have been prohibitively expensive.

A Food Policy Orientation

Many food-deficient, poor countries urgently need higher real food grain prices as an incentive to millions of small farmers to raise their agricultural productivity through adoption of modern technology. But those same higher, incentive food grain prices will have a disproportionate impact on food consumption of the poor. Many of these people are already suffering from inadequate protein–calorie intake, and further reduction in their food consumption may mean serious malnutrition or death.

This food policy dilemma has been resolved historically in two ways. First, food grain imports are used to fill the gap between inadequate domestic production and consumption levels generated by low food prices. Second, in some countries prices of the preferred food grain have been raised as an incentive to domestic farmers while secondary grains and root crops have been kept cheap, even subsidized, to protect the poor. The "substitute opportunities" increase a government's degrees of freedom to deal with this fundamental food policy dilemma.

Policy analysis in multi-staple-food economies is obviously much more complex than in single food grain economies. The consumption picture becomes more complicated because of the need to know multiple own-price effects by income class, and cross-price effects also become important. The production side is made more complicated by the substitute possibilities if they are produced domestically. Planning intensification programs for rice, for example, when maize, wheat, or barley are alternatives, requires a complex balancing of output price incentives, input subsidies, credit programs, and development of suitable seed and production technologies. Attempts to raise rice prices to increase production while keeping maize prices low to protect poor consumers may simply be frustrated by the substitution options and the level of alternative technologies unless dual price systems with extensive subsidies can be implemented.

The complications extend to the import and domestic marketing areas. Planning food grain imports, especially if much of the grain will be available under food aid terms, is far more complicated if several grains are being imported (or some exported) and changes at the margin in their rate of substitution are being attempted. On the domestic side, the marketing structure for the preferred grain, typically rice or wheat, is usually much more fully developed than that for secondary grains and root crops. The latter are frequently treated as inferior foods, produced primarily for subsistence, that deserve little government attention to production, marketing, or consumption.

A number of important countries with large populations now seem unable to increase the availability of favored food grains fast enough to meet market demand at constant prices, not to mention the latent nutritional demand that would be forthcoming at significantly lower prices. In the absence of massive food aid transfers, these countries will have to seek food grain substitutes for the poorest parts of their populations until long-term investment in agricultural infrastructure, made profitable by higher incentive prices for the preferred food grain, begins to transform the domestic production outlook.

A differential price policy by commodity, even if it includes direct subsidies on those foodstuffs, such as cassava and maize, that are consumed primarily by the poor as a means of implementing the policy, offers the potential to "target" the nutritional impact without many of the associated enforcement costs and leakages of target-oriented programs using more preferred foods. Such a strategy calls for high political commitment to increasing the access of the poor to adequate food, but it may also be the only financially feasible way of coping with protein-calorie malnutrition over the next several decades.

The high analytical costs of such a multicommodity price policy must be compared with the costs of subsidizing food consumption for much of the population, or attempting to manage target-oriented food distributions. The combination of high analytical and political costs is not attractive, but neither are the alternatives.

REFERENCES

1. Schultz, T. W. (Ed.). *Distortions of Agricultural Incentives.* Indiana University Press, Bloomington, Indiana, 1978.
2. Krishna, R. Agricultural price policy. In: *Agricultural Development and Economic Growth,* H. M. Southworth and B. F. Johnston (Eds.). Cornell University Press, Ithaca, New York, 1967.
3. Hayami, Y., and V. Ruttan. *Agricultural Development: An International Perspective.* Johns Hopkins University Press, Baltimore, Maryland, 1971.
4. Timmer, C. P., and W. P. Falcon. The political economy of rice production and trade in Asia. In: *Agriculture in Development Theory,* L. Reynolds (Ed.). Yale University Press, New Haven, Connecticut, 1975.
5. Timmer, C. P., and W. P. Falcon. The impact of price on rice trade in Asia. In: *Trade, Agriculture and Development,* G. S. Tolley and P. A. Zadrozny (Eds.). Ballinger Publishing, Cambridge, Massachusetts, 1975.
6. Lyons, D. C., and R. L. Thompson. The Effect of Relative Prices on Corn Productivity and Exports: A Cross-Country Study. Draft Journal Article, Department of Agricultural Economics, Boston University, November, 1977.
7. Peterson, W. International farm prices and the social cost of cheap food policies. *Am. J. Agric. Econ.* 61 (1):12, 1979.

8. Timmer, C. P. Food prices and food policy analysis. *Food Policy*, August, 1980.
9. Pinstrup-Andersen, P., N. R. de Londoño, and E. Hoover. The impact of increasing food supply on human nutrition: Implications for commodity priorities in agricultural research and policy. *Am. J. Agric. Econ.* **58**:131, 1976.
10. Pinstrup-Andersen, P., and E. Caicedo. The potential impact of changes in income distribution on food demand and human nutrition. *Am. J. Agric. Econ.* **60**:402, 1978.
11. McCarthy, F. D., and L. Taylor, Macro food policy planning: A general equilibrium model for Pakistan. *Rev. Econ. Statist.* **62** (1):107, 1980.
12. Taylor, L. Price Policy and the Food People Consume. Mimeo, Massachusetts Institute of Technology, Cambridge, Massachusetts, 1978.
13. Timmer, C. P. Food price policy and protein–calorie intake: Issues and methodology. Mimeograph, 1978.
14. Reutlinger, S., and M. Selowsky. *Malnutrition and Poverty: Magnitude and Policy Options.* World Bank Staff Occasional Papers No. 23, Johns Hopkins University Press, Baltimore, Maryland, 1976.
15. Alderman, H., and C. P. Timmer. Food price policy and protein–calorie intake: Estimating consumption parameters for Indonesia. In: *Development Issues in Indonesia*, S. M. Gillis and C. P. Timmer (Eds.). OGH Publishers, Cambridge, Massachusetts (in press).
16. Timmer, C. P., and H. Alderman. Estimating consumption parameters for food policy analysis. *Am. J. Agric. Econ.* **61**:982, 1979.
17. Frisch, R. A complete scheme for computing all direct and cross-demand elasticities in a model with many sectors. *Econometrica* **27** (2):1959.
18. Timmer, C. P. Is there "curvature" in the Slutsky matrix? *Rev. Econ. Statist.* **62**(3):395–402.
19. Payne, P. R. Safe protein–calorie ratios in diets: The relative importance of protein and energy intake as causal factors in malnutrition. *Am. J. Clin. Nutr.* **28**:281, 1975.
20. International Bank for Reconstruction and Development (World Bank). *Nutrition and Basic Needs.* World Bank, Washington, D.C., July, 1979.
21. Ahmed, R. *Foodgrain Supply, Distribution, and Consumption Policies within a Dual Pricing Mechanism: A Case Study of Bangladesh.* International Food Policy Research Institute (IFPRI) Research Report No. 8, Washington, D.C., May 1979.
22. Gavan, J. The Calorie Energy Gap in Bangladesh and Strategies for Reducing It. Paper read at the Conference on Nutrition-Oriented Food Policies and Programs, Bellagio, Italy, August 1977.
23. George, P. S. *Public Distribution of Foodgrains in Kerala—Income Distribution Implications and Effectiveness.* International Food Policy Research Institute (IFPRI) Report No. 7, March 1979.
24. Kumar, S. K. *Impact of Subsidized Rice on Food Consumption and Nutrition in Kerala.* International Food Policy Research Institute (IFPRI) Report No. 5, January 1979.
25. Rogers, B., and F. J. Levinson. *Subsidized Food Consumption in Low-Income Countries: The Pakistan Experience.* International Nutrition Planning Program, Discussion Paper No. 6, Massachusetts Institute of Technology, Cambridge, Massachusetts, April 1976.
26. Swamy, G. Public Food Distribution in India. AGREP Division Working Paper, International Bank for Reconstruction and Development (World Bank) Working Paper, July 1979. World Bank, Washington, D.C.
27. Timmer, C. P. Food policy in China. *Food Research Institute Studies* **16**:1, 1976.
28. Griffin, K., and J. James. Supply Management Problems in the Context of a Basic Needs Strategy. Unpublished draft, IBRD, 1979.

Consumer Food Price Subsidies in Pakistan

BEATRICE LORGE ROGERS

INTRODUCTION

Consumer food price subsidies have been a feature of Pakistan's economy since World War II. They operate through a system of government-licensed, privately owned ration shops that sell fixed quantities of wheat and sugar. They were initiated, not in response to an existing nutritional need, but as a way of allocating essential consumer items in the face of wartime shortages of goods and transport. The system has persisted to the present, however, with beneficial results for the level of food consumption of the population.

The Pakistani system of food price subsidies provides a useful demonstration of the fact that price subsidies in themselves are neither bad nor good, useless or beneficial, wasteful or cost-effective. Rather, these aspects of a program of subsidies vary according to the characteristics of the subsidized foods, the mechanism by which the subsidy is provided, and the manner in which the subsidized food is distributed and marketed.

In this chapter, Pakistan's consumer food price subsidy system will be used as an example to show, first, how the design of a program can

The results reported in this paper are based on data collected as part of the Pakistan Micronutrient Survey of 1976, a national-level nutrition survey undertaken by the Nutrition Cell, Planning Division, Government of Pakistan, using funds from the Planning Division and from the U.S. Agency for International Development. A more complete presentation of these results may be found in references 1 and 2.

BEATRICE LORGE ROGERS • International Nutrition Program, Massachusetts Institute of Technology, Cambridge, Massachusetts.

affect its cost and its effectiveness and, second, that a policy that was not adopted for nutritional reasons can nonetheless have considerable effect on nutrition. First, a brief history of the program will be presented; then the program will be described, and the design features of interest to planners will be discussed. Finally, the effect of the subsidy on food consumption and nutritional status will be estimated.

HISTORY OF THE RATION SHOP SYSTEM[*]

The ration system was established in Pakistan by the British in 1942 to deal with shortages of goods caused by the war. Fixed quantities of certain staple consumption items, including wheat, sugar, tea, matches, kerosene, yarn, and cotton cloth were sold through ration shops that were privately owned and operated, but supplied by means of government procurement. Because the shops were not set up as a welfare measure, no criteria of eligibility for the ration were established. Quantities that could be purchased were fixed on a per capita basis, without regard to income or other indicators of need. This feature of the ration system has not changed, and is probably one source of its political strength.

After partition in 1947, the ration system was continued as a means of controlling hoarding and profiteering on goods that were still scarce. Between 1947 and 1950 food grains were in plentiful supply. Wheat prices fell, and rationing was abandoned. At the same time, a minimum support price was set to benefit farmers, and the wheat that the government procured through this guaranteed price scheme was distributed through the ration system. During this period, the government controlled all trade in food grains; private sales were not allowed.

Later in the 1950s, grain became scarce as domestic production failed to keep pace with population growth. The ration system was still operating, and rationing was reintroduced. This cycle has been repeated: in the early 1960s, grain was plentiful and there was no quantity limit on ration shop sales of wheat; later in that decade supplies became scarce and rationing was once again imposed.

In 1959, as an incentive to grain production, the government abandoned its monopoly on the grain trade. From then until the present, a free market in wheat has coexisted with the ration system: the government enters the market competitively as a buyer of domestically produced wheat.

Distribution of sugar through the ration shops was started during

[*]This information is presented in greater detail in reference 3.

the Korean War, when high demand for textile fibers shifted domestic production away from sugar, creating a shortage. In 1972, the government took control of the sugar market, prohibiting exports in order to keep supplies in the country, and prohibiting imports to prevent the drain of foreign exchange. The ration system has been used to ensure equitable distribution of the limited amount of sugar available in the country. No free trade in sugar is allowed.

In 1972 and 1973, the ration shops were used to distribute vegetable oil at fixed prices, in response to a severe shortage. Oil is now freely available on the open market.

The point to note in this brief history is that the ration system has served a number of different purposes. When there was no need for market intervention, the system operated simply as another set of retail food stores. During periods of scarcity or high price, the government was able to make use of the shops to administer its policies of rationing and price control. The flexibility of the ration system, which has handled varying commodities, changing prices, and different quantity limits, has contributed both to its usefulness and to its viability.

At present, the ration system embodies a considerable amount of administrative expertise; the logistics of supply and distribution are well established; shops are widely available throughout the country. Furthermore, the ration and subsidy program is highly visible and has a strong political constituency. For all these reasons, it is worthwhile to investigate the program to determine what its benefits are and whether there may be ways to improve it, because it is unlikely to be disbanded, and has the potential for reaching a large proportion of Pakistan's population.

PRESENT OPERATION OF THE RATION SHOPS

MANAGEMENT

The ration shops are privately owned and run. Shop owners are licensed by the provincial government. They obtain their supplies from provincial warehouses, and they may purchase only enough to fill the quotas of the number of households registered with their shops. They buy at fixed prices and sell at a fixed mark-up. Interestingly, most of the profit the shop owners make is derived from the sale of the bags in which the wheat and sugar are supplied. These are provided free by the central government. Obviously, shop owners have an incentive to pad their lists of registered recipients, since the more they sell, the more they earn.

There is evidence that considerable padding does take place. For example, in 1974 the city of Karachi had a registered ration population of 5.1 million and a census population of only about 3.5 million (4).

Procurement of wheat and sugar for the ration system is a central government responsibility, and it is the central government that provides the price subsidy, but the operation of the ration system is controlled by the provincial governments. The central government purchases supplies at the support price and releases them to the provinces at the subsidized price. The provinces distribute supplies among their warehouses, where they are sold to shop owners for retail distribution.

The advantage of this system is that operation of the shops is decentralized; each shop owner is responsible for setting up and staffing his own shop and managing his own inventory, so demands on the administrative capacity of the government are reduced. Also, the incentives of the ration system, like those of the free market, encourage people to set up shops in underserved areas where they will have more customers, and to provide for the convenience of customers by means of adequate staff and hours of operation.

Licensing of shop owners is a political favor, because the potential for profit as a shop owner is high. This is probably another reason for the large number and wide distribution of shops, since it is to the benefit of locally influential politicians to dispense such favors as often as they can.

As a result of these incentives, coverage of the population by the ration shop system is remarkably high. In urban areas, better than 99% of the population has a ration shop within an hour's walking distance; well over 90% can reach a shop in less than an hour. There are some rural areas in which no ration shop is available, and the people there are deprived of the benefits of the subsidy. These areas tend to be the most remote and difficult to reach, which probably means that the people living there are among the neediest as well.

On the whole, though, coverage is excellent. Although government policy is to have one shop for every 3000 people, average availability is higher than that, ranging from one shop for 1326 people (urban Northwest Frontier) to one shop for 1878 people (rural Sind). These figures are based on number of shops compared with census figures for the region, not on the registered ration recipients, so the number of potential recipients should not be overstated.

RATIONED COMMODITIES

Two commodities are distributed by the ration system: whole wheat flour (called atta) and refined sugar. These commodities provide a sharp contrast, both in terms of their consumption patterns by the population and in terms of their distribution. In fact, one could almost think of the distribution of rationed wheat and sugar as two distinct systems, even though they use the same shops and procurement mechanisms.

Wheat and Atta

Wheat, consumed mainly in the form of unleavened bread called chapatis, is the dietary staple of Pakistan. It provides low-income households (lowest 5% of the population; those with monthly incomes under Rs. 100 or U.S. $10.00) with 51% of their calories and 66% of their protein, and absorbs 36% of their income (5). Even at high-income levels, wheat consumption predominates: per capita consumption is not much different in above or below median-income groups. As is characteristic of a food staple, however, the income share devoted to wheat falls off as income rises. The price and income elasticities* of demand for wheat are relatively high in low-income groups, but fall with rising income. At a household income level of Rs 900 per month (U.S. $90), well above the median, income elasticity of demand for wheat is negative. This means that, at this level, people actually reduce their consumption of wheat if they have more money. The reason for this behavior is that wheat has some of the characteristics of an inferior good: those who can afford to prefer to buy other foods (meat, poultry, and milk, for example) rather than to consume more wheat.

This is an advantage from the point of view of the nutrition planner. Presumably the target group for a food price subsidy is the low-income population, since the poor are most likely to be nutritionally needy. To control the cost of a subsidy program, one would like the benefits to reach the target group, but not the nonneedy population. To the extent that the relatively well-off population chooses not to consume a subsidized food, leakages are minimized, and the cost-effectiveness ratio of

---

*Elasticities of demand are a measure of how responsive demand for a good is to changes in price or income. The price elasticity of demand is the percent by which demand changes in response to a 1% change in price. Price elasticities are usually negative, since when prices go up demand usually goes down. Similarly, income elasticity of demand measures changes in response to a 1% change in income. For most goods, income elasticities are positive, because when incomes go up people can and do buy more. Income elasticities are negative, however, for inferior goods, because as soon as people can afford to, they stop buying the inferior good and start to buy a higher-quality substitute. The concept of elasticity of demand was developed to deal with aggregate demand figures, not household demand. It is a relative, not an absolute, measure. If very little of an item is consumed, then even if income elasticity is very high and the quantity demanded doubles with a given income change, the absolute amount consumed may still be very small.

the program is improved. The same effect can be achieved by restricting eligibility for the program to those with incomes below a given level, but this entails complex administration and opens the door to corruption. Also, such restriction is likely to be politically unpopular in a program that was once open to all. These problems may be avoided if the commodity chosen for subsidy leads to voluntary targeting.

Wheat itself shows this characteristic only mildly. Even at high-income levels, substantial quantities of wheat are consumed. The whole-wheat flour distributed in the ration shops, however, is perceived to be of lower quality than that available from other sources. This perception is not related to poor nutritional quality; in fact, in most years rationed atta has had a higher protein content than commercially available flour because much of it has been imported (some on concessional terms from the United States), and the imported wheat has been a different, higher-protein variety. The higher protein content, though, is associated with more gluten in the flour, and this, according to Pakistani taste, produces a "rubbery" chapati. Another reason why ration wheat is considered inferior is that consumers tend to suspect that preground flour is adulterated, and they prefer to buy whole wheat and have it ground privately.

As a result of this consumer perception, ration atta demonstrates some degree of targeting toward the low-income population, even though there is no restriction on who may buy it. The expenditure elasticity of demand for ration atta is negative in above-median-income households, but positive in those below the median.

In order to measure the equity of distribution of a good in a population, the concept of intensity of consumption has been developed. This is the ratio of the proportion of the total population represented by a group to the proportion of the total supply of a good that group consumes. If the ratio is greater than 1.00, this means that the group consumes more than the share it would have under strictly equitable distribution. If it is less than 1.00, this means the group is consuming less than its fair share. For example, say the city of Karachi represents 5% of Pakistan's population, and that 20% of all automobiles in Pakistan are bought and used in Karachi. The intensity of consumption of automobiles by the population in Karachi is 0.20/0.05, or 4.00.

The intensity of consumption of wheat by the below-median income population is 0.95, indicating that the poor consume somewhat less than their share of the total wheat supply in the country. By contrast, the intensity of consumption of ration atta by this group is 1.11 in urban areas, indicating that the poor consume a larger share of this commodity. However, it should be noted that this degree of targeting is not very strong. In this discussion, households of below-median income have been considered the target group. Since in Pakistan, low-income households on average have fewer members, this group represents 39% of the population. Their intensity of consumption indicates that they consume 43% of available ration atta. This means that more than half the subsidized atta is "leaking" to the better-off households. If the quality differential between the ration food and its market substitutes were greater, the degree of targeting would undoubtedly also be greater.

Although ration shops are widely available throughout the country, ration atta is sold only in urban areas. In wheat-deficit rural areas, the ration shops distribute whole wheat, which, of course, does not show the same self-targeting effect as the atta does because whole wheat is not considered an inferior good. In rural areas that do not have a wheat deficit (that is, as much or more wheat is produced in the area as is consumed there), the ration shops do not sell wheat. The assumption is that people grow their own wheat and do not require a price subsidy because they do not enter the market. However, the Micronutrient Survey (6) found that, in these areas, the average household purchased 61% of its wheat from the market; this degree of dependence on the market was even higher in low-income households. This indicates that a price subsidy that is intended to reach all the needy should probably extend to rural areas as well.

Sugar

In marked contrast to ration atta, the sugar distributed by the ration system is far from an inferior good. In fact, refined sugar is strongly demanded by all income groups. The income elasticity of income share devoted to sugar, while naturally falling off somewhat with increased income, remains significantly positive even at higher income levels. It is 0.46 at Rs. 300 per month, and 0.35 at Rs. 900 (5). Sugar does not have the nutritional significance that wheat has in the Pakistani diet. It contributes about 6 % of average caloric intake. (This value is almost the same at household income levels of Rs. 100, 600, 900 per month. Of course, the same percentage contribution of calories represents a considerably larger absolute quantity consumed at higher incomes, since total caloric intake is much higher.) Nonetheless, consumers apparently consider sugar to be virtually an essential commodity, at least in some quantity. At an income level of Rs. 100 per month, households devote an average of 12.8% of their income, a substantial proportion, to the purchase of refined sugar (5). Since available supply is limited, one function of the ration system is to regulate demand in order to prevent upper-income households from bidding up the price, and to ensure access to the supply even by low-income groups. The system does serve to make the consumption of sugar more egalitarian: intensity of comsumption of ration sugar by below-median households is 0.93, while that for all refined sugar (ration and black market) is only 0.78.

MARKET CONTROL

A free market in wheat (whole wheat and atta) coexists with the ration system in Pakistan. Those who wish to may supplement their ration allotment from the market; those who do not like the ration atta may turn to the market for their whole supply of wheat. There are several advantages to allowing free trade in a commodity that is also distributed at a subsidized price. One advantage is that it reduces the cost of the program, since the government may subsidize only a portion of the supply of the good rather than all of it. If the quota is high enough to meet the nutritional needs of the poor (which is not the case in Pakistan), or if there are several distinguishable qualities of the food, then a premium can even be charged on open market sales that can be used to pay for the subsidy. This can work particularly well if a large difference prevails between the quality of the subsidized food and that of the food whose price is held high on the free market. In such a case, the premium is charged on a food that is likely to be purchased exclusively by the relatively well-off, who will not suffer nutritionally from the higher price.

Another advantage is that the incentive is reduced for diversion of subsidized food supplies to the black market. People are unlikely to pay high black market prices for atta when they can buy it legally on the open market. Black markets flourish in situations of scarcity; if supplies are plentiful, black marketeering is reduced.

In contrast, there is no legal trade in refined sugar outside the ration system. Of course, the circumstances of sugar rationing are different from those for atta. In the case of sugar, rationing was established precisely because supplies were scarce, and the government was unwilling to support the foreign exchange cost of meeting demand through imports. There is no explicit government subsidy on sugar; the price is kept low by rationing, which reduces demand, and by government-mandated producer prices, not by direct government expenditure. As a result, it is the sugar producer who pays for the subsidy in terms of income foregone.

The government monopoly on sugar, combined with the fact that sugar is in high demand at all income levels, has led to a lively black market in sugar. In any village or town, people are able to quote black market sugar prices that are about twice the ration shop price.

One result of the attempt at government control of the sugar trade, and its consequent black market, is that supplies of sugar are more likely to be diverted from the ration shop than are supplies of atta. In urban areas, only 2% of households have reported that the ration shops run out of atta, while 4% have said the shops were out of sugar at more than one out of four visits. In rural areas, 8% of households have reported that shops run out of wheat more than one in four visits; the figure for sugar is 29% (1). Of course, this situation may be the result of the higher demand for sugar, not solely of diversion to the black market.

NUTRITIONAL IMPACT OF THE RATION SYSTEM

The nutritional impact of a subsidy is determined by the size of the quota, the size of the difference between the subsidized and the free market price,* the price and income elasticities of demand for subsidized food, and the substitution between consumption of the subsidized food and of other foods.

The size of the quota, the amount purchased, and the magnitude of the price difference determine the increment in real income that can be obtained from the subsidy. Note that the size of the price difference is not determined by how much the government spends on the subsidy, but by the forces that affect the free market price of the food or its closest substitute.

The effect of a price subsidy on food consumption may be measured by the price elasticity of demand for the subsidized food and the cross-price elasticity of demand for other foods only in cases where the subsidized food is not rationed, or the ration is not a constraint on consumption. This is because price elasticity measures changes in consumption at the margin, when the consumer considers purchase of an additional unit of a given food. Price elasticity measures the sum of two effects: the income effect (change in behavior due to the increase in real income represented by the price subsidy) and the substitution effect (shift in preference toward the food because of its new, lower price relative to other foods, irrespective of income changes). If the subsidized food is also rationed, and if the consumer buys more than the ration

---

*This is the difference between the subsidized price and the free market price that would prevail in the absence of a subsidy system. In this discussion we have used the prevailing free market price as a proxy, since the true free market price is not observable.

quantity, the price he faces at the margin of consumption is not the subsidized price, but rather the prevailing free market price.

In such cases, it has been maintained that the consumption effect of the subsidy is limited to that of the real income increment obtained, measurable by the income elasticities of demand for foods (6). However, there is recent empirical research (7,8) indicating that the income received from a food subsidy may be disproportionately devoted to food. This behavior is not immediately explainable by economic theory, but may have to do with which household member controls spending of the subsidy income. If such behavior with respect to food subsidy income is general, then the effect on food consumption of a food price subsidy, even with rationing, will be greater than is suggested by the size of the income increment.

Measuring changes in household consumption is not the same as measuring nutritional effect. Increased consumption will influence nutritional status only if it is the nutritionally deficient individual whose consumption is increased. This depends not only on household food supply, but also on how the food is allocated among household members. Furthermore, the effect of increased food intake may be offset by other factors such as infection or parasitic infestation.

QUOTA SIZE

The urban quota of ration atta is one seer (940g) per "unit" per week. Adults (over age 12) represent two units, while children and infants represent one unit each. The adult quota is therefore 7.5 kg per month, and the child's is half that. The adult quota of wheat, if it is all consumed, represents an average daily intake of 825 cal and 26 g of protein (9). This amount constitutes roughly one-third of the average caloric requirement for adults, and more than half the protein requirement (although the wheat protein in the quantities normally consumed is incomplete without a suitable pulse or animal protein complement) (10). In recent years, since there has been no shortage of wheat, children have been receiving the adult quota in most places. The rural quota is the same, when it is given; in many areas wheat is given only at certain times of the year (e.g., before harvest), and since many people take only their sugar ration, more than enough wheat is available to give as much as is wanted to those who use it. In some rural areas the quota is lower; in a few areas the quota may be reduced because supplies are unavailable.

The quota of sugar is the same for adults and children. In urban areas it is 940 g per person per month in Sind and Punjab, 1400g in the Northwest Frontier province, and 700 g in Baluchistan. Rural quotas are less, ranging from 235 g in Punjab and the Northwest Frontier to 470 g in Baluchistan. These quantities can make only a negligible daily caloric contribution to the diet, although they may represent a substantial income transfer due to the high black market price of sugar.

RELATIVE PRICES

The official price of ration atta in 1976 and 1977 was Rs. 0.93 (U.S. $0.09) per seer (940 g). That for ration sugar was Rs. 4.50 (U.S. $0.45). The Micronutrient Survey found some variation in the price charged, and, not surprisingly, considerable variation in the open market prices of substitutes. Table 1 shows the range of prices observed during the course of the Micronutrient Survey (September to December 1976). Whole wheat is a high-quality substitute for atta, while gur, or unrefined brown sugar, is a low-quality substitute for refined sugar. The price of whole wheat is low because it does not include the cost of milling. It should be noted also that substitutes are not always available in the market. Gur is sometimes not found in urban markets, and atta or whole wheat, or both, may be unavailable in various regions and seasons. The Micronutrient Survey found whole wheat for sale in only 40% of urban Punjab markets, and atta sold in only 25% of rural markets, for example. Therefore, in some

TABLE 1. Price Ranges for Ration Commodities and Their Substitutes (Rupees per Seer)[a,b]

Food	Mean	High	Low	(N)
Urban				
Whole wheat	1.21	1.55	0.55	145
Ration atta	0.92	1.13	0.87	265
Market atta	1.32	2.25	1.00	249
Unrefined sugar	2.92	6.00	2.00	270
Ration sugar	4.27	5.00	4.00	176
Black market sugar	9.13	10.00	5.50	20
Rural				
Whole wheat	1.08	1.50	0.87	500
Ration atta	0.95	1.13	0.80	255
Market atta	1.29	1.75	1.00	413
Unrefined sugar	2.53	5.00	1.25	777
Ration sugar	4.18	5.00	3.00	358
Black market sugar	7.35	10.00	5.50	183

[a] U.S. $1.00 = Rs. 9.90. 1 seer = 940 g.
[b] Source: Reference 1.

cases the relevant price differential is not between ration and market atta, but between ration atta and its closest available substitute.

An important finding of the Micronutrient Survey was that households whose consumption of protein and calories was below the median faced higher food prices than those whose consumption was above the median. The differences were substantial: 8% for wheat (all sources), 6% for pulses, 9% for sugar (5). This indicates the importance prices may have in affecting food consumption levels. It also means that the nutritionally needier groups derive greater benefit from the subsidy (because of the larger price difference) than those who consume more food.

EFFECT ON FOOD CONSUMPTION

Quantifying the increment in food consumption that can be attributed to Pakistan's ration and subsidy program poses several difficulties. First, the idea of measuring an increase in consumption implies a change in a population's dietary behavior, yet the ration system has been in operation for a generation, and people have undoubtedly adapted their comsumption patterns to the expectation of continuing availability of subsidized wheat and rationed sugar. One can look at income elasticities and guess that a given income increment would increase consumption by some fixed amount, but the suggestion that removing the subsidy after such a long time would cause an equivalent decrease in consumption is not necessarily correct (11). Furthermore, income elasticities are

TABLE 2. Mean Income Increment Due to
Consumption of Ration Wheat and Sugar
for Urban and Rural Households above and
below Median Expenditure (Percent of
Household Income)[a]

	Rural		Urban	
	Below	Above	Below	Above
Wheat	0.1993	0.1191	3.4641	1.3819
(N)	(229)	(250)	(95)	(118)
Sugar	0.9809	0.4761	7.4079	2.9971
(N)	(343)	(353)	(128)	(134)
Total	1.1802	0.5952	10.8720	4.3790

[a] Source: Computation by the author, using data from the
Pakistan Micronutrient Survey 1976–1977, performed
by the Nutrition Cell, Planning Division, Government
of Pakistan.

TABLE 3. Expenditure Elasticities of Demand for Foods by Income Group and Urban vs. Rural Location[a-c]

Food	Rural		Urban	
	Below	Above	Below	Above
Wheat	0.3975	0.5406	0.5313	0.2343
Rice	1.0923	0.5008	0.3805	0.6340
Maize	−0.1161*	0.1186*	0.1116*	0.1124*
Other cereals	−0.1218*	−0.0339*	0.0339*	0.0582
Pulses	0.4226	0.6470	0.4022	0.1497*
Meat, fish, chicken	0.8128	0.6221	0.5326	0.7470
Milk	1.7352	0.9721	0.8688	0.8849
Eggs	0.9016	1.5245	0.9297	1.8000
Vegetables	0.8066	0.7866	0.7166	0.6500
Vegetable oil	0.2967	0.0457*	0.5255	0.1950*
Sugar	0.4630	0.6808	0.3775	0.2720
Unrefined sugar	0.5097	0.8942	0.1973	−0.0016*

[a] Computed according to the following equation:

$$\log \text{Consumption} = a + B_1 (\log \text{Exp}) + B_2 (\log \text{HH}) + B_3 (\text{Bal}) + B_4 (\text{Sind}) + B_5 (\text{NWFP})$$

where Consumption is monthly household consumption, Exp is total household monthly expenditure, HH is household size (number of resident members), Bal is a dummy variable for Baluchistan, Sind is a dummy variable for Sind, and NWFP is a dummy variable for the Northwest Frontier Province.
[b] All elasticities are significant by F-test at 0.05 or better unless marked with an asterisk (*).
[c] Source: Computation by the author, using data from the Pakistan Micronutrient Survey 1976–1977.

here computed based on cross-sectional data for income from all sources. As we have mentioned, income from food subsidies may cause different behavior, and income changes over time may not be exactly comparable with cross-sectional variations (12).

In spite of these problems, we have attempted to estimate the effects of the ration system on food consumption. This has been done by measuring the expenditure elasticity of demand (used as a proxy for income elasticity) for 12 major foods in the Pakistani diet and computing the average income increment obtained through the ration system. The income increment was computed using the difference between the ration price and the local free market price of each rationed food, multiplied by the amount purchased, as a proportion of household income. The use of prevailing market prices as a proxy for those that would obtain in the absence of the ration system introduces a further element of inaccuracy. Income elasticities are used rather than price elasticities, since the quotas for both wheat and sugar are inframarginal for well over 90% of those who purchase these commodities.

The calculations have been made separately for urban and rural populations. In rural areas, about 80% of the population is served by a ration shop. Most of these shops sell only sugar; less than 13% of rural households can regularly buy ration wheat, and 83% never have access to it. The rural sugar ration, as we have mentioned, is less than that in urban areas. The average increment in income from the ration system in rural areas is quite small, since it includes so many areas where reduced benefits, or none at all, are available. If only areas receiving both wheat and sugar from the ration shops had been included, the average increment would, of course, have been much higher.

Populations with household expenditure levels above and below the median were also treated separately, to account for the known variation in income elasticity by income level. This makes it possible to compare the benefits of the ration system for the presumed target group (below-median households) with those for the relatively better-off population.

Table 2 shows the mean income increment in each group attributable to the purchase of ration commodities. Table 3 shows the expenditure elasticities of demand for the major contributors of calories and protein to the Pakistani diet. Using these elasticities—the food subsidy income increment for each household and the amount consumed of each of the foods—it was possible to calculate the changes in consumption that, subject to the reservations discussed above, might be attributed to the subsidy program. These were converted into their calorie and protein content to derive the figures in Table 4, the net increase in protein and calorie intake permitted by the subsidy. These figures assume equal distribution of food among household members, a necessary assumption in the absence of better information. If indeed food subsidy income tends to be disproportionately spent on food, then these figures underestimate the consumption effects of the program. Another possible source of such

TABLE 4. Average per Capita Daily Increase in Calories and Protein Consumption Due to Ration Distribution[a]

	Rural		Urban	
	Below	Above	Below	Above
Calories/person per day	16.1	11.2	113.8	36.7
Protein (g)/person per day	0.59	0.39	3.84	1.34

[a] Source: Computation by the author (see text for complete explanation), using data from the Pakistan Micronutrient Survey 1976–1977.

understatement is that the computations are based on average monthly consumption. One important contribution of the ration system may be to provide a reliable source of low-cost food at times when seasonal price increases would otherwise precipitate clinical malnutrition in a marginally nourished population. The nutritional significance of such a "floor" on consumption would be greater than these average figures suggest.

Nutritional Impact

The relationship between household food consumption and individual nutritional status is indirect. The Micronutrient Survey collected anthropometric data on children under five; this was the only direct measurement of nutritional status. To test the influence of the wheat subsidy on nutritional status, regressions were run using the degree of malnutrition of the most seriously affected child as the dependent variable. (Only households with children under five were included.) Malnutrition was measured by the methods of Waterlow (13) and McLaren and Read (14). In the regression for urban areas, neither the total quantity of ration atta consumed by the household, nor the percent of total grain consumption that was ration atta, showed a significant relation to the presence of a malnourished child, when income and number of household members were entered first in the regression equations. This is probably because per capita consumption of grain showed a small but statistically significant negative relation with the percent of ration atta consumed. Per capita grain consumption was most strongly positively related to income, and negatively to the number of household members.

These findings do not indicate that the ration system has no effect on grain consumption or nutritional status. On the average, ration atta represents 45.5% of total grain consumption of urban households; this percentage is higher in low-income groups. Total grain consumption is negatively related to the percent of ration atta because those who can afford to consume more grain also rely less heavily on the ration system. It appears that the ration system in urban areas provides a kind of minimum level of consumption, with the relatively better-off population purchasing larger additional quantities of food on the open market.

The effect of ration atta consumption is not seen in superior growth levels of children because the per-person monthly ration does not provide sufficient calories and protein to meet nutritional requirements, but can act only as a supplement to the diet. Intrafamilial food distribution patterns might also reduce the actual incremental nutrients going to the preschoolers, thereby reducing nutritional impact. One cannot compare equivalent low-income families who do and do not consume ration atta, because consumption of ration atta is almost universal among the urban poor. Nevertheless, it is likely that, in the absence of the wheat subsidy, food consumption by poor families would decline.

In rural areas, a relatively small number of ration shops sell subsidized wheat. Considering only those areas where wheat is sold, there was a small positive relationship between percent of ration atta consumed and nutritional status as measured by the McLaren and Read method, when income and provincial variation were controlled. This may indicate that the availability of ration atta enabled the household to consume more food than would otherwise have been possible. Income is more strongly related to household and per capita grain consumption levels in rural than in urban areas, and the consumption of ration atta shows a stronger inverse relation to income. Even with income controlled, in rural areas the availability of home-produced wheat shows a significant inverse relation to the use of ration wheat. This means that the ration is used by the relatively needy and by those who do not, or cannot, produce their own grain. In rural regions where ration wheat is available, it constitutes 27% of total grain consumption on the average. These findings indicate that the subsidy probably plays a positive role in maintaining existing levels of consumption in some rural areas.

PROGRAM COST

The budgetary costs of the wheat subsidy and ration program are made up of the following components: the cost of the wheat itself, less the net price paid for it by the consumers; the costs of procurement, transportation, and storage of the wheat in warehouses, as well as the relatively minor administrative costs of maintaining offices and staff to oversee program operation; and the costs of the bags in which the wheat and sugar are delivered to the ration shops. Milling charges for wheat are included in the price paid by the consumer, and the costs of transport from the warehouse and distribution at the retail level are covered by the shop owners. In the case of sugar, the government pays for procurement, processing, and storage, but these costs are supposed to be fully covered in the retail price, so that the entire subsidy consists of the cost of the bags.

The major cost—that of the wheat itself—fluctuates with the world market price, the quantity imported, and the quantity available as foreign aid. This is not subject to the government's control. Within the limits of political feasibility, costs can be controlled by raising the retail price, reducing the ration size, or reducing the number of recipients of subsidized wheat. In recent years, the only strategy used by the government has been to raise the price.

Still, the cost of the program has fallen in recent years, largely because of several excellent harvests in Pakistan that have allowed the system to reduce its dependence on the world market for supplies of wheat.

In 1974–1975, about 50% of the wheat procured by the government was imported. In that year, it was estimated that the cost of subsidized ration wheat distribution was U.S. $143 million, which represented 10.8% of the government's operating budget (3). In 1976–1977, imported wheat constituted about a third of ration wheat distribution (816,000 tons, compared with 1.58 million tons of domestically produced wheat). The estimated cost of the program was U.S. $135 million, a figure representing 5.9% of projected government revenues (2). Considering the effect of inflation, this cost is substantially lower than the earlier figure. Of course, an increase in world prices, or a shortfall in domestic production, would reverse this trend.

SUMMARY AND CONCLUSIONS

Pakistan's ration system demonstrates how variations in the design of a subsidy can alter the effectiveness and the cost of the program. The particular features we have discussed are (1) commodity selection; (2) degree of market control, and (3) degree of private management. We have shown that a subsidy program can be targeted, albeit imperfectly, to the low-income population, if the subsidized food is perceived to be of low quality, and therefore not consumed by the nonneedy. Such a low-prestige food also will not be very saleable on the black market. Black marketeering is also reduced if the government does not attempt to exercise monopoly control over the subsidized food. Allowing a free market to coexist with the price-controlled one has the additional advantage that costs can be minimized, since the government does not have to subsidize all of the available supply of that food. We have suggested that the very high level of accessibility of ration shops and the reliability of supply are at least in part the result of their decentralized management and private ownership: The government's financial and administrative resources are not strained to set up large numbers of distribution centres and coordinate their supply.

The ration system was not established for purposes of improving the nutritional status of the population. Nonetheless, the subsidized wheat distribution appears to have a positive impact on the food consumption of the poor. In a nutritionally marginal population, increased food consumption is likely to improve nutritional status. However, changes in the system could be made that would improve its effectiveness and reduce its costs. Leakages at present are more than 50%. This could be reduced by increasing the quality differential between ration and open market atta, by selecting a less desirable food grain (such as sorghum) for subsidy, or by limiting eligibility bureaucratically. One area in which nutritional effectiveness might be improved would be the extension of the wheat program to more rural areas, since many low-income rural dwellers depend on the market for their food. Another might be to subsidize foods in addition to wheat. Improved targeting might make this economically feasible.

While the cost of the program is substantial, its visibility and political strength make it unlikely that it will be eliminated. Therefore, further efforts to evaluate the subsidies and to reduce their costs and improve their effectiveness are certainly warranted.

REFERENCES

1. Rogers, B. L. *Consumer Food Price Subsidies and Subsidized Food Distribution Systems in Pakistan.* MIT-INP Discussion Paper No. 13. Massachusetts Institute of Technology, Cambridge, Massachusetts, March 1978.
2. Rogers, B. L., C. Overholt, F. Sanchez-Carillo, A. Chavez, C. P. Timmer, and T. Beldins, Consumer price subsidies, in: Special Study VI in AID Series, *Nutrition Intervention in Developing Countries*, Oelgeschlager, Gunn, and Hain, Cambridge, Massachusetts, 1980.
3. Rogers, B. L., and F. J. Levinson. *Subsidized Food Consumption in Low-Income Countries: The Pakistan Experience.* MIT-INP Discussion Paper No. 6. Massachusetts Institute of Technology, Cambridge, Massachusetts, April 1976.
4. MICAS Associates, Ltd. *Roti: Appendices to the Feasibility Study*, Report prepared for the Government of Pakistan, Planning Division, Karachi, Pakistan, 1974.
5. Hammer, J. *Determinants of Malnutrition in Pakistan.* Ph.D. Thesis, Department of Economics, Massachusetts Institute of Technology, Cambridge, Massachusetts, 1979.
6. Selowsky, M. Lecture delivered at the International Nutrition Program, Massachusetts Institute of Technology, Cambridge, Massachusetts, Winter 1979.
7. Kumar, S. K. Impact of Subsidized Rice on Food Consumption and Nutrition in Kerala. International Food policy Research Institute (IFPRI) Report No. 5, Washington, D.C. 1979.
8. Gavan, J. D., and Chandrasekra, I. S. The Impact of Public Foodgrain Distribution on Food Consumption and Welfare in Sri Lanka. International Food Policy Research Institute (IFPRI) Report No. 13, Washington, D.C. 1979.
9. United States Department of Health, Education and Welfare, and Food and Agriculture Organization of the United Nations, *Food Composition Table for Use in East Asia.* National Institutes of Health, Bethesda, Maryland, December 1972.

10. World Health Organization. *Handbook on Human Nutritional Requirements*. WHO Monograph Series No. 61, WHO, Geneva/FAO, Rome, 1974.
11. Hogarty, T. F., and R. J. MacKay. Some implications of the "new theory of consumer behavior" for interpreting estimated demand elasticities. *Am. J. Agric. Econ.* **57:**340–343, 1975.
12. Sinha, R. P. An analysis of food expenditure in India. *J. Farm Econ.* **48:**113–123, 1966.
13. Waterlow, J. C. Note on the assessment and classification of protein–energy malnutrition in children. *Lancet* **ii:**87–89, 1973.
14. McLaren, D. S., and W. W. C. Read. Classification of nutritional status in early childhood. *Lancet* **ii:**146–148, 1972.

Food Subsidies in Egypt

LANCE TAYLOR

INTRODUCTION

The Egyptian government subsidizes a very wide range of commodities and services, among them food. The subsidy system is well-established, having begun in the 1950s, but only during the 1970s did it expand to a substantial share of public spending. Along with economic importance, the political and nutritional consequences of the subsidies have waxed in recent years. A general sketch of these developments is all that can be presented in this brief survey chapter, along with some indication of how proposed changes in the subsidy system might affect the economic and nutritional well-being of poor Egyptians.

HISTORY AND MAGNITUDE

By the standards of many countries, Egypt does not, on the average, suffer from deprivation of food. Per capita energy availability is about 3000 cal, though half comes from only three staples—wheat and wheat flour, rice, and vegetable oil. Almost all the wheat (along with substantial proportions of other foods) is imported. Together with domestic political pressures, this import dependence is a major factor giving rise to Egypt's large food subsidies in recent years, as explained shortly.

Foods are subsidized in various ways. For example, common (or baladi) bread is available to all consumers in unlimited quantity at a unified price, while sugar, tea, and edible oils are sold in limited quantities con-

LANCE TAYLOR • Department of Economics and International Nutrition Program, Massachusetts Institute of Technology, Cambridge, Massachusetts.

TABLE 1. Budgetary Allocations for Major "Supply"
Commodities (£E million)

Item	1973	1974	1975	1976	1977	1978 (projected)
Wheat	70.8	194.1	135.1	152.3	117.5	127.6
Flour	8.2	27.0	27.6	25.8	31.6	19.6
Corn	4.4	16.5	29.2	23.1	40.6	49.2
Lentils	0.6	2.2	6.3	9.0	9.4	14.6
Beans	0.3	0.7	5.2	6.0	2.0	6.0
Fats and oils	20.7	59.4	91.2	57.4	84.9	95.9
Frozen meat	—	—	0.5	—	20.4	37.0
Frozen fish	0.5	—	2.0	0.2	0.4	2.3
Tea	—	—	—	—	18.3	45.6

trolled by ration cards. Frozen meat, cheese, and dairy products are available on a "first come, first served" basis, sometimes in connection with major festivals or holidays.

As mentioned above, direct subsidies appeared as a separate item in the expenditure budget soon after the 1952 revolution, but in small amounts—in 1960 the outlay was £E 9 million.* At that time, only a few basic consumer goods such as wheat, kerosene, and sugar were included in the subsidy scheme. Total payments increased slowly to a level of about £E 20 million in 1970. The dramatic increase in the subsidy bill occurred after 1973, when world food prices rose steeply, multiplying severalfold the difference between costs and sale prices of a large volume of food imports. The direct subsidy bill in 1975 was about £E 622 million. Despite a decline in dollar prices of foodstuffs since the mid-1970s, total outlays in domestic currency kept increasing along with a rising volume of imports and a falling exchange rate. The direct subsidy cost in 1978 was about £E 680 million, concentrated on a dozen or so "supply commodities."

Tables 1 and 2 present budgetary data on the costs of subsidies for the major supply commodities and the tonnages involved. Note that there is a steep rise in supply of most items, i.e., wheat went up 50% between 1973 and 1978, flour by 80%, lentils by 150%, and edible oils by 180%. Also, new items such as frozen meat and tea entered the subsidy list.

*The Egyptian pound (£E) is currently worth U.S. $1.43. It has been devalued through a series of parallel rates from a 1973 value of U.S. $2.56.

TABLE 2. Quantities of Major Subsidized Commodities
(Thousands of Metric Tons)

Item	1973	1974	1975	1976	1977	1978
Wheat						
Imported	2373	2877	2950	2758	3297	3560
Domestic	211	318	332	269	87	150
First-rate flour	452	395	701	541	655	837
Imported corn	609	457	506	435	676	690
Beans						
Imported	—	22	116	83	25	35
Domestic	14	16	26	49	50	50
Lentils						
Imported	12	16	50	17	44	50
Domestic	12	3	1	12	11	10
Oil						
Imported	138	162	242	222	225	250
Domestic	—	—	—	—	—	125
Fats	28	127	150	163	127	179
Frozen meat	—	3	—	—	65	70
Frozen fish						
Imported	32	33	40	43	31	50
Domestic	—	—	—	—	—	17
Tea	—	—	—	—	48	37

These increases clearly outstrip the rate of population growth, plus any increment in demand that could be caused by rising per capita income. The Ministry of Supply tends to attribute the increasing demand to changing consumption patterns, especially on the part of new consumers from rural areas, who are allegedly relying more on supply commodities as their prices fall relative to alternative marketed or subsistence foods. The relative cheapening of supply commodities is, in any case, likely to be a significant factor underlying the growth in demand for them. For example, a standard size cake of baladi bread (weighing 135 g) has had a stable price of £E 0.005 for years. Meanwhile, the urban consumer price index rose by 50% (probably an understatement of the true price inflation) between 1974 and 1978. With inflation at nonnegligible rates, a policy question arises as to whether the subsidy system should be operated to generate a *falling* real price for staple foods. Moreover, with nominal prices of subsidized foods held steady, average subsidy rates as a consequence must increase over time, as demonstrated in Table 3.

THE CURRENT POLICY DEBATE

This question of correct real pricing policy reflects just one of several aspects of the subsidy system that have been under intense discussion in the last year or two. As indicated above, the initial rapid rise in subsidies after 1973 was the inevitable result of a government decision to maintain internal grain prices during the world "food crisis." In fact, this decision itself had an air of political inevitability about it, as witnessed by the riots in January 1977, which forced the government into hasty reversal of announced price increases for bread and other staple foods. Whether there will be a replay of the riots in response to any future price increases is a question behind the current debate. Despite the unvoiced worries, however, a number of issues have been raised. They include the following:

1. Who exactly benefits from the subsidies? This question cannot be answered in detail, as no micro studies exist on patterns of consumption of subsidized vs. nonsubsidized commodities by income class, regions, or rural/urban breakdown. However, the periodic consumer budget surveys do provide data about purchases of relatively broad categories of commodities at the household level, as well as some information on income distribution.

TABLE 3. Average Subsidy per Ton, Major Commodities, 1973–1978
(£E/Ton)

Item	1973	1974	1975	1976	1977	1978
Wheat						
Imported	29.27	66.64	77.6	51.73	34.78	47.8
Domestic	6.43	7.42	18.53	35.57	68.78	—
First-rate flour	18.0	68.36	39.33	47.65	47.88	35.34
Imported corn	21.18	32.08	57.8	53.04	58.90	71.2
Beans						
Imported	—	22.86	42.06	58.03	81.88 ⎫	
Domestic	21.5	14.56	12.8	22.85	0.2 ⎬	70.8
Lentils						
Imported	45.58	134.62	124.08	133.89	208.9 ⎫	
Domestic	8.0	14.61	103.3	3.0	32.45 ⎬	243.6
Oil	121.43	278.77	297.97	184.5	220.03	119.32
Animal fat	105.17	107.37	127.24	100.9	292.62	285.9
Frozen meat	—	2.0	—	—	318.9	528.9
Frozen fish	16.34	54.95	50.77	3.74	14.06	104.7
Tea	—	—	—	—	482.2	1231.9

TABLE 4. Income Distribution According to 1974–1975
Household Survey[a]

	Urban	Rural
Share of bottom 20% of households	0.0586	0.0570
Share of bottom 20% of persons	0.0919	0.1128
Share of top 10% of households	0.3118	0.3181
Share of top 10% of persons	0.2733	0.2532
Gini coefficient for households	0.40	0.40
Gini coefficient for persons	0.33	0.27

[a] "Blown up" to match size of population and corrected for savings and direct
tax incidence.

If we start by analyzing distribution as a decisive factor underlying
food consumption patterns, then the 1974–1975 household survey suggests moderate income concentration for Egypt, as Table 4 indicates.

Note that urban and rural *household* distributions are quite similar,
although as might be expected, mean household income in urban areas
is higher (£E 716 and £E 386 are mean annual urban and rural household incomes, respectively). Personal income distributions are more egalitarian than household distributions, especially for rural incomes. The
reason is that household size, at least as defined by the expenditure survey, rises sharply with income. How much this household size increase
is due to the role of servants, possibly higher fertility or lower mortality
at higher levels, and extended family living patterns is unclear, but its
net effect is income-equalizing on average.

Given the low levels of per capita income in Egypt and the country's
not unusual degree of income inequality, it should not be surprising that
a large share of the expenditures of the poor is for staple foods. The patterns for three representative ranges of annual household expenditure
levels are shown in Table 5.

Noteworthy in this set of numbers are the falling shares, as income
goes up, of grains and starches, and sugar and sweets. Insofar as the food
subsidy program is directed toward such items, it benefits the poor. Peru-
sal of Tables 1 and 2 suggests that this is the case.* The major problem

---

*An exception to this generalization is the increase in subsidies for meat in recent years.
The food consumption patterns given in the text imply that the income elasticity of
demand for meat products (and also dairy products and fats and oils) is close to one. As
such, meats are not an ideal target for a good subsidy, which ought to concentrate on
products with relatively high demand elasticities for the poor and low ones for the better-off. The nutritional cost-effectiveness of the subsidy system may therefore have
declined in light of recent trends.

that available data do not resolve is the extent to which rural households purchase subsidized bread or flour on the one hand or use home-produced maize and wheat on the other. Bits of evidence, such as an observed decline of rural pellagra (a deficiency disease associated with high-maize diets) and the recent rapid growth of wheat consumption, suggest that people in the countryside have been making increasing use of subsidized bakeries.

All in all, these data show that despite its low overall per capita income level (perhaps $300), Egypt has a relatively egalitarian income distribution, and that the food subsidy system benefits at least certain classes of the poor. These assertions do not add up to an affirmation that subsidies benefit *nutrition*. There would be small nutritional benefits (though there would be distributional ones) if a substantial share of subsidized commodities were resold in the market by the poor to gain money for other purposes. No one knows what volume such resales reach, although it is certain that they occur.

2. The major doubts about the cost-effectiveness of the subsidy system arise from the fact that it incorporates no effective "means test." For bread especially, the fact that anyone can obtain unlimited quantities at the official price opens opportunities for profitable commodity arbitrage. A major problem that the Egyptian government must sooner or later face is the redesign of the system to minimize the possibilities, not just for speculation, but for guaranteed profits for the relatively well-off from commodity resale. Several possibilities present themselves, including enforcement of rations on sales of commodities besides sugar, edible oils, and tea. Or, if quantity rations could not be enforced, transactions costs for the well-to-do could be increased via queuing, removal of luxury con-

TABLE 5. Shares in Total Household Expenditure of Several Food Classes

	Grains and starches	Sugar and sweets	Meat, fish, eggs	Fruits
Rural households				
£E 100–150	0.2674	0.0378	0.1341	0.0230
£E 350–400	0.2073	0.0403	0.1369	0.0270
£E 1400–2000	0.1227	0.0356	0.1319	0.0408
Urban households				
£E 100–150	0.1793	0.0429	0.1258	0.0287
£E 350–400	0.1324	0.0323	0.1265	0.0355
£E 1400–2000	0.0914	0.0179	0.1243	0.0345

sumer goods such as fine flour and meat from the subsidy list, and similar devices. The presumption is that if the poor do have access to the subsidy system, they benefit. The problem is to design policies to keep the non-poor from benefitting excessively.

3. In discussing the overall role of the subsidies, it is essential to distinguish their macro-economic impact from how effectively they are targeted. For example, subsidies could be abolished while the overall level of economic activity was maintained by increases in some other public expenditure item (e.g., public investment). But what would be the micro-nutritional impacts of such a policy change? Previous calculations made by the author* suggest that food consumption per capita among the poor might drop by 100 to 200 cal/day under a program of subsidy reductions coupled with compensating macro-policies. (Of course, the consumption decreases would be far more severe if compensating policies were not applied.) For groups at major risk, such as small children and pregnant or lactating mothers, such population-wide reductions in *average* calorie intake could easily translate into acute undernutrition. Wholesale abolition of subsidies is clearly not in the cards for Egypt, for nutritional as well as political reasons.

4. Nonetheless, there remains the question hinted at above as to whether or not the real value of the subsidized commodities should continue to fall in the face of continuing inflation. Price indexing of subsidized commodities would itself be inflationary, but budget deficits (and the wrath of international lenders) will grow steadily along the lines of Table 3 if prices of subsidized goods and services are held constant while all other prices go up. In such circumstances, "corrective" inflation of the subsidized commodities is finally impossible to avoid. Doing it gradually via indexation instead of at once in a large shock impacting directly on the poor is a policy option that the Egyptian authorities might want to put into effect.

POLICY PROSPECTS

It seems reasonably clear that the Egyptian subsidy system will be gradually revised, if only to respond to continuing pressures from aid donors and international organizations such as the International Mone-

---

*See Lance Taylor, *Macro Models for Developing Countries*. McGraw-Hill, New York, 1979, Chapter 4.

tary Fund. Such nutritional benefits as the existing system may offer can be retained (or even enhanced) if the revisions are sensible. Some of the alternatives suggested above include:

- Incorporation of a means test and rationing to discriminate against volume sales of subsidized commodities for profit by people wealthy enough to finance the transaction.
- Concentration of the subsidies on foods where their cost-effectiveness is likely to be highest, e.g., on foods to which the poor devote a high share of their budgets and for which the price elasticity is relatively high.
- Incorporation of some sort of indexing of subsidized prices to the general rate of inflation, to preclude a drastic but otherwise inevitable upward price revision at some point in the future.
- Modification of the subsidy system with due regard to the macroeconomic repercussions, especially as they affect the purchasing power of the poor.

Attention to these considerations could help make the future benefits accruing to the system even higher than they have been in the past.

ACKNOWLEDGMENTS. Research support by the Cairo University/Massachusetts Institute of Technology Technological Planning Program is gratefully acknowledged. Neither the Program nor the United States Agency for International Development (which finances it) bears responsibility for the contents of this paper.

Strategies and Mechanisms for Urban and Rural Subsidization
The Case of CONASUPO

JAMES E. AUSTIN

INTRODUCTION

Almost all governments have explicit or implicit strategies and direct or indirect mechanisms for subsidizing certain groups within their societies. All subsidies effect income either by decreasing the cost of inputs (production supplies or consumption goods) or by increasing the price paid for outputs.

The general rationale for subsidization usually falls into one or a combination of three categories:

1. *Political,* favoring certain groups to achieve political goals, e.g., subsidies to certain powerful economic groups in exchange for their support, or subsidies to urban masses to reduce the cost of living and minimize the chances of political unrest due to economic pressures.
2. *Economic,* creating financial incentives to increase production or stimulate investments in certain areas, e.g., farm price supports or reduced prices on farm inputs for crops that the country needs in greater quantities (perhaps to decrease imports and save foreign exchange), or tax relief or subsidized interest rates for plants built in more remote regions.

JAMES E. AUSTIN • Harvard University Graduate School of Business Administration, Boston, Massachusetts.

3. *Social*, channeling added resources to deprived groups in order to improve their welfare, e.g., distribution free, or at reduced prices, of basic staples to ensure access to a minimally adequate diet, or free health services through a social security or other system.

Nutritional improvement has seldom been the principal, explicit goal of subsidization schemes. This is understandable because subsidization is a policy instrument that can be used to achieve many different development objectives. Furthermore, it has only been in recent years that combating malnutrition directly has emerged as a more central concern and focus of development efforts. In this context, one of the major challenges facing policy makers is how to reorient the subsidization strategies and mechanisms to increase their impact on the malnutrition problem in their countries.

This chapter will examine the efforts of the Mexican government through its national marketing agency, CONASUPO, to develop strategies and instruments to meet the basic needs of low-income groups. Although the Mexican government employs various subsidization mechanisms throughout its economy, from the nutrition perspective CONASUPO merits particular attention because it deals primarily with food, has grown tremendously in the last 10 years, and has been the government's primary institutional vehicle for subsidies in the food system. The chapter will first provide a description of CONASUPO's activities and then discuss their implications for the formulation and implementation of subsidization strategies.

CONASUPO: HISTORICAL PERSPECTIVE

The regulation of the marketing of basic foodstuffs has a long history in Mexico.* The first order to regulate the price of maize and wheat was issued in 1525 during the colonial period; throughout this epoch various mechanisms were used, such as maximum prices, margin limitations, and direct procurement and sale by the government.

After independence, the management of the grain marketing system largely returned to the hands of the large haciendas and private intermediaries. However, subsequent to the Revolution in 1913, interest in government intervention to protect the small farmer was rekindled. In 1934 the first government institution with agricultural regulatory func-

---

*These historical data are derived from Gustavo Esteva, La Experiencia Regulardora de Los Mercados de Subsistencias en el Período 70–76, undated mimeograph, Mexico City.

tions was formed: Almacenes Nacionales de Deposito, S.A. (ANDSA). The fundamental purpose of ANDSA was to regulate grain commerce to prevent speculative activities.

In 1938 the Regulatory Committee for the Basic Goods Market (Comité Regulador del Mercado de las Subsistencias) was formed to combat a dramatic rise in the prices of basic goods. The Committee recognized the fundamental conflict of needing to ensure remunerative prices to farmers while at the same time protecting urban consumers from excessive prices. The Committee put pressure on intermediaries to buy from farmers at more just prices, and also put up 30 of its own retail outlets and at the same time encouraged the organization of consumer stores by cooperatives and unions. The Committees's actions were attacked by affected intermediaries as interference with freedom of commerce, and by others who saw as unwarranted the government's intervention in this and other social areas.

The Committee was subsequently replaced by two public enterprises—one (CEIMSA) in charge of importing foods in short supply and exporting surpluses, and the other (NADYRSA) engaged in distributing basic goods in urban areas through its own and other outlets. During the 1950s, the government used these organizations to provide incentives to efficient, large farmers through support prices. These prices were paid even when above the world prices. Surpluses were exported by the government at a loss (subsidy). The subsidies, in effect, were used to reduce the farmers' risks and accelerate the development of a modern agricultural subsector. Small, traditional farmers were not a primary target group. During this period emphasis was also on keeping food prices in the city low in order to keep the costs and wages for labor down, thereby enhancing the basic development strategy of industrialization.

In 1961 these entities were replaced by another public enterprise, CONASUPO. During the 1960s, CONASUPO adjusted the policy by stabilizing the support price for basic grains in order to shift the commercial farmers to export crops. Agricultural production in basic crops stagnated and grain imports began to rise. Unrest among small farmers began to mount. Income disparities between the rich and poor were increasing. Thus, when Luis Echeverría Alvarez assumed the presidency in 1970, pressures were mounting to rethink the country's rural development strategy.

The new managers of CONASUPO played a critical role in diagnosing the underlying structural problems in the country's food system and were consequently given major political and economic backing to undertake a new and more aggressive approach to their activities. As a result, CONASUPO experienced dramatic growth during the period 1970–1975. The expansion was such that by 1976 CONASUPO was the second largest economic enterprise in Mexico, with sales of U.S. $715 million and assets of U.S. $1.051 billion.* CONASUPO's growth was halted subsequent to 1976 as part of the new Lopez Portillo administration's austerity and consolidation program. However, expansion is currently under way again.

For the purposes of this chapter, I will concentrate on the period 1970–1976 when the most dramatic changes occurred. I will examine the following dimensions of CONASUPO's experience during this period: objectives and strategy, growth, subsidies, and organization and operations.

OBJECTIVES AND STRATEGY

The 1965 decree that formed CONASUPO (as an expanded version of the 1961 Compañia Nacional de Subsistencies Populares, S.A.) set forth CONASUPO's objectives, function, and organizational structure, all of which have undergone subsequent changes. Around 1971 or 1972, a significant strategy shift occurred; it was asserted that CONASUPO's programs had succeeded in increasing production and improving marketing channels, but that the distribution of the resultant benefits had been quite unequal. Consequently, CONASUPO reformulated its objectives to focus more sharply on the lower-income segments of society, especially in the rural sector.

CONASUPO set forth three basic objectives:

- To regulate the basic goods market.
- To increase the income of poor farmers.
- To increase the ability of low-income consumers to acquire basic goods.

More specifically, the target groups were producers with annual incomes below M $12,000 (U.S. $960), and families with monthly incomes less than M $2000 (U.S. $160). Approximately 94% of the farms have annual sales of less than M $12,000, but they account for only about 33% of the total agricultural output. In effect, CONASUPO was targeting its programs toward the subsistence and small-farmer segments. In 1972 these low-income urban and rural consumer groups constituted 57% of the population. Of those families with annual incomes under M $7200, 61% lived in the rural areas; of those with incomes less than M $12,000, 56% were in the rural sector.

Preliminary data based on a national survey by CONASUPO of 3570

---

*Las 500 empresas mas importantes de Mexico. *Expansión*, August 30, 1978, p. 74; PEMEX, the Government's oil enterprise, is number one in sales and assets.

small, traditional farmers provided guiding data in the formulation of the new strategy for CONASUPO's rural development effort. The study revealed that in this traditional segment of the agricultural sector, 68% of the land was "ejidal"*, 22% privately owned, and 10% communally owned. This constituted 87% of the traditional segment, with the other 13% being rented or sharecropped. Modern inputs were used on a limited basis. Only 13% used herbicides, 16% improved seeds, 23% insecticides, and 26% fertilizers. This sector was also relatively neglected by government agencies: only 19% received formal credit and a mere 4% received technical assistance. The bulk of the farmers primarily grew corn†; approximately 45% of the land was dedicated to corn. Of the corn produced, 70% was for human consumption, 20% for animal feed, 8% for industrialization, and 2% for seed. The small farmers retained about 69% of their crop for on-farm consumption. Forty percent of the farmers sold some or all of their crop. Approximately 17% of the corn they sold went to CONASUPO. The reason for selling to CONASUPO was stated, by 79%, to be the better prices. The major reasons given for not selling to CONASUPO were distance (30%), crop promised to others (23%), and lack of information (15%).

CONASUPO's rural development strategy was based on the dynamics of the rural economy that pointed to structural factors in the economic interaction between farmers and external groups as being the primary cause of stagnation in the development of the rural sectors. More specifically, the rural dwellers paid too much for the goods they bought and received too little for the produce they sold, because their suppliers and buyers were exploitative and/or inefficient. The exploitation may not have been a conscious phenomenon, as is often implied in stereotyping intermediaries, but rather a consequence of an inefficient intermediary filling a void in the economic system in order to earn a living. The local store owner or corn buyer may have been a fellow villager with an entrepreneurial flair, simply trying to eke out a meager income by means other than tilling the soil. When farmers were able to increase their production, this potential economic gain was drained off by unfavorable prices from store owners, from corn buyers, or from nonproductive expenditures.

Credit played a key role in the maintenance of these unfavorable terms of trade. The farmers were unable to accumulate capital reserves and, therefore, did not have enough funds to support their families for

---

*The use of state land was ceded to individual farmers (ejiditarios) in the agrarian reform for their perpetual use, but the land cannot be sold.
†Seventy-seven percent own animals of some kind.

the entire period between harvests. Consequently, the farmers were frequently obliged to seek credit for the purchase of staples. The two primary sources were either rural storekeepers who sold on credit or intermediaries who loaned to the farmers in return for a promise to sell their crop to the intermediaries at a preset price lower than the government's guaranteed price. According to CONASUPO studies, approximately half of the small-farmer sales were in exchange for consumer credit, and an estimated 40–60% of rural purchases were on credit.* CONASUPO's studies also indicated that the average prices of goods in rural stores were 20–23% higher than the prices charged in CONASUPO stores.† The difference is attributable to the greater efficiency and lower profit margins of CONASUPO.

Credit was not the only mechanism by which intermediaries obtained the farmers' crops at relatively lower prices. For example, the lack of transportation, storage, shellers, or bags often pushed the farmer into selling to intermediaries who had these facilities or services. These economic relationships represented structural barriers that would not necessarily be altered by channeling increasing amounts of funds into the traditional areas of crop financing, production infrastructure, and technical assistance. Structural weaknesses must be addressed directly if maximum benefit is to be obtained from investments in other areas.

Based on the foregoing perception of the rural environment, CONASUPO set forth the following general strategy for its rural development efforts: enable the farmer to increase his income, retain it, and invest it in productive means. A probable short-run effect of this strategy was to be the direct welfare benefit accruing through an increase in effective purchasing power and in consumption. It was assumed that this incremental consumption would most likely be in food, and hence the possibility of enhancing the nutritional level of the rural populace. Nonetheless, it is important to emphasize that the thrust of the strategy was toward increasing the productivity of farmers rather than just improving their immediate standard of living. The concept was to generate sustained self-development rather than simply adjust income distribution.

CONASUPO designed an integrated strategy aimed at altering the structural relationships in the rural economies by combining various related services and activities in a specific area; the idea was to produce a synergistic effect of sufficient magnitude between resources and ser-

---

*Studies by the Banco Agropecuario produced similar figures.
†This price differential was corroborated by direct observation in the field by the author in February 1974.

vices to break some of the key constraints on rural development. The major components of the CONASUPO strategy were the following:

1. Regulate the national food system through a vertically integrated procurement, processing, and distribution system that included facilities, ownership, and operation at each stage.
2. Provide improved marketing opportunities to farmers through guaranteed prices, storage facilities, and ancillary procurement services such as transportation and shelling.
3. Improve consumer purchasing power and access to basic goods through direct distribution at subsidized prices and on credit to rural and urban consumers.
4. Increase rural productivity through enhanced incomes and market opportunities, input provision, and training.

GROWTH

This new strategy was implemented aggressively and resulted in a rapid growth of CONASUPO's operations. Table 1 presents key statistics that reveal the expansion that took place during the period 1970–1975.

As can be seen from Table 2, CONASUPO financed this growth by increasing its equity (capital allocations from the federal government)

TABLE 1. CONASUPO Growth[a,b]

	1970	1975	Percent increase
Financial			
Assets	2,355	14,770	527
Inventories	1,319	7,320	455
Equity capital	1,713	6,481	278
Bank financing	357	7,001	1,861
Operating budget	5,000	35,000	600
Purchases	3,419	15,792	354
Government subsidy	850	4,225	397
Facilities			
Retail outlets	2,000	12,000	500
Buying centers	1,109	2,434	119
Storage capacity (tons)	1,033,250	1,511,500	46
Grains purchased (tons)	2,677,082	5,703,326	113
Fertilizer sales (tons)	11,700	212,000	1,700

[a] The prevailing exchange rate through mid-1976 was M $12.50 = U.S. $1.00
[b] Source: CONASUPO.

and its borrowings. Increased reliance on debt financing and supplier credit was the cornerstone of the financial strategy. In 1970 these sources accounted for 27% of CONASUPO's capital; by 1975 they represented 56%. Approximately 36% of the loans had a maturity of 1–5 years. The increased capital requirements were largely due to CONASUPO's expanded procurement operations with a concommitant increase in inventories.

SUBSIDIES

The growing operating deficits of CONASUPO were covered by direct annual subsidies from the federal budget. CONASUPO's basic financial strategy for its subsidiaries was that they operate on at least a break-even basis. For example, in the urban areas CONASUPO's supermarkets generated a profit that was used to offset the losses incurred by the small rural stores. The large deficits occurred because of subsidized prices to farmers and consumers rather than operational inefficiencies. Table 3 reveals that almost two-thirds of the M $4.2 billion (U.S. $376 million) deficit in 1975 was due to the subsidies on basic grains, particularly maize, wheat, and beans. The comparison in Table 4 shows that the support price paid to the farmers was both above and below the import price, but in later years exceeded the import price for maize. Similarly, Table 5 shows that CON-ASUPO support prices were generally higher than those prices prevailing in the local market. These differences roughly represent the farmer sub-

TABLE 2. CONASUPO Balance Sheet (in Millions of Pesos)[a]

	1970	1971	1972	1973	1974	1975
Assets						
Current Assets						
Inventories	1,195	1,231	913	1,526	4,652	7,320
Other	339	556	668	2,158	2,666	3,735
Fixed Assets						
Share in Subsidiaries	339	344	346	489	1,182	2,915
Other	482	342	340	331	457	800
Total	2,355	2,473	2,267	4,504	8,957	14,770
Liabilities and Equity						
Liabilities						
Bank Loans	357	350	304	1,284	3,208	7,001
Other	285	410	250	1,507	2,511	1,288
Equity	1,713	1,713	1,713	1,713	3,238	6,481
Total	2,355	2,473	2,267	4,504	8,957	14,770

[a] Source: CONASUPO.

TABLE 3. CONASUPO Operating Results, 1975 (in M $000)[a]

Commercialization program	Cost of goods sold	Total costs	Sales revenues	Program (deficits) or surplus
Maize	$ 4,578,249	$ 5,561,338	$ 3,967,218	$(1,594,120)
Wheat	2,205,054	2,252,897	1,832,133	(420,764)
Beans	988,471	1,859,980	909,958	(950,022)
Rice	384,701	421,031	360,126	(60,905)
Sorghum	1,284,549	1,578,988	1,239,340	(339,648)
Barley	5,111	5,646	5,143	(503)
Powdered milk	629,684	677,743	759,480	81,737
Tallow	137,678	149,748	203,842	54,094
Oilseeds	1,128,584	1,312,523	1,167,708	(144,815)
Crude oil	307,349	330,648	249,937	(80,711)
Refined oil	21,664	27,883	18,373	(9,510)
Oil meal	119,927	135,457	122,069	(13,388)
Other	29,280	71,001	29,671	(41,330)
Subtotal	11,820,357	14,384,883	10,864,998	(3,519,885)
Special and social action programs				(226,003)
Subsidiaries				
ACONSA (fresh vegetables)				(49,182)
ARCONSA (clothing)				(40,702)
BORUCONSA (warehousing)				(30,752)
DICONSA (distribution)				(204,470)
LICONSA (milk)				(164,257)
MACONSA (construction materials)				(17,978)
MINSA (maize)				50,637
TRICONSA (wheat)				(1,873)
ICONSA (processed foods)				15,287
Subtotal				(443,290)
Auxiliary support				
Grain containers				(38,096)
Headquarters administration				(447,577)
Subtotal				(485,673)
Other provisions				(47,849)
Other costs and revenues				138,910
Finance costs and revenues				(595,311)
Federal subsidy				4,200,000
TOTAL				(978,101)[b]

[a] Source: CONASUPO.
[b] The operating deficit for the period 1/1/76–7/31/76 was M $ 1599 and the federal subsidy was M $ 1450.

TABLE 4. CONASUPO Import[a] and Domestic Purchasing Prices (in M $ per Metric Ton)[b]

	1970	1971	1972	1973	1974	1975	1976
Maize							
Import	$ 913	$ 738	$ 940	$1319	$1961	$1813	$1622
Guarantee	940	940	940	1200	1500	1900	1900
Difference	$ (27)	$ (202)	$ 0	$ 119	$ 461	$ (87)	$ (278)
Wheat							
Import	$ 809	$ 843	$ 925	$1346	$2389	$2130	$1615
Guarantee	800	800	870	1200	1300	1750	1750
Difference	$ 9	$ 43	$ 55	$ 146	$1089	$ 380	$ (135)
Beans							
Import	$2849	—	—	—	$9535	$8411	—
Guarantee	1750	1750	1750	5000	6000	6000	4500
Difference	$1099				$3535	$2411	
Sorghum							
Import	$ 736	$ 824	$ 790	$1395	$1797	$1449	$1525
Guarantee	625	625	740	$ 775	1100	1420	1600
Difference	$ 111	$ 199	$ 50	$ 620	$ 697	$ 29	$ 75
Rice (palay)							
Import	$1452	—	$1839	$3615	$5045	$4988	—
Guarantee	1100	1100	1100	1100	3000	3000	2500
Difference	$ 352		$ 739	$2515	2045	1988	

[a] Average annual prices including transport and insurance delivered to Mexico.
[b] Source: Comisión Coordinador del Sector Agropecuario.

sidy (see Table 3). These subsidy profiles and their increased size are important in that they reveal, in quantitative terms, the government's priorities toward small farmers and low-income urban and rural consumers. The consumer subsidies on basic staples have been significant, averaging 25% below costs. The direct farmer subsidies appear much smaller relative to local or import market prices, but cloak the indirect intervention's effects on private buyer prices in CONASUPO's marketing operations.

ORGANIZATION AND OPERATIONS

In order to carry out the new strategy, CONASUPO made several important changes in its organizational structure and administrative systems during the period 1970–1976. One such major change was decentralization, which aimed at increasing CONASUPO's abilities to cover broader areas, especially in the rural sector. CONASUPO discovered in 1973 that it did not have the capacity to support the rapidly expanding network of rural stores from a Mexico City base with a distribution system traditionally oriented toward the urban sector. Consequently, the distribution subsidiary (DICONSA) was divided into six new regional subsidiaries, each with its own capital, responsible for stocking and supervising the CONASUPO stores in their different zones. This system gave CONASUPO more flexibility and presumably greater responsiveness to local needs. The general policies on, for example, pricing and regional budgets were set in the Central Office in Mexico City, but operating decisions were decentralized.*

Accompanying this operating decentralization was the establish-

*There is a National Procurement Committee that makes direct supply arrangements with factories. If a regional office can get a better price from local factories, it is free to do so.

TABLE 5. CONASUPO Average and Rural Prices (in M $ per Metric Ton)

	1970	1971	1972	1973	1974	1975	1976
Maize							
Local[a]	$ 905	$ 900	$ 900	$1110	$1460	$1860	$2250
Guarantee	940	940	940	1200	1500	1900	1900
Difference	$ (35)	$ (40)	$ (40)	$ (90)	$ (40)	$ (40)	$ 350
Wheat							
Local	$ 842	$ 860	$ 850	$ 890	$1340	$1720	$1900
Guarantee	800	800	870	1200	1300	1750	1750
Difference	$ 42	$ 60	$ (20)	$ (310)	$ 40	$ (30)	$ 150
Beans							
Local	$1848	$1980	$2030	$2990	$5600	$5260	$5100
Guarantee	1750	1750	1750	5000	6000	6000	4500
Difference	$ 98	$ 230	$ 280	($2010)	$ (400)	$ (740)	$ 600
Sorghum							
Local	$ 646	$ 680	$ 735	$ 850	$1270	$1580	$1900
Guarantee	625	675	740	775	1100	1420	1600
Difference	$ 21	$ 5	$ (5)	$ 75	$ 170	$ 160	$ 300
Rice (palay)							
Local	$1190	$1230	$1127	$1608	$2690	$2820	$2900
Guarantee	1100	1100	1100	1100	3000	3000	2500
Difference	$ 90	$ 130	$ 27	$ 508	$ (310)	$ (180)	$ 400

[a] Source: Dirección General de Economía Agricola.

ment of CONASUPO state delegates (one per state). These individuals served three main functions: (1) to coordinate CONASUPO's different activities in the state, (2) to link CONASUPO into the local political and power structure, and (3) to help create joint programs with other government institutions. The state delegate was basically a coordinator and troubleshooter. If all was going well, he had no hierarchical authority over the managers of the CONASUPO subsidiaries in the state. However, the Central Office could give him specific supervisory authority over all or part of the CONASUPO operations if circumstances warranted. Subdelegates existed in 17 states to provide further coordination and supervision within the states. One primary criterion used in selecting these delegates was their knowledge of and access to, yet independence from, the local political structure, which was critical to CONASUPO's success in the state.* The role of the delegates was further enhanced by building central facilities to house the offices of the CONASUPO subsidiaries, with the delegates being the nominal heads of these facilities. In effect, this was a form of centralization within the decentralized structure. It permitted improved coordination among the CONASUPO affiliates.

In addition to decentralization, CONASUPO underwent further vertical and horizontal integration. On the supply side it broadened its procurement, farm input, and training activities, and on the distribution side it expanded its warehousing services and large discount stores. It also expanded its processing operations to new products through the acquisition of a private firm that produced oil, shortening, soups, pastas, animal feed, and flour. These products were added to the existing line of wheat, maize, and milk products. Some consolidation also occurred. Affiliates that had been formed to procure and distribute clothing and fresh vegetables (ARCONSA and ACONSA) were fused into the main distribution subsidiary (DICONSA). The ANDSA warehousing system, which was operated independently, was integrated into CONASUPO's BORUCONSA system. A community development program (Development Micro Poles) was largely terminated as a separate activity, with many of its functions being absorbed by the warehouse subsidiary (BORUCONSA) and the training affiliate (CECONCA).

These organizational changes resulted in a broadened spectrum of activities and operating entities (see Fig. 1). CONASUPO stands out among government agricultural marketing organizations in Latin America because it developed a vertically integrated system ranging from input supply, produce procurement (with price supports), storage, food pro-

---

*The 31 delegates then serving were selected from a list of 2500 candidates.

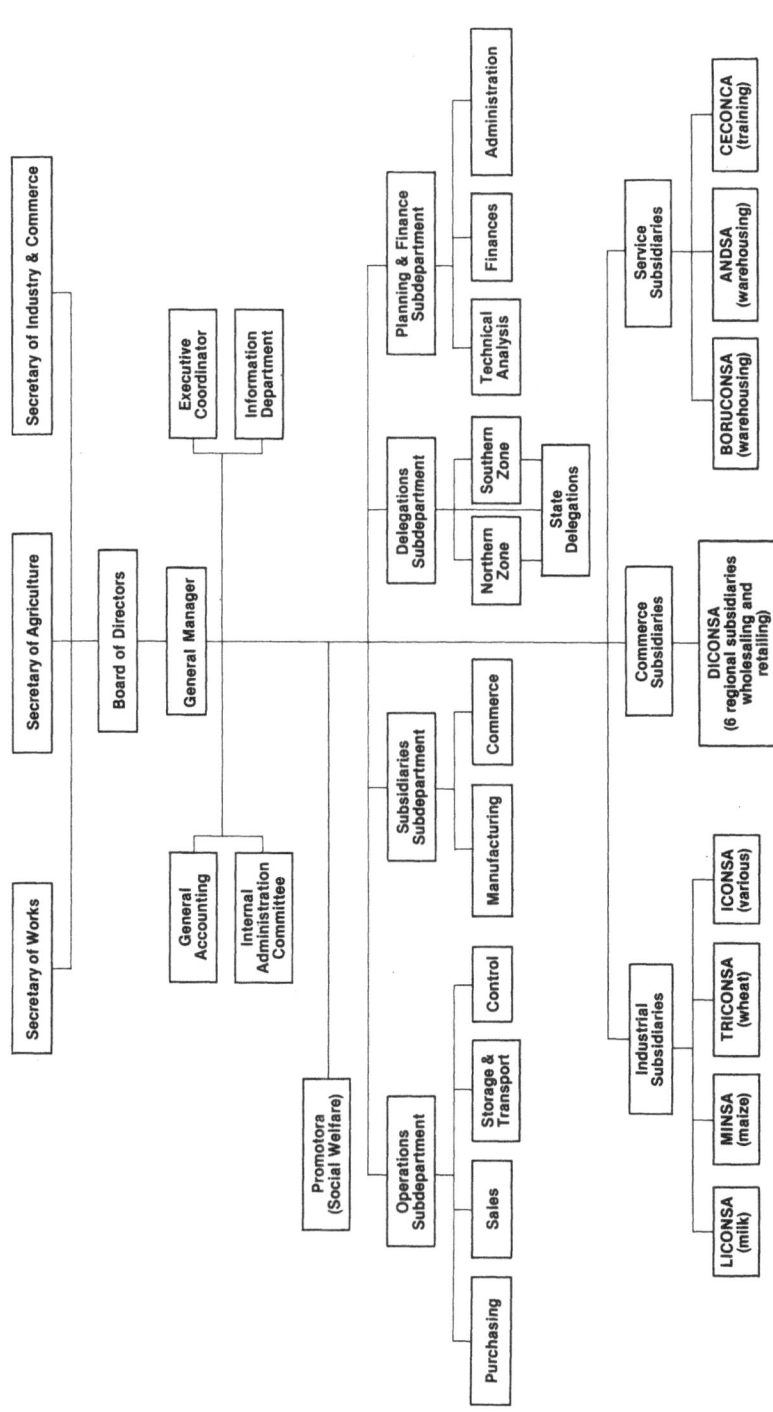

FIGURE 1. CONASUPO organizational chart.

cessing, and wholesaling to retail distribution. This organizational structure increased the points in the seed-to-consumer food system at which CONASUPO could exercise leverage. Each of these CONASUPO operations will be briefly described*:

1. BORUCONSA handled the administration of 1257 rural warehouses and the procurement price support program that utilized the warehouses for storage; it also sold staples at 1126 of its warehouses.
2. DICONSA operated CONASUPO's network of 11,769 urban supermarkets, neighborhood stores, rural stores, and mobile stores.
3. CECONCA was in charge of training the BORUCONSA warehouse operators as well as campesinos in specific skill areas; its programs were reaching over 50,000 campesinos annually.
4. TRICONSA processed wheat into flour and bread, which, in turn, was distributed to DICONSA; annual production was about 276 million pieces.
5. MINSA processed corn into flour that was primarily used for making tortillas; annual production was approximately 120,000 tons.
6. LICONSA imported low-fat powdered milk and reconstituted† and fortified it for distribution at subsidized prices in a ration system, primarily in Mexico City; it also bought and processed some domestic whole milk. Annual production was about 256 million liters.
7. ICONSA had seven plants in six states with a combined annual capacity of 931,000 tons for vegetable oils and their subproducts, maize and wheat flour, soup, pastas, and animal feed.

IMPLICATIONS FOR SUBSIDIZATION STRATEGIES AND IMPLEMENTATION

From the CONASUPO experience, we can draw several instructive conclusions regarding the formulation and implementation of subsidization strategies for nutritional purposes. A caveat, however, is that each subsidization scheme must be tailored to the particular political, economic, social, and administrative circumstances prevailing in the country. Certain concepts, and even implementation mechanisms, of one country

---

*A fuller description may be found in J. Austin, CONASUPO and Rural Development: Program Description, Analysis and Recommendations, report submitted to the World Bank, December 1976.
†LICONSA is the only institution with permission to reconstitute milk sold to the public.

may be applicable in another, but adjustments are generally needed. The salient dimensions that will be discussed are nutrition evaluation, multiple instruments, organizational structures, financing mechanisms, and political support.

NUTRITION EVALUATION

Despite the large resource allocation, including the federal subsidy to CONASUPO's operations, its nutritional impact has not been documented. There may be several reasons for this, including the absence of nutritional improvement as a central goal, limited technical skills in carrying out the research, and financial constraints.* One partial cross-sectional study of CONASUPO's subsidized milk ration program concluded that the nutritional status of participants was not superior to that of the control group, but that intrafamilial food distribution of the participants was affected in favor of the preschoolers.† It appeared that greater impact would be possible if even lower income groups were incorporated into the program. The income and purchasing power effects of the other subsidies can be estimated. For example, if the farmer sells his crop to CONASUPO, he might receive prices about 10–40% higher than he had been paid elsewhere. Similarly, if the families buy at CONASUPO stores, the lower prices would increase their purchasing power by 10–50%. Thus, purchasing power for urban and rural low-income groups can be significantly increased. The nutritional impact of this augmented purchasing power is not known precisely, but is likely to have been positive. Thus, to the extent that policy makers want to know and maximize the nutritional impact of their subsidization efforts, they should employ a nutritional status monitoring system as an integral part of their program.

MULTIPLE INSTRUMENTS

Central to CONASUPO's strategy was the recognition that several constraints enveloped the economic behavior of the small farmer. The use of a single instrument, price supports, was not sufficient to remove the

*For a fuller discussion of constraints and approaches to nutrition evaluation, see J. Austin, The perilous journey of nutrition evaluation. *Am. J. Clin. Nutr.* 31 (12):2324–2338, 1978.
†See Chapter 5 in: *Consumer Price Subsidies*, B. Rogers, C. Overholt, F. Sanchez-Carillo, A. Chavez, C. P. Timmer, and T. Belding. Special Study VI in AID Series *Nutrition Intervention in Developing Countries.* Oelgeschlager, Gunn, and Hain, Cambridge, Massachusetts, 1981.

constraints and allow the target group access to the subsidization benefit. Originally, farmers did not sell to CONASUPO because: the buying centers were too distant (a transportation constraint), they did not have bags or shellers (an input constraint), they did not know about CONASUPO's higher prices (a communications constraint), or they had presold their crop to intermediaries in exchange for consumer credit (a capital constraint). It was only by employing a full range of instruments aimed at each of these constraints that the original price support instrument was able to realize its potential impact.

On a broader scale, CONASUPO used this same multifaceted focus in developing its vertically integrated system. This allowed CONASUPO to intervene directly or indirectly on inputs or outputs throughout the food system. Clearly, this increased the government's control and flexibility; it was able to buy at high prices and sell at lower prices as well as adjust margins throughout the distribution system. At the same time, this administrative structure required greater capital and administrative competency.

CONASUPO used several mechanisms for targeting. On the retail side it located its stores in low-income neighborhoods, but did not restrict who could patronize the stores. For the subsidized milk centers, however, it used an income criterion and ration card system. In the rural areas it located its buying centers and stores in the zones where small farmers predominated. Still, the lack of nutritional criteria and needs assessment limited the precision of its targeting efforts.

ORGANIZATIONAL STRUCTURES

One of the revealing points in CONASUPO's experience was that its strategic decision to place greater emphasis on reaching the low-income rural producers and consumers could not be implemented within the existing organizational structures. Strategy changes generally require structural adjustments in order to equip the organization to carry out its new mandate. Such adjustments will, of course, depend on the nature of the strategy. In CONASUPO's instance, the key organizational change was decentralization. Because CONASUPO's activities included direct service delivery, it could not just employ the existing market mechanisms or the old urban-oriented CONASUPO system. The crucial balancing act with decentralization is how to delegate responsibility and authority while still maintaining adequate control. CONASUPO used the policy, budgetary, information, and personnel mechanisms to achieve this balance. It also attempted, although with limited effectiveness, to balance its "top-down" approach with village-level participation in the supervision and operation of local activities.

FINANCING MECHANISMS

CONASUPO's subsidization strategy required significant funds from the Federal treasury: U.S. $338 million in 1975, which represented 4.6% of the federal government's public investment that year, or 2.1% of total federal expenditures. However, it should also be pointed out that these percentages are far less than in some other countries, such as Sri Lanka or Egypt.

One of the interesting self-financing mechanisms used by CONASUPO was the cross-store subsidization. Most of CONASUPO's urban supermarkets and discount stores are quite profitable. They sell their goods at prices generally somewhat below private supermarket prices, but they are often patronized by middle-income or lower-middle-income consumers. One could criticize CONASUPO for not using these stores to reach the lower-income groups. However, the profits from these stores help offset the losses incurred in smaller urban and rural stores. This helps keep the overall operation on a break-even basis, thus reducing the fiscal burden and enhancing sustainability. A similar cross-subsidization approach can be used for items within the total product line. Certain scarce products preferred by higher-income groups could be sold at larger profit margins to permit thinner or negative margins on those items of greater nutritional significance to needier groups.

POLITICAL SUPPORT

CONASUPO would not have been able to expand and implement its strategy without strong political support. In Mexico's highly centralized and largely single-party system, this meant presidential backing. President Echeverría lent this support because CONASUPO's multifaceted strategy and mechanisms for subsidization represented the best administrative vehicle available to pursue the President's expressed desire to benefit the rural and urban poor.

During the initial years (1977–1978) of the new López Portillo administration, CONASUPO retained strong presidential support, but it was a period of austerity and retrenchment. Subsidies were reduced as was the retail outlet network. However, during 1978–1979, CONASUPO began to expand its retail network once again. In addition, its top management expressed an intensified interest in designing means of increasing the impact of its operations on nutritional problems in Mexico. It is clear that CONASUPO's size, multiple intervention points, decentralized structure, distinctive financing mechanisms, and strong political support place it in a position to use the subsidization intervention in ways that could significantly enhance the nutritional well-being of deprived groups. It is also clear, however, that CONASUPO's instruments can be used in ways that do not really benefit the neediest groups. Thus, perhaps the major challenge facing CONASUPO is to respecify clearly the lowest-income consumers and producers as the primary target beneficiaries, and to review continuously the design and implementation of each policy instrument to ensure that it is maximizing the impact on these neediest groups. Mexico has the human, natural, and financial resources to eliminate malnutrition by the turn of the century, and CONASUPO could play a major role in that task if the political commitment is present.

Comment

ALBERTO CARVALHO DA SILVA

My comments are based on the assumption that implementation of nutrition intervention must follow a period of planning, pretesting, and project demonstration so that the government may incorporate the intervention as a part of regular health and nutrition planning. Some funding might come from nongovernment resources, but most should be a part of the government budget, thus ensuring continuity without the need for external support.

Implementation has at least three fundamental requirements: political decision, technical support, and structural and manpower resources. The following discussion will illustrate four cases of nutrition intervention in which one or more of these factors proved decisive. They also prove that academic groups are essential to prepare program-oriented research and analysis and to plan for actual implementation. Three examples come from Brazil; the fourth is from the Republic of Indonesia.

THE THREE BRAZILIAN CASE STUDIES

Since 1973, Brazil has had a National Food and Nutrition Program (PRONAN), planned and implemented by the Food and Nutrition Institute (INAN), a federal agency affiliated with the Ministry of Health, acting in cooperation with the Ministries of Education, Agriculture, Labor, Social Welfare, and Planning. PRONAN has selected a target population—families living on minimum salaries or less*—comprised of approximately 50% of 120 million inhabitants.

*A minimum salary is equivalent to approximately U.S. $78 per month (December 1979).

ALBERTO CARVALHO DA SILVA • Programa Multidisciplinar de Nutriçao, The Ford Foundation, Rio de Janeiro, Brazil.

PRONAN has two fundamental program components: food supplementation and stimulation of food production. Food supplementation, delivered through the health system, is provided for (1) vulnerable groups—pregnant and nursing women and children under 6 years of age, (2) children 7–14 years old, supplemented through school lunch programs under the aegis of the Ministry of Education, and (3) low-wage industrial workers, in the form of subsidized meals supported by the Ministry of Labor.

Support for food production provides assistance to small farmers, who receive credit and technical inputs to strengthen their capacity for increasing production and marketing their products.

In addition to PRONAN, INAN has a second, parallel program, the Brazil Nutrition Project, supported by a loan from the World Bank. Its purposes are to (1) strengthen the capacity for nutrition planning, implementation, and evaluation; (2) experiment with alternative strategies and delivery systems for nutrition intervention; and (3) support applied research on relevant topics, such as the interrelations between agricultural policies and nutrition.

The following three programs illustrate different aspects of the problem of implementing nutrition planning:

SUBSIDIZED MEALS FOR LOW-WAGE LABORERS

The purpose of this program is to supply one subsidized meal per day, 5 or 6 days per week, to low-wage industrial workers. It was included in PRONAN but implemented by the Ministry of Labor, under the leadership of a former INAN nutrition planner.* It was put in place directly by private organizations without preparatory pilot studies or pretesting. By July 1979, 800,000 workers were covered. They pay 20% of the cost of the meal, and employers and government pay the balance. Part of the costs borne by the private sector are reduced by income tax deductions.

Five important factors contributed to successful and rapid implementation in this case:

- A clear, simple project strategy, shared between the private sector and only the Ministry of Labor; no other government agencies are involved.

*Dr. David Boianowski, a former professor of nutrition, University of Brasilia, who received training as a student in the International Nutrition Program at the Massachusetts Institute of Technology in 1974.

- A firm political decision made by the ministry directly responsible for program implementation.
- A well-developed, flexible delivery system provided by private companies.
- Strong technical and managerial input contributed by a competent nutrition planner.
- No conflict with social structures.

In conclusion, except for the costs largely borne by the government both directly and as an income tax subsidy, the project represents a straightforward intervention. Implementation followed a firm political decision and the private sector supplied managerial expertise.

CONSUMER PRICE SUBSIDY FOR BASIC FOOD COMMODITIES

This project is being tested in the city of Recife, where INAN's target population (maximum family income equal to two minimum salaries per month) has an average daily energy intake of from 64 to 80% of normal requirements and an average daily protein intake of 30–41 g, 80% of it from vegetable sources.

Initially, the project subsidized consumer prices for four food commodities: 2.5 kg rice, 0.5 kg corn meal, 2.0 kg beans, and 0.5 kg dry milk per person per month. This added 590 cal per day for a total of 10,000 families in a poor section of Recife,* meeting from 75 to 130% of the average daily energy deficit in the target population. These families were divided into four groups composed of 2500 families each. Price subsidies in relation to average market prices were: group 1, 60%; group 2, 30%; groups 3 and 4, 45%. The first three groups are free to attend the health centers, while for group 4 health services, basically maternal–child health care, are compulsory. The purpose of compulsory care was to evaluate the impact of systematic health care. Analysis of this part of the program is difficult because families in the other groups are "free" to attend the health centers if they so wish. A fifth, or control group, is comprised of 2500 families from a socially comparable area of the city not covered by the project.

Food was purchased at COBAL markets† with coupons on which

---

*The boroughs of Santo Amaro, Encruzilhada, and Beberibe, the same ones included in the PAHO infant mortality study (1968–1971).
†Companhia Brasileira de Alimentos (Brazilian Food Company, Ministry of Agriculture). COBAL buys food directly from producers, from cooperatives, and from the buffer food stocks supervised by the Production Financing Board, Ministry of Agriculture.

were printed family identification, number in family, and level of subsidy. By the end of the first year, the number of children with third-degree malnutrition decreased by 33%; those with second-degree, by 11%. Other relevant observations are:

1. Notwithstanding a considerable drop-out rate, especially among group 2 families receiving a 30% subsidy, the population assisted is reacting favorably and wishes the program to continue. They report a more regular supply of food, and the majority prefer the subsidy as food instead of in money, because money would be at least partially spent for other urgent purposes.
2. On the negative side, families complain that they are not able to accumulate enough cash to pay for 40–70% of the price once or twice a month, and this is especially true for the poorest families who benefited most from the program. For operational reasons, families were asked to purchase the monthly quota at one time.
3. Carrying home more than 30 kg of food, as is the case for large families, may involve transportation costs. For example, a family with 10 members—not unusual in the area—would be entitled to 50 kg of subsidized food per month.
4. Consumers would like to select the food commodities to be purchased at subsidized prices instead of being restricted to the four offered by COBAL and the program. Specifically, they would like dried beef included, as they firmly believe that meat is an essential item for the diet.

On the basis of the experience obtained during the first year, INAN, COBAL, and the state government of Pernambuco are complementing a food subsidy program (PROAB) by introducing the following modifications in the initial model:

1. Distribution of subsidized food will be through a network of small, private retail shops.
2. The food basket will be increased to include 11 basic food commodities.
3. A price stabilization system operated by COBAL (as purchasing agent for small producers and bulk suppliers to a voluntary chain of food retailers) will be formulated.

PROAB was first tested for 7 months in two slum areas and recently launched on a much larger basis. Other states—Bahia and Ceará—are already considering implementing this food subsidy program using the PROAB format.

This second example of implementation is obviously a much more complex program. Even though the basic idea was very simple and had previously been tested in other countries, there were several variables outside the control of the planner. These included such problems as consumer acceptance, drop-outs, purchasing capacity, participation of COBAL, coupon supervision, adequate utilization of food by the families, operational problems of food distribution and price control, and evaluation of benefits in terms of nutritional improvement of vulnerable groups in the participating families.

Solving these problems took more than a year and was possible because of strong, competent scientific and managerial leadership. The program was considerably reoriented to correct logistic, operational, and acceptability problems. Implementation is taking a stepwise course and it is expected that further modifications and regional adjustments will be required before the program can be expanded to cover other areas with comparable nutritional conditions. However, it is already clear that, should funds be available, operational problems will be solved and implementation will depend only on political decision.

INDIRECT SUBSIDIES TO IMPROVE FOOD PRODUCTION AND CONSUMPTION BY SMALL FARMERS

This project involves testing the effectiveness of interlinked agricultural and social extension services in stimulating improvement of food production and intake among the rural poor. It reaches 7500 small-farm families (45,000 persons) distributed into four categories: landowners with 0–10 hectares, those with 10–30 hectares, establishments with 30–50 hectares, and tenants. Four interventions are tested in each category:

1. Help with production and commercialization through labor and community organization; technical assistance; institutional credit; minimum prices; other rural extension services existing in the area.
2. The above plus assistance by other trained (contact) farmers.
3. The same as (1) plus advanced purchase of production.
4. All three of the above.

In addition, all four groups are offered health and nutrition services (sanitation, prenatal care, immunization, and nutrition education that covers adequate practices of breast-feeding, child-weaning, and child-feeding).

The demonstration project has been active since mid-1977. Increased productivity and food consumption have been reported for the four groups with minor differences, depending on the intervention. Interpretation of these differences is difficult because crop productivity has also been influenced by annual and statewide variation in climate. However, some unforeseen problems have emerged:

- The project is contributing to an increase in use of land for pasture (animal grazing), leaving less available for crop production.
- Extending credit to landless farmers continues to be difficult, since most of the bank agencies in the area are neither flexible nor cooperative in dealing with would-be borrowers.
- Landlords have found ways of sharing most of the benefits of the program by introducing modifications in the land-renting contracts.
- So far, advanced purchase of agricultural products has proven difficult, as COBAL and the local cooperatives lack the necessary flexibility.

Solving the above problems is particularly complex, because different ministries and government agents are involved, including the Bank of Brazil, at the central, state, and municipal level.

Also, some of the small farmers choose to use the additional income for repairing their homes and purchasing animals as a capital reserve to face future shortages instead of increasing food consumption. This may well be an economically rational decision, but it does not fulfill the nutritional objectives of increasing food production and consumption.

Unfavorable attitudes of farmers can be at least partially changed under the influence of nutrition education, but structural and social resistance is viewed with much greater concern, considering the political power of landlords and the fact that most of the bank agents responsible for loan approval and administration are relatives of the landlords and are therefore reluctant to oppose the privileges of their peers and frequently even their own families.

The Indonesian Case: The Integration of Academic Groups and Government for Program Implementation

The fourth case represents an excellent example of the need for close cooperation between academic groups and the government for effective program implementation.

For more than 10 years, the Republic of Indonesia has maintained a National Applied Nutrition Program covering, by the middle of 1979, approximately 6% of the rural population. The program is a combination of nutrition and health education, maternal–child health care with emphasis on nutrition and development of the child under 3 years of age, family planning, and agricultural extension that focuses on food production through a home garden component; it also includes preventive and curative supplementation with vitamin A, iron, and iodine.

The third Indonesian five-year plan for national development (1979–1984) states that by the end of 1984, the nutrition program should cover at least 40,000 of the 60,000 villages in the country. This, of course, requires the development of manpower to conduct the technical and managerial activities, a task to be fulfilled by the training centers under the leadership of program coordinators. Training this needed manpower will require the participation of several schools of nutrition, medicine, and agriculture. Development of the instruments required by the program (messages for nutrition and health education; formulas and technology for nutrition supplementation; viable technology packages for agricultural extension and criteria; methodology and data processing for program monitoring and evaluation) is also a responsibility assigned to the research and training centers of Indonesian universities, assisted by outside consultants.

This example shows clearly how political decision makers and academic groups complement each other, neither group alone being capable of implementing a successful, large-scale program. It is expected that once the managerial and technical problems are solved and the needed manpower is made available, program implementation will develop without unusual difficulty because it does not collide with the goals of privileged groups or call for social reforms. To the contrary, the program endeavors to increase food production and offer nutrition and health education without interfering with the current system of land ownership or the relations between landlords and tenants.

CONCLUSION

The decisive factor for implementation of nutrition programs is the political decision, usually based on nutritional analysis conducted by academic groups. Nutrition planning and evaluation fill the gap between them and make government decisions possible, provided that it is socially and politically viable. Implementation is usually successfully accomplished when objectives are clear and simple, and when remedies are available for implementation through an already existing structure. Coordination and integration involving different structures and groups usually present a serious obstacle because they require much more capacity for coordination and management than are usually found in developing societies.

More complex programs that try to correct the causes of malnutrition by influencing the current balance between economic forces and privileged classes tend to generate political resistance. This is usually the problem with rural nutrition programs that try to develop a mechanism to protect landless farmers from exploitation by landlords. On the contrary, community-oriented programs based on nutrition and health education, maternal–child health, and food supplementation are usually well accepted and may prove effective, although they are not expected to correct the *causes* of malnutrition and poverty.

Nutrition planners should be willing to analyze the social and political background of a society and formulate interventions that do not conflict with them. Nutrition interventions should be evaluated for their acceptability and the results obtained, not for their intellectual value. Nutrition interventions paving the way for social reform are highly desirable, but unless political conditions are favorable they are at risk of being rejected or ineffectively implemented.

Comment

JAMES GAVAN

It is fairly clear that in countries with inadequate food consumption levels, food subsidies do effectively address that problem. But that is not the main issue. Rather, the questions are how much are we willing to pay for such a program, and how can we make subsidy policies more reasonable?

One way to increase cost-effectiveness is to restrict access to these systems through a variety of devices. Geographic restriction to urban areas is one tool available to cities. Although criticism has been raised that subsidizing urban areas will encourage migration to the cities, I think that we have tended to condemn governments too quickly about this problem, because the alternative is often no subsidies at all. Similarly, the use of income tests, which is now being tried in Sri Lanka, will be an interesting case to follow.

However, while restrictions seem appropriate in order to make subsidy programs more cost-effective, eventually such an approach converges with a direct feeding program. As such, we must give more consideration to how food subsidy recommendations are linked with programmed food aid. For example, it is reasonable to consider a two-price system where international donors support domestic procurement, keeping prices high to farmers and low to consumers.

Finally, I would like to comment on a methodological point raised by Taylor: the question of taxing other foodstuffs to finance subsidies. In the 1960s, Sri Lanka did this quite effectively by taxing flour and sugar to help defray part of the rice subsidy. At the same time that Sri Lanka ran a system of subsidies, the government also maintained prices to farmers. From that experience, a case could be made as to how the operation of their entire food system has facilitated the rather even income distribution in Sri Lanka.

JAMES GAVAN • International Food Policy Research Institute, Washington, D.C.

Discussion

Discussion began by stressing that changes in food prices impact on the rural poor, and that this should be given primary consideration when initiating a food subsidy scheme. If food prices increase, the plight of the rural poor who grow the food improves, and rural migration to cities will be slowed or possibly even reversed. If food prices decrease, however, there will be a negative nutritional impact concurrent with greater migration to cities.

Expanding on this theme, it was argued that the major effect of government policies with respect to controlling food prices is the potential for depressing relative rural incomes, and possibly even agricultural output, as a result of the manipulation of the trade between rural and urban sectors. In other words, experience suggests that there is a propensity for government interference in price mechanisms to make prices less favorable for the rural poor.

If one wishes to ensure that an improvement in agricultural trade will benefit the poorest, one must take care that the "improvements" (and other policies) do not discourage rural production for self-support and subsistence. The poor tend to produce and consume similar products—cassava, millet, maize. Subsidies on these will undermine the market if (and only if) the poor begin to emerge as sellers. Since small farms remain relatively efficient users of scarce land and capital with a given technology, government support should best be given to production of crops grown and consumed by the poorest. Thus, if the objective is to keep food cheap, a negative nutritional impact may nevertheless be expected if this is done by depressing prices to rural growers. An overt subsidy, paid for by taxpayers in proportion to capacity to pay, and the establishment of a gap between producers' and consumers' prices would be a better approach.

Other participants noted that much of the emphasis in the presentations had been on the formal market economy. However, as much as

70–75% of basic foods do not enter the marketing channels in certain countries. While this issue of subsistence production was acknowledged, it was pointed out that even though a peasant may keep 85–90% of a commodity for home consumption and sell only a small percentage for cash needs, the selling price of the peasant's produce influences the amount of the commodity sold versus that consumed. In Asia, for example, almost all households have some significant interaction with—and are influenced by—markets, despite a high degree of subsistence consumption. Therefore, subsidy policies must also pay attention to the subsistence farmer, since his production and consumption will likewise be affected by various policy decisions.

Given that the market influences consumption in all segments of a society, including the subsistence farmer, the question was raised about just how far pricing and subsidy policies can go in improving nutritional status. It was recommended that nutrition education efforts complement pricing policies. Moreover, due to the importance and costs of food subsidy schemes, many argue that it is now time to take a more comprehensive and systematic view of these efforts.

Part of this new approach must include consideration of the opportunity costs: benefits that might have come from agricultural research and from agricultural extension to the small farmer. Similarly, attention must be devoted to the trade-offs between allocating scarce resources and capital to subsidies and the alternative of integrated nutrition, health, and family planning programs—especially since, in many countries, the rural population continues to increase. While middle-income countries like Brazil and Mexico can afford subsidies without greatly debilitating other basic needs programs, countries like India, Bangladesh, and Tanzania cannot afford subsidies without sacrificing more essential programs such as integrated health and family planning activities.

In addition to the question of opportunity costs, others mentioned that food subsidies often will not reach the poorest segments of society. This is where the food subsidy scheme must interface with direct feeding activities. Furthermore, alternatives to traditional subsidy schemes must be considered. For example, a cooked corn–cassava mix could be developed and sold to small-scale peddlers at a subsidized price. They, in turn, would go through the streets or communities selling the food product at its low, subsidized price, taking a small profit. This would produce both an income and price effect, an innovative type of approach to interventions in the economic system.

Finally, discussion centered on the need to consider the sociopolitical aspects of a subsidy program. It was pointed out, for example, that it is not possible to raise the issue of opportunity costs of a subsidy without taking a political stand. Likewise, a food subsidy is easy to start, but politically difficult to stop or even reduce. The general tendency, in fact, is for subsidies to increase over time regardless of either the availability of resources or the cost-effectiveness of the program. Therefore, greater attention must be paid to the political forces that both initiate and perpetuate such programs.

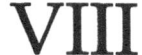

VIII

Nutrition Policy Implementation

The previous sections of this volume have examined a broad spectrum of policy issues and program experience, each representing a different kind of approach to reducing the prevalence of hunger and malnutrition. In some respects, a comparison of the relative effectiveness of one methodology versus another is rendered spurious by the great variation in political, economic, social, and technical factors inherent in each. Yet, in every case, the interface between the rhetorical statement of policy objectives and the actual start-up and operation of a tangible program— that is, the process of food and nutrition policy and implementation—has been a critical determinant of ultimate program success.

Thus, this section of the volume attempts to address the issue of implementation directly. While there is no pretension that this represents the definitive statement on the subject, the comments and discussion contained herein do point the way at least toward the formulation of an appropriate set of questions.

A summary of the most salient points raised by participants in the final plenary discussion is presented, followed by an insightful rapporteur's summary and analysis of the conference, prepared by Chafkin.

Final Discussion

The final session provided an opportunity to review major issues discussed in previous sessions and to assess what had been learned during the course of the meetings. Among the themes so identified was the need for caution in formulating nutrition policy, especially when technical expertise is provided to foreign governments. The development of a comprehensive nutrition policy is an onerous task, requiring a formidable amount of country-specific data. Moreover, even when extensive data are available and the appropriate policy analysis has been performed, it may still only be feasible, politically or financially, to address one or two main problem areas that are the causative agents of malnutrition. Therefore, it is incumbent upon individuals involved in nutrition policy to be more attuned to the competing goals and priorities of governments and to the opportunity costs of various governmental actions. Clearly, this is possible only through careful and concerted analysis of specific circumstances.

This theme was reiterated by those who stressed that a comprehensive or agreed upon set of instructions to policy makers and planners from any international meeting is both unrealistic and infeasible. No simple truths exist; there are no universally applicable frameworks for intervention. Similarly, there is no *a priori* stepwise progression for selecting and formulating policy guidelines that can be implemented by administrators, planners, or program personnel. The reason is that it is not a linear process; policy decisions must reflect the realities of the implementation process, and vice versa. In other words, the processes of policy making, providing program guidelines to fulfill those directives, and thereafter translating guidelines into action programs are, or should be, continuous and inextricably interwoven.

It was also emphasized that, despite the complexity of factors and options to be considered in food policy formulation and nutrition planning, it is vital that whatever strategies are developed be as practicable and as disaggregated as possible. Too often in the past unrealistically complex prescriptions have emanated from sophisticated policy analysis. In their preoccupation with the infinitely complex subtleties of the malnutrition problem, they ignore common sense practicality.

Perhaps the most significant change in the nutrition planning experience during the past few years has been the difficult adjustment of expectations. There has been a realization that incremental improvements are probably the most that traditional planning efforts can accomplish within the existing framework of social, political, and economic realities. At a minimum, it was agreed, nutrition planning should guard against causing further harm to the physical and social welfare of those it intends to assist.

The accumulation of experience during the past few years also suggests that there were overly optimistic expectations about what the multidisciplinary and multisectoral approach could accomplish, especially when the number of individuals trained explicity in nutrition policy and planning is small. Rather, nutritionists, economists, political scientists, physicians, and other disciplinary experts have converged on a problem that, until recently, has been plagued by a lack of textbooks, case studies, policy analyses, and similar material. Recommendations were for greater emphasis on building a body of knowledge based on past experiences. This demands careful documentation of both pilot and large-scale operational programs. The gleaning of knowledge from past experiences continues, and unraveling the complexities of implementation should help to expand political support for more effective implementation of food and nutrition policies and programs in the future.

Among the lessons extracted from recent experiences has been the notion that program implementation, as an art and a skill, has been underemphasized. While the international community has concentrated on providing technical assistance, sending biological and social scientists throughout the world, the need to develop managerial capabilities has been relatively neglected. As a consequence, good management—rather than political and resource commitment—may well represent the biggest constraint to successful planning and policy making. This is especially true in the context of the complex "systems approach" to multisectoral nutrition planning that has been so widely embraced during the past few years.

Related to the need for enhanced management capabilities was the theory that program success requires responding to the felt needs of individual communities. Although it was recognized that enlisting communitywide participation is sometimes difficult, such involvement was deemed a crucial factor in program success. Various degrees of community participation may be appropriate for different settings and phases of work in the same community. It was also acknowledged, however, that consideration must be given as well to the formidable time and social constraints limiting community participation, particularly in circumstances of extreme poverty. Nevertheless, every attempt should be made to understand and to be responsive to a community's expectations and perceptions of programs to benefit them. Ideally, nutrition programs should play a catalytic role in fostering community learning, organization, and sensitization.

The issue that received the greatest attention during the course of the summary discussion was the number of obstacles constraining expanded linkage between nutrition research and nutrition program planning and implementation. In this regard, discussion focussed on the sufficiency of existing scientific knowledge as well as the most appropriate directions for future research. The distinction was stressed between the type of knowledge required for publication in a scientific journal and that demanded to guide interventions. It was asserted, in fact, that the exacting and cautious nature of good science sometimes is an obstacle to good policy formulation and good program advocacy. Some even went so far as to agree that, in circumstances such as famine and disaster relief, nutrition research has hardly any relevance whatsoever.

Despite these distinctions, nutrition planning is often characterized as highly political and unscientific. Some felt that it is a mistake for practitioners to "water down" the scientific approach of programs in order to enable politicians to grasp their significance better. What is needed instead is for nutritionists to present politicians with the scientific facts in a confident, straightforward manner that they can understand. By the same token, the programs must be built on a solid scientific foundation in order to be convincing to politicians.

The recent experience in Nicaragua was presented to illustrate this point. A rigorous scientific evaluation of the salt iodization program was undertaken prior to the revolution and the fall of the Somoza regime. Pre- and postiodization evaluation of thyroid hormones and antibodies, goiter, and iodine-131 intakes indicated program success. Not coincidentally, salt iodization was the only nutrition program continued immediately after the revolution, precisely because of the availability of unambiguous scientific evidence. It was argued on this basis that the presentation of sound facts, and the alternatives that emanate from such knowledge, represent the most effective method for mobilizing the necessary political support, for either establishing a new program or maintaining an ongoing one.

Unfortunately, many previous efforts to reduce malnutrition have been plagued by ineffective information transfer from scientists to government planners, administrators, and implementors. The general consensus of the participants was that enough is known of nutrition science to convince leaders, in both government and the community, of the central importance of nutrition to development and human welfare. While efforts should obviously continue to fill in the gaps in scientific knowledge, more attention should be given to the problems identified by the policy makers. Translation of scientific and policy analysis into practical action is now at the forefront of the battle against malnutrition.

In much of the current literature regarding nutrition policy, either the implementation question is never asked, or it is asked only at the end of the study instead of at the beginning. It was urged that study protocols should include an implementation hypothesis, not as an afterthought, but rather as an integral part of the end research. Journal editors and other opinion makers should recognize that problems of implementation are respectable subjects of research. In this way, investigators will have the support and criticism necessary to develop rigorous methods and to study and publish about implementation problems. Yet, the group also concluded that the problem of writing frankly about sensitive political issues will remain unsolved. Nevertheless, understanding the *art* of implementation remains a difficult but indispensable aspect of the efficient translation of nutrition science to policy and policy to implementation.

The last major area of discussion involved the relationship between nutrition planning, in terms of the political motivations and ideological orientations of governments, and socioeconomic development. Attention must be given to the question of just how far policy makers, planners, nutritionists, and implementors can go within the limitations of the social and economic constraints in which they operate. For example, it was agreed that the problem of improving nutrition is *not* simply one of nutrition policy or implementation *per se;* it is also a function of such factors as better crop mixes, more evenly distributed agricultural output, and greater production on small farms.

Although academics cannot assume the role of armchair revolutionaries, they can advocate better distribution of land and water resources, availability of credit, and similar measures that are worthy of support and encouragement. Nutritional improvement is rooted in the outcomes and repercussions of such efforts. This is not to suggest that unless these issues are addressed all else fails. However, recognition and consideration of these factors is important in the sense of reconciling frustrations, preventing loss of confidence and spirit, and improving the quality of the effort put forth.

In a similar vein, the major bottleneck for nutrition program implementation in developing countries is the usual disregard for the political motivation associated with government decisions concerning socially oriented policies, including nutrition. In other words, political goals and expectations may be (and usually are) quite different from the goals and expectations of nutrition planners. It is only natural, therefore, for nutrition programs to suffer considerable readjustment when moving from project proposal to social and political reality. Nutrition planners should be prepared to anticipate these changes, taking them into account when formulating their projects.

One participant asserted that prior efforts may have erred by limiting major goals of nutrition programs to measurable biological responses. An important contribution of such programs to human welfare would be to create awareness and social responsibility. Part of the results would be a growing commitment of a society to correct the distortions responsible for poverty and malnutrition. Within this approach, nutrition programs will continue to be needed urgently in developing societies. They should include not only nutrition education activities, but also a strong component of social education at all levels in order to create awareness of the problem.

While the long-term integration of nutrition goals and programs into general development strategies was given high priority by workshop participants, special nutrition projects were deemed a present necessity. Despite rhetoric to the contrary, development efforts often do not aid the families of malnourished children as much as they help those families best prepared by education, wealth, and status to profit from them. The result may be, therefore, to increase the gap between the poorest of the poor and the slightly better-off. The children of the abjectly poor remain malnourished while those of the better-off are shown as evidence of the success of development. Development activities that include special efforts to assist the most seriously poor require many years to achieve results. In the meantime, the group concluded that children must be fed and that feeding them will probably require special nutrition programs.

Summary Comments

SOL H. CHAFKIN

The conference gained momentum as it went along. The agenda was sufficiently untidy to permit a liveliness in searching for some common ground on which everyone could stand in viewing the promise and the problems in moving from the rhetoric (not rhetoric in a pejorative sense) of concepts, plans, and policies to the realities of implementation. We began properly by asking ourselves what was bothering us. Why were we searching for solutions to nutrition problems? And we did this, I thought, through a very helpful discussion of the functional significance of malnutrition.

We have learned more and more over the past several years about the consequences for life, learning, and the behavior of individuals, and, in return, for communities and societies, of what does or does not go into the mouth. The presentations—together with other work in the United States and overseas—suggest that health and nutrition factors, especially those affecting central nervous system function, may play a much larger role in behavior than the psychosocial scientific community has heretofore believed. This is especially relevant as these factors interact with the social stresses faced by low-income populations in *any* country, developed or developing.

Through the mysterious logic of the agenda makers, we immediately plunged into food fortification, and Arroyave presented three of those painful, instructive lessons on how economics and politics affected implementation of a policy for fortifying a single food with an essential nutrient. I was left with a sense that, despite past disappointments, fortification is a technique—a kind of intervention—that has special cost-effectiveness potential in certain situations and with certain nutrients. Yet Arroyave's program came very close to being buried for 10 years.

SOL H. CHAFKIN • The Ford Foundation, New York, New York.

We then turned to the subject of small-farm agricultural systems. Case studies were presented in rich detail and considerable perceptiveness by Fiester and Okigbo. I must confess that I would have had great difficulty in making the connection with relevance to the conference theme had not Lipton helped by illustrating some of the connections.

The problem of the relevance of the papers to the conference theme of implementation was intensified, I think, in the workshop on food conservation and post-harvest loss. Pariser posed the basic issue of whether reducing such losses would, in fact, benefit those at nutritional risk, and this issue was pursued further by Guggenheim and Spitz. Parpia opened up the managerial and technological possibilities derived from his knowledge and experience. But Koga and Spitz reminded us of the characteristics of the food production and processing chain, namely, that prices and profits may have more to do with determining investment decisions in post-harvest technology than an abstraction called "appropriate technology."

My qualms of Tuesday were replaced on Wednesday by new ones as we turned to the subject of supplemental feeding programs and formulated foods. Here, at last, was a subject directly connected to the nutrition policy–implementation interface. But the picture drawn by Scrimshaw, Allen and Koval, and Ghassemi was generally dismal. They suggested that supplemental feeding is often very ineffective with uncertain benefits. Only Tandon brightened the outlook by offering some rather impressive results of India's sustained—and I emphasize sustained—investment in, and periodic improvement or modification of, supplemental feeding interventions.

The third afternoon brought us to what our unfortunate jargon calls integrated, multisectoral village interventions, and it also brought us to the cases of the large-scale programs in Indonesia, Colombia, and the Philippines. I will express my reservations about the *multi* syndrome later, but here not only was it relevant in terms of theme, but there were actually *implementors* standing before us. In a similar fashion, we listened Thursday morning to the description and analysis of large-scale interventions in the form of food price subsidies. I finally began to feel better about how the conference was progressing, as I became aware of the kind of weight and importance that such interventions have in distributional terms, although they are somewhat more murky in terms of nutritional results.

With the benefit of a productive roundtable discussion, plus hindsight, we did build up to a set of issues, clearer than I had expected them to be, that seemed highly relevant to the policy–implementation interface, the theme of the conference. I detected a few important points, some of which were touched on during the final part of the conference, that suggest the need to revise, modestly and quietly, some of our concepts about nutrition policy and its implementation. The first point is that there is a need to redeploy some energy and attention from constructing the *multis*, that is, the multisectoral, multiagency, and multidisciplinary national nutrition planning style, to *subnational* jurisdictions, including the village level. Also, I am persuaded that coordination is doable at the local level. This shift of attention is already beginning, I am glad to report, at INCAP, which had one of the more elaborate exercises in national nutrition planning. They have now recognized not only the need to shift to subnational units, but also the need to shift, perhaps, to single-agency implementation modes.

The second point is that there is a need to attach greater importance to simplifying, or decomplexifying, some of our approaches. I was delighted when Hendrata said, "We stopped using the words 'nutrition status.' We say 'weight gain.' That is a message we can transmit and understand. It is not going to please everybody, but it is good enough for what we want to do." There is also, despite the other kinds of complexities, a simplicity regarding food price subsidies, e.g., when Timmer suggested that it is useful to look at one commodity at a time and its relationship to other things. There, of course, you have simplicity in terms of administration; at least the kind of "heavy lifting" that has to be done administratively when programs have to be operated or goods and/or services have to be dispensed, is avoided. But there are risks, because you may start altering one policy only to discover that the nature of the business is such that you must change four other policies at the same time. It is a lot to ask a government to change one important macroeconomic policy, much less four.

The third point is that the significance of this simplifying, or making less complex, the concept of implementation is matched by the significance of the scale of the implementation machinery. Here, largeness itself seems to me of immense importance in future decisions about nutrition. The significance of what the World Bank did in Brazil was, I believe, the result of its obtaining a very large commitment from the government, creating overnight a constituency and a continuing claim against budgetary resources of the government. There are pressures that will continue the program; they will multiply; people will get new ideas.

The fourth point concerns structure. Once you have the machine, i.e., a coherent policy, you can put all kinds of programs through it, *including* the results of research. It is true, of course, that the larger the structure, the longer it takes to make changes. Thus, if you start with a good program for that large structure, it will persist. If you begin with a bad policy that must be changed, you may have some problems. But adjustments are possible, as Florentino pointed out.

The largest interventions, for example, food price subsidies, whether food stamps in the United States or the subsidy systems in developing countries, were created for reasons that were *not* aimed primarily at improving nutritional status. Like programs of supplemental feeding, which are not aimed primarily at nutritional status, this should not be viewed with disapproval, nor should it be ignored. What is significant in this area is that there is a need for a fresh look at various types of financing techniques to meet that recurring cost for central government budgets. There may be possibilities for some local self-financing of at least part of that burden. The kind of tax techniques employed by CONASUPO in Mexico aim at the high-income consumer so that those with lower incomes can be subsidized.

Fifth, there is another set of concerns requiring attention. One thing that has not changed very much in recent years is the dominance of the public health–physician–pediatrician approach to these problems. It is easy to rely on health improvements as the reason for doing something. I would suggest that we think about a problem that is larger than public health, and what appeals to me very much as an anchor to help make these choices is: Where do we want to be 10 years from now with respect to child development? I am not referring to nutritional status or even food consumption. Rather, I mean what can be done to help children to be born well enough to survive and grow so that they can function both as children (in terms of learning), and later as adults in the work force? Then, let *that* determine what the interventions, policy, or program ought to be. This is not a new thought by any means, but it has been missing throughout our discussion.

There has been, in the past 20 or 25 years, an astounding growth in investment in primary school education in developing countries without a concomitant improvement in the performance of children. We have given educators a chance to perfect the educational system, especially at the primary school level, and it is entirely possible, in the light of their failure, that the problem is not with education but with the students. There may be nutritional deprivation, health deprivation, and what Brozek called psychoeducational deprivation, that are outside the educational system. I raise this point about the functional significance of child growth and development and education because I would commend this kind of process to those involved in research or policy analysis. This is the significance of assessing various choices of interventions, because the particular interventions will, of course, vary according to the country, the political opportunity, and different budgetary situations.

We need, ultimately, to build some kind of an inventory of successful implementation models to help the implementors. The implementor wants to know who does what for whom next, and for how much. It is clear that we cannot even agree on midday school feeding, much less the details of who should do what for whom. Understanding all the causes, and all the interactions, all the mechanisms, is not necessarily the most cost-effective approach to acting. Indeed, there have been many intractable problems that have been faced in many societies where the approach was, "We may never fully understand this, but let us try a few things and see what works."

Finally, there is no question that policy analysis ought to be a continuing activity. We have examined here the implications of both the present and proposed new policies. This must continue, even though it may take a long time before there are any results. There likely will be all kinds of political resistance, even to conducting the analysis, but it must be done.

Concluding Afterthoughts

The volume concludes with a number of cogent afterthoughts on the subject of implementation, contributed by some of the conference participants shortly after the termination of the meeting.

ALAN BERG

1. Opportunities exist in many countries to reform government services in ways that help people more effectively meet their nutritional needs.

2. Some interventions *do* work, but practical and definitive evaluations are not easy. We probably will have to be satisfied with less-than-precise measurements of impacts.

3. The key to the successful launching of any nutrition policy is the catalyst/entrepreneur, qualities that must be actively sought and that must be maintained in the replication or bureaucratization of pilot efforts.

4. The major constraint to successful, operational nutrition programs is the shortage of capable management.

5. Poor internal project communications have seriously inhibited the effectiveness of some efforts.

6. The major financial need for most nutrition activities is to meet recurrent expenses. Similarly, the greatest concern of national officials is how to sustain large, recurrent expenses once they are begun.

7. Large-scale nutrition interventions have demonstrated the power to sensitize policy makers and institutionalize attention in ways that lead

to programs much larger than the project. Such programs have the effect of mobilizing a constituency and institutionalizing large, recurrent costs in an acceptable way.

8. Large-scale projects may initially be disorganized, but the need is to get on with such projects; they will be refined in operation. Because of the need to capitalize on political interests that are often temporary, such projects are unlikely to emerge if dependent on a drawn-out planning period.

9. The proposed time frame for most nutrition undertakings has been unrealistically short. Large-scale operational projects should be thought of in some instances in a 7- to 10-year time frame.

10. Certain efforts have been hampered by their complexity. Nutrition programs should strive toward simplicity. They should, for instance, be designed in ways that limit needs for managerial skills.

11. Unanticipated opportunities emerge during implementation. Sufficient flexibility should be built into programs to allow substantial modifications while in progress.

12. The earlier acclaimed multiministerial mechanisms to promote national nutrition policy and implementation have not proved to be particularly promising in accelerating actions. The single-agency implementation mode is generally more acceptable. However, more coordination appears to be needed at subnational levels.

13. Initial implementation is not enough; vigilance is needed to make sure that projects continue to operate efficiently.

14. The earlier infatuation with sophisticated food technology to help solve major nutrition problems appears to have been somewhat misguided.

15. Strong political commitment is essential if large-scale impact is to be achieved. However, important contributions can be made with only nominal commitment, by developing manpower and institutional capability and testing delivery systems, so that all will be in place for a major intervention when there is commitment.

MERRILL S. READ

In reviewing the scope of material presented in this conference, it is quite apparent that there are varieties of strategies that may be employed within the philosophy of national development that may result in nutritional improvement. However, in reviewing this wealth of alternatives, it is easy to lose sight of the overall objective of intervening. It therefore seems vital to redirect our attention to this point. As was clearly apparent in the data summarized on the first day of the conference, there are significant functional consequences of malnutrition that have important ramifications for the health, performance, and societal well-being of children and adults.

It is particularly important to comment on the behavioral outcome of malnutrition, an area with which I have been associated for more than a dozen years. I believe that Pollitt has been overly conservative in his interpretations of the available data. It seems amply clear from longitudinal studies that prolonged, severe protein–energy malnutrition in early life leads to irreversible alterations in behavioral and psychological development; the consequences are greater if the mother, too, was undernourished during pregnancy. Similarly, most of the data from studies of chronic undernutrition in childhood sufficient to lead to marked growth retardation also indicate subsequent impaired behavioral development, depending, however, on the nature of the social environment in which the child lives.

Studies of educational rehabilitation following malnutrition do not support the blanket contention that the deficits can be overcome or reversed by stimulatory interventions. As one example, in the Cali, Colombia, study, a massive preschool-based educational effort, coupled with a nutritional supplementation program for growth-retarded young children, resulted in improvements in scores on a battery of behavioral tests. Nevertheless, these children continued to live in their impoverished home environments and never achieved the test performance of age-matched children who were not malnourished and who lived in middle-class homes. The interplay between malnutrition and social setting clearly is important and both must be taken into account in designing suitable interventions.

The potential role of deficiencies in other nutrients must also be taken into consideration. Viteri's report on apathy and decreased physical performance in iron-deficient working adult males is fascinatingly similar in many ways to observations of changes in motivation and behavior of iron-deficient preschool children and school-age children, as has been shown by Pollitt and others. In both situations behavioral alterations appear to be reversible through iron repletion. Whether there is long-term impairment in learning ability of the children requires clarification.

Based on the above, it seems to me that the goal of any nutrition, food, or economic development policy must be to improve the health and life potential for the next generation of children. Depending on the specific situation in each country or community, interventions may be directed toward the pregnant mother so as to improve infant birth weight and subsequent child health and growth, or to the young child during the very early years when morbidity is highest. In either case, a healthier child is likely to be a more active one, demanding more attention, and benefiting from a wider variety of stimulating experiences, which in turn sharpens social competence and psychological or intellectual development.

The approaches for intervening are as varied as the countries, cultures, and communities experiencing malnutrition. They range from economic reinforcement for the family to specific programs to benefit individuals at greatest risk. Many alternatives have been outlined and discussed during this meeting. It is neither possible nor desirable to attempt to put them in a priority order for implementation, nor to suggest that any have higher or lower potential for success; the ultimate choice will depend on the circumstances and politics found in specific situations. However, it would seem desirable to keep in mind that organizing, implementing, evaluating, and modifying an intervention will be more easily accomplished if efforts begin on a modest scale and are expanded as success dictates.

Another point that has not been adequately discussed is the problem of identifying "at-risk" groups and communities and the methods for assessment of the nature and magnitude of nutrition problems. Similarly, some system is needed for estimating the impact of any intervention undertaken. Most countries have the needed data on the first point, at least in broad terms. What is needed is ongoing nutritional surveillance for the latter. Here I am not referring to complex multidisciplinary surveillance, but rather to comparatively simple surveillance using a limited number of indices derived from existing data and responsive to hoped-for improvements from the interventions. In this way, pilot interventions may be evaluated and modified as indicated.

Badri N. Tandon

I interpreted the title "Interface between Nutrition Policy and Its Implementation" as a multisectoral subject. Nutrition policy in any country can be developed meaningfully only with the joint efforts of several departments, viz., health, social sciences, agriculture, economics, rural development, housing, water supply, and education. Whenever several departments are involved in developing a policy, there are always difficulties in arriving at an agreed-upon approach. Somehow, finally, a policy is framed, but then the real difficulty starts in its implementation. Every department tries to pull the string in its own direction, or it loses interest in active involvement. Thus, there are a number of interface problems that need identification and appropriate solution.

The problem is very straightforward; however, arrival at the correct answer—particularly the practical application of the correct answer—is very difficult. It may sound simple that a government should establish an intersectoral group, including not only administrators but also specialists who have been involved with field studies, to review critically the results of the research projects and to utilize the information to form the guidelines for nutrition policy. The guidelines can be listed, giving priorities to the more pressing problems and phasing them in in accordance with available human and material resources. The formulation of nutrition policy from the guidelines should be undertaken by the same intersectoral group, but involving many more persons belonging to related disciplines and working at more peripheral points.

This statement can be clarified by citing the example of a large country like India. Our administrative structure is such that we have a central government, with its head office in New Delhi, and state governments with their head offices in their respective capital cities. Our state is divided into regions called commissionaries that have the smallest administrative units, known as districts. While it is possible to draw out the guidelines for nutrition policy at the central level with the help of studies carried out in different states, it will be necessary to involve the state authorities in framing the final nutrition policy. Unfortunately, this process is not in practice. A nutrition policy should have sufficient flexibility for adaptation to different regions in a big country.

I have had modest experience with a few large-scale nutrition programs in India. We do not have a national nutrition policy, but we have a number of programs aiming toward nutrition. I have been pleading for quite some time with the Planning Commission to develop a national nutrition policy, but I believe that we do not have the right type of system through which such a policy could be implemented successfully. At present, neither the bureaucratic system, nor the technocrats' temperament, nor the academicians' commitment, are helpful for the implementation of a nutrition policy. It is futile to blame the politicians when the key functionaries themselves are unable to change.

Some of the main points I would emphasize for successful policy implementation are the following:

1. The components of nutrition policy should become the felt needs of the community so that they participate fully in the program. This can be achieved by sustained efforts in nutrition education. Although I believe community participation is absolutely essential, mere slogans from the central office will not achieve community participation. We have learned from the father of our nation, "Gandhiji," that community participation can be achieved only if functionaries become part of the community. As long as the functionaries maintain a large gap between themselves and the community, it is futile to expect the community to participate. We need to change the present system and move closer to the communities, if possible becoming part of them.

2. The grass-roots functionaries should not feel isolated; they should be specially trained and have the opportunity for continued education, timely rewards, and appropriate supportive supervision. The supervisory staff should be fully trained and committed to the program. There should be a good system of monitoring, midcourse corrections, leadership, and links with the policy makers and project evaluators. Observation of supervisory staff should receive full consideration at the time of program review.

3. The top-level persons should be committed to the program rather than simply involved because the program helps one or the other government hierarchy to project its image among the poor people.

4. The program should be evaluated frequently, and the results analyzed critically for the purpose of modifying nutrition policy if desirable.

Most of the points I have listed above may sound theoretical, but I am afraid that, unless we attempt to change the present system and bring it closer to the above ideal, there will continue to be a large gap between policy and its implementation.

MICHAEL LIPTON

Although it may be some years before we have sufficient technical information to create policy, there is already much information that can be transformed into policy. In fact, I do not think the real problem is "implementation." We *know* about the effects of formula foods when bought by people who cannot afford enough of them or who cannot treat them hygienically, but who are persuaded to use these foods to replace breast milk; yet the widespread promotion of these foods continues almost unabated. We *know* that an enormous amount of money, scientific talent, land, and time have been devoted to nutritionally specific varieties of numerous crops, especially maize, with little if any serious effort to discover whether these specific nutrients (for which breeding is taking place at the expense of yield and frequently of robustness) are actually in short supply in the diets of persons consuming these particular cereal crops as a main staple. Yet these distortions of research continue, with the heroic exception of ICRISAT (International Crops Research Institute for the Semi-Arid Tropics).

We *know* that decision on the crop mix—both decisions by farmers as influenced by price relatives and extension priorities, and decisions by governments on investments and regional resource allocation—influence enormously the ability of the poorest groups to produce and eat enough basic calories. Yet policy continues to be oriented toward higher-value cereals, and frequently toward dairy products and vegetables, with demonstrably far less pay-off in terms of the nutrition of those at risk.

In these three areas, what we need is much more work on how to get policies put into effect. Perhaps it is a question of persuasion. More probably, it is a question of understanding, pressure, and power. How many of the world's undernourished persons recognize, themselves, the consequences for their diets of government and aid agency decisions directly affecting the output mix in agriculture? Of course, once the poor groups do become aware of what is going on, they will still need organization and power in order to make their views felt, whether in a democratic environment or otherwise. But knowledge is a necessary condition, though not a sufficient one, for progress by them.

That is not to say that I go along with the fashionable notion that semiliterate communities, rural or urban, can or should design their own packages of nutritional or general health improvements. It might be ideal if that were possible, but it is not. True, agronomists must not be allowed to skew the system toward rich men's foods, economists toward growth-centered policies that ignore politics, medical men toward concentration of research and treatment upon "interesting" as opposed to important and widely spread sicknesses or nutritional problems, and so forth. But to move from this undoubted truth about the dangers of professionalism to a sort of pop Maoist belief in the untutored capacity of poor, powerless, largely uneducated, and exploited people to make complex techno-economic systemic decisions on their own is to move much too far.

Recent nutrition programs have gone wrong in ways very well analyzed in the course of this conference. Too many nutrition studies have indeed been repetitive efforts, designed to get papers into learned journals. But we do need more surveys, preferably within *communities* where some baseline data already exist, designed specifically to look at the least-cost ways of bringing about improvements. The divorce of economic analysis from nutritional materials, and of information about individuals and "averages" from information about groups and classes within specific communities (e.g., villages, urban slums), constitutes the main barrier toward developing the information base needed for sensible nutrition policies.

Several people raised the question of why there was not more interest in implementation. Most of us are not unconcerned with implementation in our work. Even researchers on issues like water management and crop improvement do their best to implement; so, of course, do medical specialists. I think the problem is that most of us feel, explicity or implicitly, that the implementation of nutritional improvement has rather little to do with "nutrition policy" in most of the senses being discussed here. There really is no substitute for getting more command over income, power, and resources to the poor, who largely overlap with the undernourished.

If natural and social scientists think that better nutrition is going to be achieved principally through the redistribution of access to land and water rights (and I do feel fairly certain of this), then they must say so and propose cost-effective ways for doing this. The international aid agencies, especially those concerned with poverty reduction and with nutritional improvement, should explicitly make aid available to compensate the losers, as well as to assist in the provision of ancillary services to the gainers, from the direct redistribution of land and water to the poorest rural groups. This not only has interesting applications for social and economic analysis, it also has direct implications for nutritional analysis and research, not least via the likely impact on the mixture and timing of crop outputs.

In the final analysis, I do not think that the problem is the "interface between policy and implementation." I think that it is mainly a problem of getting the policy right, based on existing knowledge. Clearly, there are fascinating opportunities for improving the state of knowledge, and some of the "purer" bases for these opportunities were brilliantly presented. It is very important to all but a naive revolutionist to know, for example, how a very poor, landless laborer's family can structure the intrahousehold and intertemporal patterns of meals and snacks, and perhaps other things, to minimize the risk of lasting nutritional damage, or reduction in work performance when work is at its peak at harvest time but before output becomes plentiful.

The problem is not to go from studies to policy guidelines. The problem is to go from policy guidelines to policy. That is a matter of convincing the people who are being damaged that the damage is happening, and explaining how it is happening. "Implementation" is a scapegoat. A "good" policy that cannot be implemented effectively is really a bad policy.

MITCHEL B. WALLERSTEIN AND NEVIN S. SCRIMSHAW

One of the most significant outcomes of the conference, in our view, was the explicit recognition by those in attendance of the difficulty they encountered in addressing the topic: "Interface Problems between Nutrition Policy and Its Implementation." While this was disappointing, it also is illustrative of certain more fundamental difficulties inherent in food and nutrition policy making. Why was it that a group of internationally recognized experts in nutrition, economics, public policy analysis, and program operation found difficulty in dealing, in an explicit fashion, with the subtleties and complexities of moving from "paper plans" to pilot projects and, ultimately, to the successful implementation of large-scale programs? Certainly it was not for lack of appropriate training or field experience. But perhaps it was the result of implicit conceptual "blinders": limitations that facilitated probing analysis of problems but constrained feasible prescription for solutions.

Some have suggested that the "wrong" participants had been invited to the meeting. According to this view, more of the audience should have consisted of those actually involved in the administration of programs at the national, regional, and local levels in the developing world—people who could speak from first-hand experience about the "dos and dont's" of successfully implementing nutrition programs. Although such individuals were represented in the workshop, there is undoubtedly some retrospective wisdom to this argument. But the lack of international attention to the interface between policy and planning, on the one hand, and program implementation and operation on the other—as reflected in both the paucity of the literature and the absence of relevant case examples—suggests a problem more profound than the nature of the individual representatives at the workshop whose proceedings are presented in this volume.

What is really at issue is whether there is, in fact, an identifiable set of norms, procedures, and techniques that may be associated with activities undertaken to deliver meaningful services to those at nutritional risk. Or, phrased somewhat differently, is nutrition program implementation more a science or an art? If it is the former, then it should be possible to delineate a methodology that, given a repeatable set of circumstances, will increase the likelihood that a particular program will transcend the "paper plan" stage (i.e., will become embodied) and will be operated long enough to have a measurable impact on an identifiable target population. If, on the other hand, it is more the latter, then discussions of implementation must remain speculative, situation-specific, and dependent on the intuitive judgments of individual program advocates.

We are inclined to believe, however, that successful nutrition program implementation is *Both* art and science. Clearly, the more empirical, scientific aspects of the problem have been seriously underemphasized from all of the relevant disciplinary perspectives (i.e., nutrition, political science, economics). But even those aspects related more to the "art" of implementation—namely, how a particular program is carried forward from the stage of preliminary political rhetoric, defended from its detractors and competitors, established and made physically accessible to the target group, and maintained over time—are relatively unknown beyond the limited world of practitioners intimately involved in specific nutrition-related activities.

While recognizing the danger of generalizations and prescriptions, it still seems reasonable to assume that, as with most other human endeavors, there is a learning curve associated with nutrition program implementation. We are concerned, therefore, that, while much attention has been devoted over the last 10 years to notable program *failures*, virtually no effort has been devoted to understanding and making known more widely the reason or reasons why certain initiatives have *succeeded*. How were the various obstacles, constraints, and pitfalls avoided? How were political momentum and financial support maintained? Were there any lessons that might have application beyond the specific context in which the program developed? We would argue that these are the types of questions and concerns that those involved in, and/or responsible for, the critical policy–implementation interface must examine and confront directly.

There are signs within the international community that the existence of the critical knowledge gap is now being recognized. We are encouraged, for example, by the attention devoted to the problems of nutrition program implementation at the meeting of the Subcommittee on Nutrition of the United Nations Administrative Committee on Coordination, held in Colombo, Sri Lanka. But in view of the severe and, in many cases, rapidly worsening, funding situation now faced by both the bilateral and multilateral development aid agencies, there is a particularly urgent need to disseminate information on how to implement programs already approved or extant with greater speed and effectiveness.

We fear that the *failure* to generate a substantial number of solid "success stories" within the next few years may lead to increasing fatigue and frustration on the part of developing country governments and external agencies and to mounting social dissatisfaction and political tension, in addition to deteriorating nutritional and health status on the part of the urban and rural poor. We conclude, therefore, with a plea to social and physical scientists alike, as well as to those involved in policy analysis and program administration, to redouble their efforts to identify the ingredients of successful nutrition program implementation and to disseminate that information widely and speedily to those in a position to make a difference.

Participants

C. ADORNA
Nutrition Center of the Philippines
Makati, Metro-Manila, Philippines

STEPHEN R. ALLEN
Catholic Relief Services
Cairo, Egypt

GUILLERMO ARROYAVE
Division of Biology and Human
    Nutrition
Institute of Nutrition of Central
    America and Panama
Guatemala City, Guatemala

JAMES E. AUSTIN
Harvard School of Business
    Administration
Boston, Massachusetts

SOLON L. BARRACLOUGH
United Nations Research Institute for
    Social Development
Geneva, Switzerland

ALAN BERG
The World Bank
Washington, D.C.

GRETCHEN BERGGREN
Department of Population Sciences
Harvard School of Public Health
Boston, Massachusetts

WARREN BERGGREN
Department of Tropical Public Health
Harvard School of Public Health
Boston, Massachusetts

RICARDO BRESSANI
Division of Agricultural and Food
    Sciences
Institute of Nutrition of Central
    America and Panama
Guatemala City, Guatemala

JOSEF BROŽEK
University of Würzburg
Würzburg, Federal Republic of
    Germany, and United Nations
    University World Hunger
    Programme
Department of Psychology
Lehigh University
Bethlehem, Pennsylvania

ALBERTO CARVALHO DA SILVA
Programa Multidisciplinar de
    Nutriçao
The Ford Foundation
Rio de Janeiro, Brazil

SOL H. CHAFKIN
The Ford Foundation
New York, New York

RANJIT CHANDRA
Clinical Research Center
Massachusetts Institute of Technology
Cambridge, Massachusetts

RICHARD S. ECKAUS
Department of Economics
Massachusetts Institute of Technology
Cambridge, Massachusetts

LUIS FAJARDO
Universidad del Valle
Cali, Colombia

JOHN O. FIELD
Department of Political Science
The Nutrition Institute
Tufts University
Medford, Massachusetts

DONALD R. FIESTER
Regional Office for Central American
    Programs
Agency for International
    Development
Guatemala City, Guatemala
Present address: Office of Agriculture
Development Support Bureau
Agency for International
    Development
Washington, D.C.

RODOLFO FLORENTINO
Nutrition Center of the Philippines
Makati, Metro-Manila, Philippines

JAMES GAVAN
International Food Policy Research
    Institute
Washington, D.C.

STANLEY N. GERSHOFF
Nutrition Institute
Tufts University
Medford, Massachusetts

HOSSEIN GHASSEMI
UNICEF
United Nations Headquarters
New York, New York

HANS GUGGENHEIM
The Wunderman Foundation
Boston, Massachusetts

LUKAS HENDRATA
Yayasan Indonesia Sejahtera
Jakarta, Indonesia

HARRY L. JACOBS
Behavioral Sciences Division
Department of the Army
U.S. Army Natick Research and
    Development Command
Natick, Massachusetts

BRUCE F. JOHNSTON
Food Research Institute
Stanford University
Stanford, California

GERALD T. KEUSCH
Division of Geographic Medicine
Tufts University Medical Center
Boston, Massachusetts

YASUMASA KOGA
Overseas Merchandise Inspection
    Company, Ltd.
Chuo-ku, Tokyo, Japan

ANDREW J. KOVAL
Catholic Relief Services
Cairo, Egypt

MIGUEL LAYRISSE
Universidad Central de Venezuela and
Instituto Venezolano de
    Investigaciones Científicas
Caracas, Venezuela

MICHAEL LIPTON
The Institute for Development Studies
University of Sussex
Brighton, England

LOWELL E. LYNCH
Morgan–Newman Associates, Inc.
Washington, D.C.

MAX MILNER
American Institute of Nutrition
Bethesda, Maryland

JOSE O. MORA
Harvard School of Public Health
Boston, Massachusetts

BEDE N. OKIGBO
Farming Systems Programme
International Institute of Tropical
 Agriculture
Ibadan, Nigeria

E. R. PARISER
Sea Grant Program
Massachusetts Institute of Technology
Cambridge, Massachusetts

H. A. B. PARPIA
Research Development Centre
Agriculture Department
Food and Agriculture Organization
Rome, Italy

JAMES PINES
Transcentury Foundation
Washington, D.C.

JOHN A. PINO
Agricultural Sciences
Rockefeller Foundation
New York, New York

ERNESTO POLLITT
University of Texas
Health Science Center at Houston
School of Public Health
Houston, Texas

MERRILL S. READ
Fogarty International Center
National Institutes of Health
Bethesda, Maryland

BEATRICE LORGE ROGERS*
International Nutrition Program
Massachusetts Institute of
 Technology
Cambridge, Massachusetts

JON ELIOT ROHDE†
Gadjah Mada University
Yogyakarta, Indonesia
Present address: c/o Agency for
 International Development
Department of State
Washington, D.C.

GEORGE ROPES
International Nutrition Program
Massachusetts Institute of Technology
Cambridge, Massachusetts

RICARDO L. SANCHEZ
Department of Nutrition
Harvard School of Public Health
Boston, Massachusetts

NEVIN S. SCRIMSHAW
International Nutrition Program
Massachusetts Institute of Technology
Cambridge, Massachusetts, and World
 Hunger Programme
United Nations University
Tokyo, Japan

F. Solon
Nutrition Center of the Philippines
Makati, Metro-Manila, Philippines

PIERRE SPITZ
United Nations Research Institute for
 Social Development
Geneva, Switzerland

BADRI N. TANDON
Department of Gastroenterology and
 Human Nutrition Unit
All-India Institute of Medical Sciences
New Delhi, India

LANCE TAYLOR
Department of Economics and
 International Nutrition Program
Massachusetts Institute of Technology
Cambridge, Massachusetts

*Unable to be present. Paper presented by Lowell Lynch.
†Unable to be present. Paper presented by Lukas Hendrata.

C. PETER TIMMER
Harvard Business School
Boston, Massachusetts

FERNANDO E. VITERI
Division of Human Nutrition and
    Biology
Institute of Nutrition of Central
    America and Panama
Guatemala City, Guatemala

MITCHEL B. WALLERSTEIN
International Nutrition Program
Massachusetts Institute of
    Technology
Cambridge, Massachusetts

JOE D. WRAY
Office of International Health
Harvard School of Public Health
Boston, Massachusetts

Index

Absolute aerobic power (V_{O_2} max), and height, 8
Adorna, C. L., 248, 261
Aerobic power: *See* Absolute aerobic power; Maximal aerobic power
Africa, labor force participation in, 182, 185: *See also* Egypt; Kenya; Nigeria
Agencies, private, and weaning foods, 106
Agency for International Development (AID), U.S., 65, 121, 291, 338: *See also* PL 480 programs
Agrawal, N. S., 363
Agricultural development
 impact of research on, 189
 India's dependence on, 182–183
 in Kenya, 185–186
 in Nigeria, 307–316
 and nutrition planning, 177
 and policy making, 186
 post-harvest processing in, 415
 processing problems, 385–416
 and reduction of malnutrition, 192–198
 regional approach to, 289–305
 ROCAP regional agricultural program, 292–299
 strategies for, 198–200
 and technological innovation, 186–187
 See also Farm production
Agricultural and Food Produce Trade Corporation (AFPTC), Burma, 407–408
Agricultural production, 47: *See also* Farm production; Processing

Agro-industrial complex, rural multifaceted, 404–406
Amino acid fortification, in developing countries, 64–65: *See also* Fortification
Anemia
 iron deficiency, 65
 and work performance, 10
 See also Iron fortification
Anthropometric measurements, 161
Ascorbic acid, and iron absorption, 74, 90
At-risk, identification of population, 129: *See also* Targeting
Atta, in Pakistan's ration system, 67–68, 457–459, 467

Bahia, weaning programs in, 113
Balahar, in Indian supplementary feeding programs, 143–146
Balint, A. B., 363
Bangladesh
 farm holdings in, 183
 post-harvest technology in, 426–427
Barakat, M. R., 123
Barangay Nutrition Committees (BNCs), of Philippines, 258
Barnes, 32
Bean-hardening, 430
Beans
 and animal protein in diet, 156, 158
 and iron absorption, 92
 and protein complementary effect of maize, 153–155
 See also Legumes